# HYPERACTIVITY:

## RESEARCH, THEORY, AND ACTION.

DOROTHEA M. ROSS

*University of California*
*San Francisco, California*

SHEILA A. ROSS

*Palo Alto Medical Research Foundation*
*Palo Alto, California*

A WILEY-INTERSCIENCE PUBLICATION

JOHN WILEY & SONS, New York • London • Sydney • Toronto

Copyright © 1976 by John Wiley & Sons, Inc.

**Library of Congress Cataloging in Publication Data:**

Ross, Dorothea.
  Hyperactivity: research, theory, and action.

  (Wiley series on personality processes)
  "A Wiley-Interscience publication."
  Includes indexes.
  1. Hyperactive children.  I. Ross, Sheila A., joint
author.  II. Title.
RJ506.H9R67    618.9'28'58    76-6125
ISBN 0-471-73678-3

Printed in the United States of America

10 9 8 7 6 5 4 3 2 1

To a real stalwart whose warmth, wisdom, and steadfast refusal to accept the school's negative appraisals as final gave a very hyperactive child the support he needed in his troubled early years.

The stalwart: Mrs. Everest, an English nanny
The child: Winston Churchill

# Series Preface

This series of books is addressed to behavioral scientists interested in the nature of human personality. Its scope should prove pertinent to personality theorists and researchers as well as to clinicians concerned with applying an understanding of personality processes to the amelioration of emotional difficulties in living. To this end, the series provides a scholarly integration of theoretical formulations, empirical data, and practical recommendations.

Six major aspects of studying and learning about human personality can be designated: personality theory, personality structure and dynamics, personality development, personality assessment, personality change, and personality adjustment. In exploring these aspects of personality, the books in the series discuss a number of distinct but related subject areas: the nature and implications of various theories of personality; personality characteristics that account for consistencies and variations in human behavior; the emergence of personality processes in children and adolescents; the use of interviewing and testing procedures to evaluate individual differences in personality; efforts to modify personality styles through psychotherapy, counseling, behavior therapy, and other methods of influence; and patterns of abnormal personality functioning that impair individual competence.

IRVING B. WEINER

*Case Western Reserve University*
*Cleveland, Ohio*

# *Preface*

Hyperactivity is one of the major childhood behavior disorders of our time. It is the single most common behavior disorder seen by child psychiatrists, a problem frequently presented to pediatricians, and a major problem in the elementary school system. Although there are no firm statistical data, conservative estimates by experts place its lower-limit incidence at 5 percent of the elementary school population. By contrast, the incidence of cerebral palsy and epilepsy is at the 0.5 percent level, and the upper-limit estimate for mental retardation is at 3 percent. As recently as the late 1960s there was a paucity of methodologically sound research on this disorder. However, during the past decade, and particularly in the last five years, there has been a substantial increase in the quality, quantity, and diversity of research on hyperactivity. Theory has assumed a more prominent role in determining the direction research should take, and a concomitant improvement has occurred in the sophistication of approaches used.

This text provides a comprehensive picture of the current status of our knowledge of hyperactivity, and places that picture within the context of a behavioral rather than a medical problem. This approach entails a discussion of research on etiology and prognosis, as well as the delineation of established fact, speculation, and unresolved problems in the field. A realistic view is taken of the problems of management, the aim being to acquaint the reader with the essential ideas underlying some of the established facts and techniques in psychotherapy, pharmacotherapy, and education, as well as *potentially* useful intervention procedures in these areas. Special emphasis has been given to two aspects of this complex spectrum of behavior that have received relatively little attention in contemporary treatments of hyperactivity: one is the prevention of hyperactivity, the other is hyperactivity from the viewpoint of the hyperactive child.

This text is intended for professionals in the fields of medicine, psychology, and education who are in contact with hyperactive children and their parents, researchers in the field of hyperactivity, students in graduate courses in the medical and behavioral sciences, and advanced undergraduates in education and psychology. Because it is addressed to an interdisciplinary group the text is written in such a way that specific training in any one field is not essential to understanding it. Although it should also be of value to the intelligent layman who seeks authentic information on hyperactivity, it is *not* a guide to rearing the hyperactive child. (An outstanding book written for parents of hyperactive children is already available. Readers seeking this type of information should see *Raising a hyperactive child* by Mark A. Stewart and Sally W. Olds.)

The task of writing this text was considerably lightened by the help, cooperation, and interest of a number of our colleagues and friends. Special thanks are due to Virginia I. Douglas, William H. Gaddes, and L. Alan Sroufe, each of whom read a preliminary version of this manuscript and offered many constructive suggestions. We are indebted to John Weakland and Richard Fisch for their contribution to the section on their brief therapy and for the case history illustrating their therapeutic method, and to a number of principal investigators who generously sent us research reports prior to their publication. We also wish to thank three members of the staff at the Palo Alto Medical Research Foundation: Eileen Cassidy, who helped us to locate many books and articles on hyperactivity, and Marilyn Bowen and Mrs. Win Vetter who typed the manuscript in its various forms with skill and enthusiasm. The material in the book was greatly enhanced by the inclusion of case studies, data, and particularly the verbatim comments of a number of hyperactive children. We express our appreciation to the authors, publishers, pediatricians, and parents who permitted us to reproduce these otherwise unobtainable materials.

DOROTHEA M. ROSS
SHEILA A. ROSS

*San Francisco, California*
*Palo Alto, California*
*December 1975*

# Contents

# HYPERACTIVITY

# CHAPTER 1

# *Overview*

In our society the restless, overactive child elicits negative reactions from socialization agents far more often than does the inactive child. This phenomenon is apparent in the dismay that maternity nurses typically express about the continually restless neonate, the approval parents show the infant who is quiet during his waking hours, the anxiety that mothers express in letters seeking advice and reassurance concerning overactivity, the tendency of baby sitters to equate successful caretaking with a low level of activity in their charges, and the favorable evaluations that preschool and school personnel accord the passive child. That parents react negatively to such behavior is well-documented by reports stating that overactivity is one of the most frequent complaints made by parents about their children (Chess, 1960; Lapouse & Monk, 1958), by historical and fictional accounts of child rearing attesting to the fact that overactivity in children has been troublesome to parents for centuries (Aries, 1962; Hoffman, 1845), and by contemporary research findings showing hyperactivity high on the list of behavior problems in children (Dielman, Cattell, & Lepper, 1971). Empirical evidence of the negative reaction of parents to overactivity as compared with average and underactivity is provided in a study by Stevens-Long (1973). Parents of elementary school children were shown videotaped sequences in each of which a boy exhibited one of the aforementioned three levels of activity. At intervals throughout the screening the tape was stopped and the parent indicated how he would respond to the child's behavior at that point if he had complete responsibility for the child. Half of these disciplinary decisions were made immediately after the parents had seen the boy aggressively reject an adult's overtures to participate in his play activity, and the remaining half of the decisions occurred at points in the videotaped sequence that were not preceded by any child-adult interaction. The parent pressed one of four keys giving a choice of disciplinary action and one of three keys indicating his affective reaction. Overactivity elicited a significantly more severe disciplinary response than either of the other two levels, and deviations from the norm in *both* directions elicited more negative affect responses than did average activity.

Even when the children are highly intelligent, creative, and from families of high social status, overactivity elicits negative reactions from socialization agents, according to an extensive study of the early environments and childhoods of eminent men and women (Goertzel & Goertzel, 1962). The positive qualities of these children did not cancel out the effects of their overactivity and accompanying disturbing behaviors. Consequently, the overactive children in the Goertzels' study generally had great difficulty, particularly during their school years. For example, Huey Long, governor of Louisiana and later United States Senator, exhibited an unusually high level of activity from birth and as soon as he walked (at 9 months) exhausted his mother and caretakers with his rapid mobility and exploratory behavior. He was described as a superactive preschool child who was always on the go, very bright, and enormously interested in everything. Although his high level of intelligence was apparent from the moment of his entry into school, his teachers disapproved of a child with almost abnormal energy combined with an encompassing curiosity, and they gave him poor grades in conduct. Thomas Edison was constantly in trouble with most of the adults in his environment. He was always into everything, asking questions, and conducting creative situational tests of his ideas, many of which resulted in minor disasters. His energetic explorations were punished or dismissed as "addled behavior," and his teachers were so derogatory that his mother withdrew him from school and taught him herself. Winston Churchill's continual overactivity and its consequences so infuriated his first governess that she resigned, angrily denouncing him as an impossible and incorrigible child. With the exception of his nurse, Mrs. Everest, the young Winston alienated a succession of teachers and other socialization agents with his high level of activity. In one school his despairing teachers resorted to a cathartic approach to modifying his overactivity by allowing him to leave the classroom at regular intervals to run around the school grounds.

Negative evaluations of restlessness and overactivity continue to be a major complaint in the school setting. A survey of the entire elementary public school population of Des Moines showed that 53 percent of the boys and 30 percent of the girls were considered by their teachers to have problems with restlessness (Stone, Wilson, Spence, & Gibson, 1969). Children who are overactive in the classroom and who are unable to inhibit this behavior on command constitute a management problem for their teachers, who view the unusually lively and active child with a disfavor seldom lessened by the fact that he is often very capable. In contrast, teachers view the quiet child with considerable approval, even though he may also be quite dull. In fact, many dull children with inadequate academic achievement are promoted each year because their good behavior exerts a halo effect on assessments of their academic progress. The concern about overactivity is notable in educational conferences and texts on classroom management, which typically devote considerable attention to the handling of this problem while showing little concern for the unusually quiet child whose pattern of hypoactivity may represent a potentially far more serious problem. In the late nineteenth century and in the early decades of this century a high level of activity in school elicited consistently negative and punitive actions ranging from isolation and physical punishment to suspension and expulsion. In the period since World War II the status of this behavior has undergone a major change from that of a conduct problem to a behavior disorder requiring a combination of medical, psychotherapeutic, and educational measures rather than disciplinary action. With this change in status, adjectives such as unruly, incorrigible, and rebellious have been replaced by the term *hyperactive,* a descriptor implying a characteristic level of activity that differs qualitatively and quantitatively from that of the child's same-age, same-sex peers and typically is accompanied by other behavior difficulties.

Hyperactivity is often defined as if it were solely a *quantitative* dimension of behavior. For example, Werry (1968, p. 487) defines hyperactivity as:

. . . a level of daily motor activity which is clearly greater (ideally by more than two standard deviations from the mean) than that occurring in children of similar sex, mental age, socioeconomic and cultural background.

One serious flaw in a purely quantitative concept of hyperactivity is its lack of validity: there are *no* activity level norms for children. The lack of norms is not the result of disinterest in activity level research or unavailability of quantitative measuring instruments. Activity level has been a topic of research interest for almost a century. In 1885 Galton proposed a fidget measure as an index of audience boredom and urged his fellow scientists to while away the time at dull meetings by "estimating the frequency, amplitude and duration of the fidgets of their fellow sufferers" (Webb, Campbell, Schwartz, & Sechrest, 1966, p. 175). Many measuring devices have since been developed, including electromagnetic movement meters (Kretsinger, 1959), actometers (Bell, 1968; Schulman & Reisman, 1959), photoelectric counters (Ellis & Pryer, 1959), ballistographic devices (Foshee, 1958; Sprague & Toppe, 1966), and FM telemetric devices (Herron & Ramsden, 1967). (Descriptions of these and other devices for measuring activity level are contained in the Appendix.) Nor should the lack of activity norms be attributed, as Werry (1968) has suggested, to the sheer technological difficulty of obtaining measures of activity level without distorting the child's normal behavior while he is wearing one of these often complex instruments. Wade and Ellis (1971) report a study in which an electrocardiograph telemetry system was used successfully to measure the free-range activity of kindergarten children. Each child was required to wear a telemeter and a pair of electrodes attached to his sternum. Far from being inhibited or distressed with these attachments, the subjects played vigorously and (p. 1460):

. . . displayed a remarkable nonchalance about the electrodes, placement of them, and the wearing of the telemeter. Many were familiar with the principles involved via the televised commentaries on the National Aeronautics and Space Administration's Apollo program, and once the device was connected showed little or no concern.

The authors have often seen children enthusiastically wearing the Holter apparatus for long-term measures of heart performance, radio monitors for recording verbalizations, or electrode attachments for monitoring sleep. These devices were often worn for long periods of time during which the children went about their normal activities with no complaints that the apparatus either inhibited or distracted them. The attachments in these cases were presented as a "Superman" speed-box or a "Batman" space helmet radio, and a practice day preceded formal measurement. Children will be willing and even eager to wear such attachments if the initial presentation of the task is done with ingenuity.

There are no activity level norms because quantitative measures of activity are of value only if an investigator is interested in the total energy output of a child over some significant period of time. Most investigators have not been interested in this aspect of motor activity, but instead have pursued such research interests as the relationship between activity level and such factors as maternal deprivation (Schaffer, 1966), body build (Bullen, Reed, & Mayer, 1964; Rose & Mayer, 1968; Stunkard & Pestka, 1962), degree of hospital restraint (Bass & Schulman, 1967), intellectual functioning (Massari, Hayweiser, & Meyer, 1969), peer model behavior (Kaspar & Lowenstein, 1971), and teacher ratings (Victor, Halverson, Inoff, & Buczkowski, 1973), as well as the genetic aspects of activity level (Willerman, 1973; Willerman & Plomin, 1973). One of the few studies of the total amount of diurnal movement was that of Schulman, Kaspar, and Throne (1965) who proposed a homeostatic model of activity level with the individual seen as having a controlling mechanism that tends to regulate his total bodily daily movement or energy output. According to this model, each individual is characterized by an activity level within his daily routines that is optimal for him (the term *modal* is used and defined as the mean optimum daily activity level); at the same time he exhibits deviations from this modal point from one situation to another. The homeostatic model also assumes marked interindividual differences within a specific situation. In an empirical investigation of this construct, modified automatically winding wristwatches called actometers were used to provide a direct measure of the activity levels of normal and mentally retarded boys. Over a significant period of time individual children did exhibit characteristic activity levels with considerable intraindividual variation across situations and substantial interindividual variation within specific situations. Recent research has confirmed the occurrence in the hyperactive child of intraindividual variation across situations (Schleifer, Weiss, Cohen, Elman, Cvejic, & Kruger, 1975) as well as a characteristic activity level within similar situations (Rapoport & Benoit, 1975).

A second serious flaw in a purely quantitative concept of hyperactivity is its failure to provide information about the *normality* of the activity level. In the clinical evaluation of activity level that appears to deviate markedly from the subjectively established norm, the essential information lies in the *qualitative* aspects of the activity behavior, including its relevance, goal-directedness, and appropriateness. For example, two infants may exhibit identical and high amounts of activity, but in one the overactivity may be of a playful, exploratory type, and in the other it might consist of the stereotyped, repetitive responses characteristic of early infantile autism. Or one child may exhibit a consistently high amount of goal-directed activity in informal play, but the same amount of activity in another child might consist of random, goalless running around in circles. In a demonstration of actometers two kindergarten girls scored at the hypoactive level, one because she was contentedly absorbed in a book for the entire measurement period, the other because she sat rigidly in a chair unable to participate in any phase of the ongoing free-choice activity. The behavior of the former child was clearly goal-directed and appropriate, whereas that of the latter was goalless and inappropriate, but these qualitative distinctions are not obtainable from measuring devices such as the actometer.

Although there are no empirically established norms for activity level in children, parents and teachers are quick to label a child as hyperactive and usually describe his high level of activity in terms of how it brings him into conflict with his social or nonsocial environment (Werry, 1968). A high level of activity is one of the most frequent complaints made about elementary school children. Lapouse and Monk (1958) reported that approximately half of a group of 6- to 12-year-old children, most of whom were boys, were described by their mothers as overactive, and about one-third were described as restless; Chess (1960) estimated that 10 percent of the children seen in her private practice were referred because of hyperactivity; Patterson, Jones, Whittier, and Wright (1965) found hyperactive behavior to be one of the most common reasons for referral in four child guidance clinics; and Safer (1971) reported that 40 percent of the children referred to child guidance clinics were there for hyperactivity. Studies of large groups of elementary school children in which psychiatrists and teachers have collaborated in assessing activity level illustrate the magnitude of the problem; it is estimated that from 4 to 10 percent of the children are rated as overactive (Gorin & Kramer, 1973; Huessy, 1967; Miller, Palkes, & Stewart, 1973; Stewart, Pitts, Craig, & Dieruf, 1966). These estimates are consistent with other large-scale studies of the incidence of hyperactivity, such as the Kauai follow-up study by Werner, Bierman, French, Simonian, Connor, Smith, and Campbell (1968) in which all of the children ($n = 750$) born in one year on Kauai were intensively studied. Hyperactivity was found to be prevalent in 6 percent of the children (9 percent of the boys) as rated by parents and teachers. Prevalence figures vary with the diagnostic criteria used, the method of investigation, and the personnel responsible for providing the data. They tend to be higher with teacher ratings than with either direct observation of behavior or the stipulation that hyperactivity be exhibited in an interview situation (Kenny, Clemmens, Hudson, Lentz, Cicci, & Nair, 1971).

Hyperactivity is not in itself a cause for concern; instead, experienced clinicians and researchers (Fish, 1971; McMahon, Deem, & Greenberg, 1970) view it as a *nonspecific* symptom whose significance depends on a variety of factors including age, sex, instigating social stimuli such as parental action, situational appropriateness of the behavior, ability to inhibit the hyperactive behavior on command, and presence of other physiological characteristics or behavioral symptoms. It is present in a diverse group of disturbances ranging from major medical problems through cerebral dysfunction to behavior disorders. Table 1 shows some of the disorders and conditions that must be considered when a child is hyperactive. Hyperactivity occurs normally in the infant and young preschool child, with gross motor excitement often being the latter's characteristic way of expressing exuberance, reacting to frustration, and demonstrating enjoyment of exciting events. Most elementary school children exhibit hyperactivity at times, and the fact that it may be a normal variant of psychological make-up has been demonstrated by Thomas, Chess, and Birch (1968, 1970) who identified a pattern of temperament, described as "difficult," in which a high level of activity was one of the characteristics. Hyperactivity becomes a cause for concern when it occurs frequently in situations in which it is clearly inappropriate, when the child is unable to inhibit his activity despite considerable social pressure to do so, when he often appears to be capable of only one speed of response in

**Table 1.  Disorders and Conditions Characterized by Hyperactivity**

```
Metabolic and Endocrine disorders - Hyperthyroidism
Toxic conditions - Lead poisoning
Allergy - Particularly food allergies
Sensory disorders - Deafness, blindness
Temperament - Normal variant of psychological functioning
Maturational lag - Immaturity of central nervous system
Central Nervous System Impairment - Acute encephalitis, chronic brain
     syndrome
Learned reaction - Response to environmental social stressors
Psychoneurosis - Phobia
Personality disorder - Pathological personality traits
Psychosis - Severe behavioral disturbance such as schizophrenia
```

situations in which he is clearly motivated to exhibit other response speeds, and if the hyperactivity is accompanied by related behavioral or physiological symptoms.

Stewart and his associates (Stewart & Olds, 1973; Stewart, Pitts, Craig, & Dieruf, 1966; Stewart, Thach & Freidin, 1970) have used the term *hyperactive child syndrome* to describe the child who is continually in motion, is often highly distractible, has a short attention span, is impulsive, is a disciplinary problem and sometimes in academic difficulty at school, is at odds with his peer group, and often exhibits a variety of secondary behavioral symptoms that are antisocial in nature or denote emotional immaturity. These investigators view the hyperactive child syndrome as a distinct group of behavioral signs that range from mild to severe, are definable in behavioral terms, are not generally associated with demonstrable brain damage, cannot be attributed to chronic medical or neurological disease or to severe behavioral disturbances such as childhood psychoses, and may be etiologically associated with a variety of genetic, medical, social, and nonsocial environmental factors. Their description of the hyperactive child syndrome was based on a study in which they used a standardized interview technique to obtain detailed information from mothers about the past and present symptoms, medical and developmental histories, school records, and family histories of 37 hyperactive elementary school children (M = 32, F = 5) ages 5 to 11 and of normal intelligence. A comparison of the interview data on these children with those of controls showed striking differences between the two groups in the incidence of symptoms related to the hyperactive child syndrome. The symptoms scored as present in one-third or more of the hyperactive group and the corresponding incidence of the same behaviors in the control group are shown in Table 2.

**Table 2.  Percent Positive Scores in the Patient and Control Groups for Symptoms Scored Positive by One-Third or More of the Patients**

|  | Patients | Controls |
|---|---|---|
| Overactive | 100 | 33 |
| Can't sit still | 81 | 8 |
| Restless in MD's waiting room | 38 | 3 |
| Talks too much | 68 | 20 |
| Wears out toys, furniture, etc. | 68 | 8 |
| Fidgets | 84 | 30 |
| Gets into things | 54 | 11 |
| Unpredictable | 59 | 3 |
| Leaves class without permission | 35 | 0 |
| Unpredictable show of affection | 38 | 3 |
| Constant demand for candy, etc. | 41 | 6 |
| Can't tolerate delay | 46 | 8 |
| Can't accept correction | 35 | 0 |
| Temper tantrums | 51 | 0 |
| Irritable | 49 | 3 |
| Fights | 59 | 3 |
| Teases | 59 | 22 |
| Destructive | 41 | 0 |
| Unresponsive to discipline | 57 | 0 |
| Defiant | 49 | 0 |
| Doesn't complete project | 84 | 0 |
| Doesn't stay with games | 78 | 3 |
| Doesn't listen to whole story | 49 | 0 |
| Moves from one activity to another in class | 46 | 6 |
| Doesn't follow directions | 62 | 3 |
| Hard to get to bed | 49 | 3 |
| Enuresis | 43 | 28 |
| Lies | 43 | 3 |
| Accident prone | 43 | 11 |
| Reckless | 49 | 3 |
| Unpopular with peers | 46 | 0 |

## THE SYNDROME ISSUE IN HYPERACTIVITY

Assigning syndrome status to hyperactivity is open to criticism, and this criticism is not purely semantic. The term *syndrome* has been defined by English and English (1958, p. 540) as "a number of symptoms occurring together and characteristic of a specific disease . . . a set of behaviors believed to have a common cause or basis," and by Eysenck (1960, p. 11) as "a fundamentally statistical notion based on covariation." On the basis of these and other definitions (Thomas, 1973), the two critical requirements for syndrome status are that the symptoms form a unitary cluster, and that they have a common cause or at least have major etiological factors in common. There is no evidence that the cluster of characteristics that Stewart et al. (1966) have subsumed under the label of the hyperactive child syndrome meets either of these requirements. Although the clustering of characteristics such as hyperactivity, distractibility, and impulsivity is frequently described by clinicians (Groover, 1972; Laufer & Denhoff, 1957; McMahon, Deem, & Greenberg, 1970) and is forced through subject selection in empirical investigations, few attempts have been made to demonstrate that these clusters are statistically interrelated (Sroufe, 1975).

In a discussion of the issue of syndrome status Sroufe (1975) has cited as evidence against it an empirical analysis of minimal brain dysfunction by Werry (1968a) in which the subjects were 103 chronically hyperactive, physically healthy children (M = 94, F = 9) of normal intelligence who, as subjects in a long-term study of hyperactivity, had been extensively studied and also tested on a variety of psychiatric, neurological, and psychological tests. Werry intercorrelated 67 cognitive, psychiatric, neurological, medical history, EEG, and other measures, many of which were known to discriminate hyperactive from normal children, and derived 10 orthogonal factors from the intercorrelations. The common variance was fairly evenly distributed among the 10 factors, with the heaviest loading (16 percent) on an almost pure neurological factor. Other independent factors, tentatively given labels such as impaired cognitive performance, immaturity, and poor environment, reflected basically unrelated dysfunctions each of which tended to be comprised largely of measures from one source, such as the psychiatrist, psychologist, or neurologist. Werry concluded that the pattern of results did not suggest a syndrome, that is, a single unitary dimension of minimal brain dysfunction, but rather a series of developmental dimensions each of which might reflect different etiological factors and singly, or in combination, might be impaired in minimal brain dysfunction. Furthermore, as Werry (1968; 1968a) and Werry and Sprague (1970) have noted, these findings are generally in agreement with those of Rodin, Lucas, and Simson (1963), Schulman, Kaspar, and Throne (1965), and Paine, Werry, and Quay (1968). In the Rodin et al. study of 72 children referred for behavior and learning problems there were several independent dimensions, including *motor incoordination,* which was comprised mainly of neurological indices of impaired sensorimotor coordination. Several other apparently independent dimensions were related to intellectual functioning, abnormal EEG tracings, level of maturation, hyperactivity, and antisocial behavior patterns. The lack of relationship between abnormal history data, neurological findings, EEG, intelligence, and behavioral findings led Rodin et al. to conclude that minimal brain dysfunction was the result of a unique combination of multiple etiological factors and that there was little evidence for a single homogeneous syndrome. Similarly, Sroufe (1975) has pointed out that in the Schulman, Kaspar, and Throne study (1965) hyperactivity, impulsivity, and emotional lability, all of which were operationally defined and measured, failed to intercorrelate, and that of all the major hyperactivity symptoms, only distractibility correlated with neurological and EEG measures. The results of the Schulman et al. study must be qualified by Benton's (1966) severe criticisms concerning the method of subject selection and measurement procedures used. However, the Paine, Werry, and Quay (1968) study, which was methodologically sophisticated, found no significant intercorrelations, and thus supported the Rodin et al. study. This pattern of results is not consistent with the concept of a hyperactive child syndrome. Even studies such as Conners' (1969, 1970) factor analysis of parent and teacher ratings (which should increase the probability of clustering) provide little support for a syndrome (Sroufe, 1975). Douglas (personal communication, 1975) and her colleagues reported some evidence of clustering in correlations that they ran between data on hyperactive subjects who all participated in several studies in the McGill laboratories. This finding suggests some common difficulties among the children in their studies but does not support a hyperactive child syndrome.

Similarly, there is little evidence for the second requirement for syndrome status, that the symptoms have a common cause. The low degree of interrelatedness among the dysfunctions identified by Werry (1968a) suggests either that different etiological factors are involved, or, at best, that clusters of dysfunctions reflect particular etiologies. Furthermore, the major symptoms that Stewart and his associates (1966) include in the description of the hyperactive child syndrome have been unequivocally linked to such diverse etiological factors as brain damage, exposure to radiation, allergy, child-rearing practices, metabolic dysfunction, lead poisoning, genetic transmission, school stress, and a variety of severe medical and psychiatric problems. It is unfortunate that the World Health Organization has suggested that a category such as *hyperkinetic syndrome* should be included in their classification scheme (Rutter, Lebovici, Eisenberg, Sneznevskij, Sadoun, Brooke, & Lin, 1969) since the label tends to be used without the accompanying restriction that it "should be used as a descriptive category as there was uncertainty both as to its nature and as to how far it constituted an individual clinical entity" (p. 49), and the research findings provide little evidence of a global syndrome. Instead, they suggest that there are a number of medical and behavioral disorders that have hyperactivity in common and that sometimes other behavioral symptoms develop in a child as a result of either the negative responses his hyperactivity elicits from others or his own feelings of frustration concerning his ineffective performance. It is *the association of these secondary symptoms with the hyperactivity* that is suggestive of a syndrome.

Although they have used the descriptor *hyperactive child syndrome* it is clear that Stewart and his associates recognize that in terms of underlying etiology there are many, not one, hyperactive child syndromes. In a recent text Stewart and Olds (1973) state that there is great heterogeneity in the group of children who currently are labeled as hyperactive, hyperkinetic, or minimal brain dysfunction, and they probably do not make up a medical entity at all. A number of other investigators, such as Howell, Rever, Scholl, Trowbridge, and Rutledge (1972) and Ney (1974), have specified subgroups of hyperactive children, and there are many statements in the literature accompanied by extensive research evidence that support the view that hyperactivity is a nonspecific symptom occurring in a variety of medical and behavioral disorders and associated with a heterogeneous group of etiological factors. Yet, *for the most part,* research on pharmacologic, behavioral, and educational intervention has treated hyperactive children as a homogeneous group of subjects. As the label *hyperactive child syndrome* is commonly used it implies that there is *one* kind of hyperactive child, a belief that has been detrimental to progress in research on and treatment of hyperactivity. Numerous research findings have shown that a certain percentage of hyperactive children benefited from a particular type of intervention, and there is rarely any suggestion that those who benefited might have differed from those who did not in underlying etiological factors. There are exceptions, but these are rare. In a study of the relationship of lead poisoning to hyperactivity, David, Clark, and Voeller (1972) classified subjects into four groups according to differences in etiology: (1) pure hyperactivity with no evidence of any event known to be associated with the onset of hyperactivity, (2) hyperactivity with a highly probable cause for it, (3) hyperactivity with a possible cause for it, and (4) hyperactivity with a history of lead poisoning that had been treated. Similarly, in an investigation of drug response Conners (1972) divided his sample of behavior problem children into seven subgroups. If subgroups within the population of hyperactive children were identified and research focused on the relationship between etiological factors and intervention, it is possible that a search for underlying commonalities in etiology would lead to improved and sharpened treatment procedures. More attention should be paid to classifying the very heterogeneous group of children now described as hyperactive into more specific and homogeneous subcategories. This refinement of categories will not proceed as long as a unitary concept of the hyperactive child underlies research and treatment.

In this text the term *hyperactive child* refers to a child who consistently exhibits a high level of activity in situations in which it is clearly inappropriate, is unable to inhibit his activity on command, often appears capable of only one speed of response, and is often characterized by other physiological, learning, and behavioral symptoms and problems. Some of these symptoms (e.g., impulsivity) seem to occur concomitantly with the hyperactivity; others (e.g., low self-esteem) appear to be responses to the child's own feelings of inadequacy about his performance and society's reaction to it. The child whose level of activity is sufficient to warrant the descriptor *hyperactive* but who does not exhibit any other of the problem behaviors usually associated with an excessively high level of activity (Werry, 1968) is also included. With the definition used here the primary presenting complaint is hyperactivity; children with major medical, central nervous system, sensory disorders, or severe behavioral disturbances, such as childhood psychoses, are excluded from the hyperactive child group. Thus hyperactivity is conceptualized not as a unidimensional entity but rather as a class of heterogeneous, inappropriate responses maintained or caused by a variety of social and nonsocial factors (Doubros & Daniels, 1966). The term *hyperactivity* is used to refer to any of the heterogeneous patterns of behavior that are manifested by the hyperactive individual and we emphasize here that in the past 5 years diagnostic acumen and research have established that hyperactivity is a problem that can appear early in infancy (Nichamin, 1972; Stewart & Olds, 1973) and persist through adulthood (Arnold, 1972; Huessy, 1974); it is not primarily a behavior problem of middle childhood.

## MINIMAL BRAIN DYSFUNCTION AND RELATED TERMS

There is considerable confusion in the literature because several descriptors are often used interchangeably with hyperactivity or related terms such as *hyperkinetic behavior disorder* and *hyperactive child syndrome*. The terms most often used in this way are *minimal brain dysfunction, brain damage,* and *learning disability* and we explain in this section how they are used in this text. It is our opinion that use of the term *minimal brain dysfunction* should be discontinued because it contributes more than its share to the morass of confusion in this area. Consider Clements' definition (1966, pp. 9–10):

The term 'minimal brain dysfunction syndrome' refers . . . to children of near average, average, or above average general intelligence with certain learning or behavioral disabilities ranging from mild to severe, which are associated with deviations of function of the central nervous system. These deviations may man-

ifest themselves by various combinations of impairment in perception, conceptualization, language, memory, and control of attention, impulse, or motor function . . . During the school years, a variety of learning disabilities is the most
prominent manifestation . . .

The definition is so broad that it can best be described as an "umbrella
term." It does not present a clear picture of the behavior problem it
describes and it fails to distinguish that problem from other problems. Our
objections here are to the *definition* of minimal brain dysfunction rather
than to the *existence* of the problem. Many children are characterized by
the difficulties in Clements' (1966) definition. According to one group of
experts there are 3 million such children (*Medical World News*, 1970). It is
our opinion that the school and social progress of these children would be
furthered if more precise descriptors, such as the *profile of function*
suggested by Gofman and Allmond (1971), were used to refer to the children's difficulties. In a discussion of the utility of a "precise and clean-cut"
definition, and the problems caused by "distinguished labels," Gallagher
(1966, p. 27) states:

These terms (minimal brain dysfunction, schizophrenia, infantile autism) describe
extraordinarily vague entities, explain nothing, and lead to no clear prescription as
to what should be done. They provide only a false sense of order and knowledge.

In this text we use the term *minimal brain dysfunction* only when it is the
term used in a particular study or article. We recognize that as we are using
them *hyperactive child* and *hyperactivity* are not ideal descriptors, however, we prefer the core-symptom approach that our definitions imply to
the umbrella term. Consequently, we will treat *brain damage* and *learning
disability* as core-symptom terms. As used here *brain damage* implies
demonstrable damage to the brain tissue as a result of prenatal or postnatal
trauma, but does not imply intellectual deficit. *Learning disability* refers to
learning difficulties that occur as a result of disturbances in cognition,
perception, or motor functioning and that result in performance discrepant
from apparent ability despite adequate intelligence, sensory and motor
capacity, and emotional adjustment in the child. A child with a learning
disability is assumed to have normal capacity for learning and normal
outcome is usually anticipated.

The confusion in terminology that pervades the literature has occurred
for several reasons, one being that hyperactivity has been erroneously
treated either as part of a minimal brain dysfunction syndrome despite
evidence to the contrary from multivariate analyses (Digman, 1965; Rodin,
Lucas, & Simson, 1963), or as synonymous with minimal brain dysfunction

and brain damage. At a major conference on minimal brain dysfunction (de la Cruz, Fox, & Roberts, 1973) the term minimal brain dysfunction was frequently substituted for hyperactivity even in discussions of studies in which the term hyperactivity originally had been used. Similarly, school administrators often lump these conditions together as "hyperactivity or brain damage or minimal brain dysfunction or whatever you want to call it." This lack of specificity is partly due to definitions of minimal brain dysfunction so broad that most of the behavior and learning problems occurring in the school setting fit into them quite comfortably. It can also be attributed to the overlap between the behaviors characteristic of the hyperactive child and those of children with demonstrable brain damage. The confusion has been further heightened by the proliferation of terms put forward to describe the hyperactive child and to general disagreement about both the definition of these terms and their diagnostic criteria. Delong (1972) has categorized 37 of the most frequently used terms into three groups, the first of which contains terms that imply pathology and its hypothesized basis and includes such labels as post-encephalitic behavior disorder (Levy, 1959), minimal brain damage (Tredgold, 1908), brain damage syndrome (Strauss & Lehtinen, 1947), and organic driveness (Kahn & Cohen, 1934). Another group attempts to link the behavior to an hypothesized source without a clearly defined pathological base by using terms such as cerebral dysfunction and minimal brain dysfunction (Clements & Peters, 1962). A third group refers to the kind of behavior exhibited by children with this disorder and avoids etiological implications with terms such as hyperkinetic behavior disorder (Bradley, 1957), hyperkinetic impulse disorder (Levy, 1959), and hyperactive child syndrome (Stewart, Pitts, Craig, & Dieruf, 1966).

However, the major reason for the general confusion lies in the historical events that first linked hyperactivity to brain damage and other disorders and then perpetuated and strengthened the link. The subsequent effect of these events on the accumulation of knowledge about and treatment of hyperactivity has been profound and for that reason it is worthwhile to trace these events briefly.

## AN HISTORICAL LOOK AT HYPERACTIVITY

### The First Period: 1902 to World War II

The knowledge that we have about the hyperactive child has accrued over three clearly defined periods, the first of which began in 1902 with descriptions of hyperactivity by an English pediatrician, Still, and ended with

World War II. In a series of lectures Still (1902) presented detailed descriptions of children who were hyperactive as a result of gross lesions of the brain and a variety of acute diseases, conditions, and injuries that presumably had resulted in brain damage. He also portrayed children whose hyperactivity was not linked to demonstrable brain damage and occurred without general impairment of intelligence and in the absence of central nervous system or other physical disease. The children that Still (1902) described over 70 years ago as having "defects in moral control" were remarkably similar to the hyperactive child of the 1970s: a 5-year-old boy had an ungovernable temper, scratched, bit, screamed, and threw other children's toys in the fire; a 4-year-old boy showed a marked change from his earlier docile disposition, lost all sense of obedience and became almost unmanageable, was unusually restless, spiteful, excitable, would not listen to his mother, and on occasion hit her; and a 10-year-old girl with demonstrable brain damage became extremely passionate in her likes and dislikes, was aggressive to other children, became so self-willed that her mother and teachers could not control her, and exhibited marked impulsivity and emotional lability. In this sample, hyperactivity occurred more often in boys than girls, a disproportion that Still (1902) did not consider to be accidental. It was often accompanied by peculiarities of physical conformation, sometimes appeared to be a function of temperament, often showed little relationship to the child's training and environment, and was frequently apparent early in the preschool years. Still linked hyperactivity to a variety of etiological factors, including genetic transmission and child rearing procedures, and reported that it was remarkably resistant to punishment. Regardless of whether demonstrable brain damage was present, Still (1902) viewed the behavior pattern as one to be treated with medication in a hospital or psychiatric ward and having a fair and often a poor prognosis.

The view that the hyperactive behavior pattern was linked to actual damage done to the brain received support from the events of the 1918 encephalitis epidemic in which hyperactive patterns of behavior were among the sequelae of the disease. In detailed case descriptions Hohman (1922), Ebaugh (1923), and Strecker and Ebaugh (1924) noted that children who recovered from the acute phase of encephalitis rarely showed evidence of cognitive impairment but often underwent a "catastrophic change" in personality, becoming hyperactive, distractible, irritable, antisocial, destructive, unruly, and unmanageable in school. They frequently disturbed the whole class and were regarded as quarrelsome and impulsive, often leaving the school building during class time without permission. These children were notable for their failure to respond to discipline. Further support for the validity of a link between brain damage and hyperactivity was provided by studies of epilepsy and other brain disorders that identified a wide range of behavior problems, including hyperactivity in children who had suffered demonstrable brain damage. At this time it was noticed that the same cluster of behavior problems commonly occurred in children who had suffered brain damage from head injuries and other causes, particularly anoxia during delivery, and in military personnel who had suffered head wounds in World War I.

To accommodate Still's finding (1902) that the hyperactive behavior pattern occurred in many of his patients in the *absence* of demonstrable brain damage, Tredgold (1908) hypothesized that some brain damage, such as birth injury or relatively mild anoxia, had occurred and passed unnoticed at the time but became apparent with the demands of the early school years. This explanation led to the idea that even when brain damage could not be demonstrated it could be presumed to be present and this idea laid the foundation for the concept of *minimal brain damage* (Doll, Phelps, & Melcher, 1932; Ehrenfest, 1926; and Smith, 1926). However, later in this period Childers (1935) noted that only a minor proportion of cases of hyperactivity seemed etiologically related to demonstrable brain damage or central nervous system disorder. Childers' discussion of this topic is notable for his differentiation between the hyperactive child and the brain-damaged child, the specificity of criteria he used in selecting truly hyperactive as opposed to lively, normal children to study, his emphasis on the need to develop appropriate treatment procedures, and the similarity between the hyperactive child that he described in 1935 and his 1975 counterpart.

Toward the end of the first period, Bradley (1937) prescribed benzedrine, an amphetamine, for emotionally disturbed children in a residential treatment center in an effort to rid them of severe headaches by raising their blood pressure. To his surprise the behavior and school performance of many of the children underwent a dramatic change characterized by increased interest in school work, better work habits, and a marked reduction in disruptive behavior. Bradley (1937) reported that "a large proportion became subdued without losing interest in their surroundings." The children called the benzedrine medication their "arithmetic pills" because they felt they could do problems more accurately and quickly when they were on medication, and made many comments indicating an improvement in mood, such as "I have joy in my stomach." Bradley is usually credited with discovering the effect of stimulant medication on behavior problems despite the fact that in the same month and journal in which the original Bradley article appeared, Molitch and Eccles (1937) published a report of improvement in the performance on IQ tests of subjects who were given amphetamines. However, these and other articles (see, for example, Bradley & Bowen, 1941; Lindsley & Henry, 1942; Molitch & Eccles, 1937), all indicating substantial improvement as a function of stimulant medication, aroused little interest Prior to the early 1950s only about a dozen clinical research papers appeared on this topic, possibly because doctors questioned the use of stimulants for hyperactive children (Stewart & Olds, 1973) and these children were not as available for clinical or research investigations as they are today. There were few special school arrangements during the Depression years and, for the most part, children who could not conform to the demands of the classroom were required to remain at home. Also, our society was not as drug-oriented then as it is now, particularly in respect to nonviolent behavior problems.

## The Second Period: World War II to the Middle 1960s

In this period studies of the behavioral concomitants of organic brain disorders provided further support for the validity of a causative link between brain damage and hyperactivity by identifying a wide range of behavioral, motor, perceptual, and cognitive difficulties in children who had suffered clearly demonstrable brain damage. Evidence from ablation studies in animals (Cromwell, Baumeister, & Hawkins, 1963; Davis, 1957; French & Harlow, 1955) also supported the association between hyperactivity and interference with cerebral functioning.

A substantial body of fetal and animal research strengthened the validity of the concept of *minimal brain damage* with evidence from epidemiological studies demonstrating a strong association between maternal and fetal factors and behavioral problems (Lilienfeld, Pasamanick, & Rogers, 1955; Pasamanick, Rogers, & Lilienfeld, 1956). The concept was also bolstered by research on the effects of anoxia in infants and young animals (Campbell, Cheeseman, & Kilpatrick, 1950) and observational and experimental evidence from animal studies of the relationship between behavior disorders and minimal degrees of brain damage (Cromwell, Baumeister, & Hawkins, 1963). Empirical evidence of a significant relationship between histories of anoxia and subsequent developmental deviations (Graham, Caldwell, Ernhart, Pennoyer, & Hartman, 1957), and the introduction of the concept of a continuum of degrees of damage (Knobloch & Pasamanick, 1966; Lilienfeld, Pasamanick, & Rogers, 1955) also contributed to the status of this notion.

In this period, largely as the result of the work of Strauss and his associates (Strauss & Lehtinen, 1947; Strauss & Kephart, 1955) brain damage came to be *inferred* from behavioral signs alone. Strauss and his associates conducted a series of studies on differences in the behavior patterns of brain-injured and non-brain-injured mentally retarded children. Having identified a number of behaviors, such as hyperactivity, distractability, and impulsivity, that differentiated between the two groups, they assigned to hyperactivity the status of a hard neurological sign that they considered sufficient to make the diagnosis of brain damage even in the absence of other neurological evidence. The hypothesis that all children showing hyperactivity and related characteristics were probably brain-injured was suggested very tentatively in a text published by Strauss and Lehtinen in 1947 and then stated explicitly in a second volume (Strauss & Kephart, 1955). Although this etiological hypothesis and subsequent attempts to verify it have been soundly criticized (see, for example, Sarason, 1949), the work of Strauss and his associates was once highly regarded. Despite the evidence to the contrary, many professionals accepted the assumption that some kind of organic etiology was involved in the complex spectrum of behavior exhibited by the hyperactive child and that hyperactivity was an unequivocal diagnostic sign of brain damage. The special education procedures described by Strauss and his associates (Strauss & Lehtinen, 1947; Strauss & Kephart, 1955) were widely adopted and served to perpetuate the link between brain damage and hyperactivity in the minds of many educators. Subsequent investigations of the use of the minimal stimulation programs recommended by Strauss et al., which required the elimination or modification of potentially distracting sources of environmental stimulation, yielded little empirical evidence for their efficacy (Cruickshank, Bentzen, Ratzeburg, & Tannhauser, 1961). This failure did not diminish the enthusiasm of the users, especially since for most of this period there was a dearth of special education procedures available for teachers of hyperactive children. Toward the end of the second period a conference held by the Oxford International Study Group on Child Neurology (Bax & MacKeith, 1963) recommended that the term *minimal brain dysfunction* replace minimal brain damage, the rationale for this change being that brain damage should not be inferred from behavioral signs alone; the Study Group also recommended that an attempt be made to classify the heterogeneous group of children subsumed under the minimal brain dysfunction label into more homogeneous subgroups.

In the middle 1950s the whole field of psychopharmacology entered a phase of rapid acceleration with demonstrations of the efficacy of major tranquilizers for adult psychiatric patients and antidepressants for a wide spectrum of mood problems. Concomitant with these developments in the drug treatment of behavior problems in adults was a revival of interest in the use of stimulant medication for problem children. This renewed interest can be attributed to the evidence that already existed on the efficacy of the amphetamines (Bradley, 1937) for behavior problems in children, to exaggerated statements about the improvement in learning and memory that could occur with medication, and an intensive advertising campaign in the mass media and professional literature by pharmaceutical companies. In the 1960s the use of psychoactive drugs increased dramatically and the use of drugs for behavior problems gained widespread acceptance. By the middle 1960s stimulant medication was well established as the treatment of choice for hyperactive children (Eisenberg, 1966; Werry & Sprague, 1970). Psychotherapeutic intervention was not widely used and this state of affairs was maintained to a great extent by acceptance of the results of a single, methodologically weak, study (Eisenberg, Gilbert, Cytryn, & Molling, 1961) suggesting that the hyperactive child would respond better to pharmacotherapeutic intervention than to brief psychotherapy. Although there were few follow-up studies on the hyperactive child, those that had been done (Menkes, Rowe, & Menkes, 1967) or were of peripheral relevance, were not optimistic about the long-term prognosis for the hyperactive child. Still, clinicians (Bakwin & Bakwin, 1966; Laufer & Denhoff, 1957) generally considered the prognosis to be good, with hyperactivity decreasing spontaneously as a function of increasing age. The composite picture of hyperactivity that emerged in the early 1960s was that of a brain damage syndrome to be treated with stimulant drugs, minimal stimulation classrooms, and possibly psychotherapy, and having a favorable prognosis for the adolescent years.

## The Third Period: The Middle 1960s to the Present

In the current period research findings and social forces are challenging all major bases of this composite picture. Hyperactivity is no longer viewed as a brain damage syndrome but rather as a complex spectrum of behavior in which a small number of cases have demonstrable brain damage. The World Health Organization has selected the term *hyperkinetic syndrome* to describe this symptom constellation (Rutter, Lebovici, Eisenberg, Sneznevskij, Sadoun, Brooke, & Lin, 1969), and the American Psychiatric Association (1968) lists this behavior profile under the category of *hyperkinetic reaction of childhood*.

Direct evidence of the occurrence of minimal brain damage continues to accumulate. For example, Towbin (1970) has reported clinical histories and autopsy data from a series of over 600 live and stillborn infants. From these he described three main types of central nervous system damage in the fetus and newborn, all of which were implicated in the etiology of subsequent minimal brain dysfunction or classic cerebral palsy. In a second study Towbin (1971) reported that cerebral hypoxic lesions sufficient to cause brain dysfunction were shown unequivocally to be present under exacting neuroradiological conditions. In a series of 140 premature infants, 52 percent of the brains showed minimal acute hypoxic changes. Towbin considered that these lesions were irreversible, could later affect the child with varying degrees of disability, and, because of their static nature, could continue to have an effect through adolescence and adulthood. Nevertheless, the concept of minimal brain damage remains overextended in that it is often still freely inferred solely from the presence of behavioral symptoms.

Psychoactive drugs are still the treatment of choice for the hyperactive child, however, there is growing concern over such issues as the risk of contributing to the drug culture by teaching the child to take pills as a way of solving problems, the possible use of drugs for social control, and the lack of documented evidence about both the long-term effects and the immediate side effects of drugs. The prescribing of drugs as a solution to problems that are primarily social, as for example when the demands of the classroom exceed the amount of effort that the teacher is willing to make (Safer, 1971; Sroufe & Stewart, 1973) is also disquieting. The use of drugs for classroom control was catapulted to national attention in a news report (Maynard, 1970) that between 5 and 10 percent of the 62,000 grade school children in Omaha, Nebraska were being given behavior modification drugs such as Ritalin, after being identified by their teachers as hyperactive and unmanageable. In the five years since the Omaha incident a barrage of attacks on the misuse of drugs by the schools has sustained public interest in the problem of the hyperactive child. One of the most comprehensive of these, a book entitled *The myth of the hyperactive child* (Schrag & Divoky, 1975), is certain to be of interest, particularly to parents and educators who feel that the school authorities are too prone to recommend the use of stimulant medication. At the same time, drug studies have become a focus of interest and several excellent critiques (Eisenberg, 1968; Freeman, 1966; Grant, 1962; Sroufe, 1975), view the large majority of studies as methodologically inadequate. The efficacy of psychotherapy for behavior problems has been seriously questioned by two careful reviews of the field (Levitt, 1957, 1963) and also by research demonstrating the successful use of behavior modification procedures. Other research has failed to provide support for the Strauss and Lehtinen (1947) teaching method of minimal stimulation and has challenged the major assumption underlying it (Douglas, 1972, 1974). There is a strong trend toward *mainstreaming* (putting hyperactive children and children with other problems back into the regular classroom), and this has been accompanied by an increasing demand that the school should change to fit the child rather than that the child should change to accommodate the school. Follow-up studies now dispute the prognosis that hyperactivity disappears in later years and it is clear that all is *not* well in adolescence (Maletzky, 1974; Mendelson, Johnson, & Stewart, 1971; Weiss, Minde, & Werry, 1971).

While these key developments have been raising serious questions about the composite picture of hyperactivity that had emerged in the early 1960s, a full-scale research and demonstration effort to understand hyperactivity has been underway at major university centers. Douglas and her colleagues at McGill University have conducted an extensive and methodologically sound series of investigations to determine the role of attention and cognitive style in the academic problems that the hyperactive child frequently manifests in the school setting (see, for example, Douglas, 1972, 1974), and currently are developing and evaluating remedial teaching methods for classroom use with the hyperactive child. Stewart and his associates at the University of Iowa have been studying the role of genetic factors in the transmission of hyperactivity and also the long-term prognosis for the hyperactive child (see, for example, Stewart, Mendelson, & Johnson, 1973). Sprague at the University of Illinois and Conners at the University of Pittsburgh are extending the research on pharmacotherapy. Conners is also engaged in an ongoing definitive study of the role of food additives in hyperactivity and a large group of investigators at the University of Washington is working on the problems of early identification and intervention with the hyperactive child. In the laboratories and classrooms of smaller groups of investigators a second set of projects is underway, each with its own emphasis and each representing an intensive attack on the problem of hyperactivity. Waldrop and her associates at the National Institute of Mental Health (see, for example, Waldrop & Goering, 1971) have pointed to the role of minor physical anomalies as predictors of hyperactivity; Schnackenberg (1973) and Plotnikoff (1971) are pursuing the use of milder central nervous system stimulants; Safer, Allen, and Barr (1972, 1975) have investigated new and potentially serious side effects of drugs, as have Newell and Henderson (1973); Weakland, Fisch, Watzlawick, and Bodin (1974) have developed a form of brief psychotherapy that has important applications to hyperactivity; several investigators (see, for example, Zupnick, 1974) have proposed new teaching methods; and Willerman (1973) is studying the role of genetic factors in the activity level of normal children. In addition, research conducted on other related areas, such as fetal electroencephalography (Borgstedt & Rosen, 1975) and biofeedback (Schwartz, 1973), also has clear clinical relevance to the management of the hyperactive child. An increasing number of conferences have been held on hyperactivity in the last five years and the rate of publication of research reports and texts has accelerated exponentially.

The result of the extensive research of this last decade has been to change the status of hyperactivity from a medical to a behavioral problem, provide new information about etiology, establish an urgency to the need for evaluation of the effects of medication, and set new directions for therapy and education. The purpose of this text is to provide a comprehensive review and evaluation of the current status of empirical knowledge of hyperactivity, synthesize research and clinical examples, discuss the implications of empirical knowledge for prevention and management techniques, and specify new directions for research and treatment.

# CHAPTER 2

# *Clinical Description*

In a clinical description of hyperactivity it is convenient to use as a framework the major developmental stages of infancy, the preschool years, middle childhood, adolescence, and adulthood. The use of successive chronological age stages does not mean that the problems of hyperactivity for a particular individual are continuous across all stages. Although some individuals are hyperactive from infancy or childhood through adulthood, others have symptoms that constitute problems at one stage but disappear at a subsequent stage. Patterns of behavior predictive of hyperactivity sometimes are present in the first days or weeks of postnatal life according to observations of clinicians experienced in the behavioral attributes of infancy (Nichamin, 1972; Stewart & Olds, 1973) and retrospective interviews with the parents of children diagnosed as hyperactive (Barnard & Collar, 1973; Stewart, Pitts, Craig, & Dieruf, 1966). By *predictive* we mean that infants who consistently exhibit certain behavior patterns have a higher probability of being diagnosed as hyperactive in the preschool or school years than do infants who are not characterized by these behavior patterns. We consider the former to be at risk for hyperactivity, but no definite diagnostic label should be attached at this point because the patterns of behavior that characterize hyperactivity are exhibited by all infants to some extent and may be transient ones that disappear as a function of increasing age. For some children the infancy period may be a relatively serene and untroubled one with the onset of the hyperactivity pattern coinciding with that of beginning to walk, or entry into preschool or grade school.

In itself the existence of behavior patterns indicative of hyperactivity does not automatically mean that the behaviors will cause immediate problems for the child. In some children the hyperactivity pattern is present in the preschool years but does not present any problem because the type of environmental pressures that exacerbate it to the problem level are absent, the household may be so chaotic that the behavior passes unnoticed, or the parents are so tolerant or inexperienced that the behavior is not viewed as unusual. In one such household a boy who was an only child had had an extremely high activity level almost from birth, had wriggled and rocked in

23

his crib so much that he wore out the mattress before he was a year old, was described as "slippery as a flying fish" to bathe, was constantly in motion and continually involved in minor accidents in his preschool, was impulsive and easily distracted, and was given to such abrupt changes of activity and mood that he was described at age five as "totally unpredictable, likable one minute and ghastly the next." This boy was not perceived by his parents as abnormal. Instead, they dismissed his level of activity almost proudly as evidence that he was "all boy," and regarded his other behaviors as a "tendency toward immaturity." They were astonished when, at the end of the first week of school, his kindergarten teacher stated that something would have to be done about his overactivity.

During each of the major developmental stages *quantitative* and *qualitative* differences exist between the behaviors of the hyperactive child and those of his same-age, same-sex normal peers. For example, in infancy this child often cries more than the average infant and his crying also has a quality that clearly distinguishes it from the normal crying of infancy. In the school years the hyperactive child engages in more inappropriate activity than the normally active child; this activity also has a curiously driven quality that seems to make it almost impossible for the child to stop on command to do so, and often results in adults being almost sympathetic about the misbehavior because the driven quality is usually quite apparent to them (Nichamin, 1972). The *form* of the behavior within any one response modality also changes from one developmental stage to the next, paralleling the changes in context. For example, the characteristically high level of activity may manifest itself in infancy as almost ceaseless thrashing about in the crib, in the preschool setting as dashing from one free-play activity to another, in the school years as the inability to remain seated during a seatwork period and using a variety of prosocial and antisocial reasons for leaving one's seat, and in adulthood as endless pacing up and down in a work situation in which most adults would remain seated. Distractibility may be expressed at 7 months as the inability to maintain interest in a crib mobile, and at 7 years as the inability to work steadily on a set of arithmetic problems without frequent reminders from the teacher. The *relative importance* of specific behavior problems also changes from one age period to the next, with parents viewing sleep problems and crying as the major problems in infancy, hyperactivity as the major problem in the early school years, and rebelliousness and antisocial behavior as the predominant problems in adolescence. Teachers generally are not disturbed about a short attention span in a preschool child, but begin to show concern about such a problem in the primary grade child, and consider it a serious problem requiring remedial intervention in the elementary school child. For each of the major developmental stages we have compiled descriptions of the behaviors commonly exhibited by hyperactive individuals, so that the behaviors subsumed under each age period represent a *composite* of the behaviors that may occur in the hyperactive individual of that age. It would be most unusual for a specific hyperactive individual to exhibit the entire constellation of behaviors described at any one age period, and it is unlikely that the behaviors he exhibits would all be of equal intensity. The reader should keep in mind that it is usually the *cumulative effect* of a number of difficult behaviors that leads parents and pediatricians to suspect hyperactivity. Taken individually the behaviors are likely to vary in intensity from strong to weak; it is their cumulative impact that is important.

The type of situation in which one interacts with hyperactive children largely determines the picture that one has of the behavioral characteristics of these children. Pediatricians, clinicians, and experimenters whose interactions are confined to one-to-one office or laboratory settings, frequently characterized by novelty or even a certain degree of intimidation, will see the behavior of hyperactive children as far less extreme than would be the case if they were seeing the children in their natural habitat of home, school, and neighborhood. In evaluating discrepancies between the reader's view of hyperactive children and the clinical description provided in this chapter, this experiential qualification should be kept in mind.

## INFANCY

If we were limited to a single descriptor for the infancy period, the word *difficult* might be the best choice, with one aspect of this quality being a pervasive kind of *irregularity* in both the infant's physiological and psychological functioning. He may exhibit asymmetrical reflex responses (Denhoff, 1973) and his features are sometimes asymmetrical (Durfee, 1974), a fact that in infancy often elicits negative comments from adults and later, derogation from peers. No contribution is made to this problem by attaching labels such as Wender's (1971) FLK (Funny Looking Kid) to the hyperactive child. Physical examination may reveal the presence of one or more characteristics that appear to be irregularities, such as head circumference out of the normal range, widely spaced eyes, low-seated, malformed, or asymmetrical ears, and a wide gap between the first and second toes. These are *minor physical anomalies* and their presence has been shown to be positively associated with hyperactivity in the early preschool years (Waldrop & Halverson, 1970). (These anomalies are described in more detail in the section on the physical examination of the hyperactive child in Chapter 7.) The infant may be yelling and appear to be almost apoplectic one minute then suddenly switch to a period of calm the next.

His bewildered mother reports that he will function like a normal infant for several days then abruptly turn into a monster. He is notably unpredictable, which makes it difficult for his mother to enjoy even his calm periods because she knows they are fleeting and likely to be interrupted momentarily by explosive outbursts. Furthermore, the infant's personality is often not an engaging one: he is described as hypertonic, querulous, irritable, demanding, unsatisfied, and he rarely smiles. Ambrose (1969, p. 198) attributes considerable importance to the absence of smiling and suggests that this characteristic has potentially serious implications for the mother-child relationship as well as for the infant's cognitive development:

> . . . I should like to emphasize the importance of the infant's smiling as a communication signal that has a powerful effect on the mother. In my earlier studies of this response in the natural setting I was very struck by the enormous delight shown by the mother when her baby first smiles at her face. Furthermore, if her infant doesn't smile at her when she feels it should be starting to do so, usually during the second month, some mothers go to considerable lengths in trying to elicit the response such as by tickling the sides of the mouth. When the infant's smiling responsiveness has really developed, one can see that this behavior does increase the chances that the infant will get longer durations of playful interaction with the mother. I believe that this kind of interaction provides important sensory inputs and early cognitive structuring for the infant which are not provided adequately in the feeding situation alone.

Often the infant is so active that it is difficult for even an experienced maternity nurse to hold him comfortably as he turns, twists, arches his back, wriggles, and squirms about in her arms (Brazelton, 1961). Even in the early months of life his activity level may be far beyond that of the normal infant. If he is left unattended for a few seconds on a table he is likely to roll over and often fall off. During routine care he often shows surprising strength in resisting activities that most infants appear to find pleasurable. He usually shows normal progress in growth and general development, but exhibits advanced motor activity: mothers describe him as kicking more forcefully both prenatally and postnatally and showing more strength of grip than the average infant. He often climbs out of his crib in the first year of life and sometimes wears out the crib mattress with his constant rocking about. Once he leaves the crib of his own volition he begins to crawl almost immediately and from then on his mother knows little peace. His motor behavior tends to be characterized by a jerky quality rather than by a rhythmic flow: he may be slowly moving his arms and legs and then suddenly give a start and twitch (Nichamin, 1972; Stewart & Olds, 1973).

The hyperactive infant often cries readily and it is usually either a distinctive high-pitched cry or an angry monotonic scream. In a study of the morphology of early vocalizations, Wolff (1969) notes that the cry is typically shrill and piercing, and its fundamental frequency is significantly higher (650–800 cycles per second) in comparison to the normal cry of a healthy infant (400–450 cycles per second). Distraught parents have described it as "a sound like a siren," "an animal in acute distress," and "the high thin note of static on a radio." The crying usually begins in the neonatal stage and continues for most of the first year of life. Although it is often mistaken for colic, it differs in several important respects: the time of onset is earlier, it lacks the painful piercing quality of the colicky cry, and it is not paroxysmal (Nichamin, 1972). The infant often begins screaming the instant he awakens and he cannot be comforted. He frequently awakens suddenly in the night and starts screaming. He does not become quiet when he is lifted to the feeding position, nor does he cry for food at regular temporal intervals.

The sleep patterns of the hyperactive infant may show some resemblance to those of the premature infant in that there are only very brief periods of quiet sleep, with much of the infant's sleep categorized as active or transitional rather than as quiet. *Active sleep* is characterized by rapid eye movements, irregular respirations, irregular heart rate, and many small limb and head movements, whereas in *quiet sleep* there are no eye or body movements and respiration and heart-rate are normal. *Transitional sleep* has some of the qualities of both active and quiet sleep. The amount of quiet sleep exhibited by the hyperactive infant is of interest because the area of the brain that controls quiet sleep is also involved in the maintenance of attending behavior (Barnard & Collar, 1973). The infant does not fall asleep quickly or at a regular time and he awakens easily with a startled reaction. In sleep he sometimes alternates between sighs of apparent contentment abruptly punctuated with twitches of distress (Nichamin, 1972).

The foregoing patterns of difficult behavior are ones that could be expected to strain the patience and enthusiasm of the most tolerant of mothers and would almost certainly elicit feelings of antagonism in less enthusiastic mothers. A systematic longitudinal study by Sander (1962, 1969), on mother-child relationships of young mothers and their normal first-born infants, has suggested that a potentially serious consequence of these difficult infants might be pervasive and lasting damage to the mother-child relationship. The purpose of the study was to present an objective picture of the emergence of the normal, early, mother-child relationship. Through the use of recorded mother interviews conducted at regular intervals, standardized situational and free-play observations of the infants, and periodic developmental tests, this investigator was able to identify and define a sequence of five levels of adjustment, common to all the mother-infant pairs, that occurred according to a temporally orderly sequence and for predictable durations of time in the first 18 months of life. Sander's *levels* are conceptually very close to the *developmental tasks* of Havighurst (1972) in that both investigators believe that one level or one task should be mastered if the next level or task is to be accomplished without unusual difficulty. In the Sander investigation it was found that a degree of harmony in the mother-child relationship at any level was dependent on the success-ful resolution of adaptation at the previous level. The relatively short duration of each level created problems for the mothers and infants who had difficulty achieving synchrony at a particular level because it meant that they would soon be faced with the demands of the next level while still not having accomplished the tasks of their current level. The adaptations in the first 18 months of life and the time spans for each level are contained in Table 3. These adaptations specify the behavioral changes at each level that are prerequisite to the progressively more differentiated degrees of regula-tion, reciprocation, and initiation of behavior essential for harmony in the mother-child interaction. Sander (1962) reported the major task to be accomplished in each level. In the first level the task concerned the regula-tion of the infant's rhythms of feeding, sleeping, and elimination so that a certain predictability in daily routines occurred which, in turn, resulted in feelings of confidence and competence in the mother. Occurring in the second level was the spontaneous development of smiling play and recip-rocal coordination of caretaking activities with an overlay of mutual affec-tion and wellbeing. The third level was characterized by a marked increase in the infant's initiation of social exchange and bids for attention. In the fourth level an increase in independence in the infant occurred that was facilitated by his mother's knowing when to intervene. In the final level there was an increase in genuine independence as the infant began to achieve both psychological and physiological separation from his mother. It can be readily seen that the hyperactive infant and his mother might have an exceedingly difficult time accomplishing these tasks. Some mothers of hyperactive infants have difficulty achieving the major task of the first level, regulation, and sometimes are unable to elicit a response as positive as smiling social play from their restless infants. Furthermore, hyperactive infants generally do not show the steady growth of independence reported by Sander (1969). A comparison of maternal reports of the behavior of hyperactive infants with respect to progress on the tasks in Table 3 often suggests a high degree of asynchrony and a lack of harmony in the mother-hyperactive infant relationship that is unlikely to be resolved by the events of the preschool years.

Some support for such difficulty in the early mother-child relationship has been provided by a report by Battle and Lacey (1972) of 74 adults who had participated in the Fels Longitudinal Study since birth. This normal,

**Table 3.  Sander's Five Levels of Adaptation**

| Issue | Title | Span of Months | Prominent Infant Behaviors Which Became Co-ordinated with Maternal Activities |
|---|---|---|---|
| 1 | Initial regulation | Months 1-2-3 | Basic infant activities concerned with biological processes related to feeding, sleeping, elimination, postural maintenance, etc. including stimulus needs for quieting and arousal. |
| 2 | Reciprocal exchange | Months 4-5-6 | Smiling behavior which extends to full motor and vocal involvement in sequences of affectively spontaneous back and forth exchanges. Activities of spoon feeding, dressing, etc., become reciprocally coordinated. |
| 3 | Initiative | Months 7-8-9 | Activities initiated by infant to secure a reciprocal social exchange with mother or to manipulate environment on his own selection. |
| 4 | Focalization | Months 10-11-12-13 | Activities by which infant determines the availability of mother on his specific initiative. Tends to focalize need meeting demands on the mother. |
| 5 | Self-Assertion | Months 14-20 | Activities in which infant widens the determination of his own behavior often in the face of maternal opposition. |

Reprinted, with permission, from Sander, L.W.  The longitudinal course of early mother-child interaction:  Cross-case comparison in a sample of mother-child pairs.  In B. M. Foss (Ed.), Determinants of infant behavior IV.  London:  Methuen, 1969, pp. 189-227.

nonclinical sample was observed during the period from 1939 to 1957. Of relevance here are the child and maternal correlates of hyperactivity present from early infancy. Children were categorized as *hyperactive* if their behavior placed them at the high end of the activity rating scale. The following description of activity level in the early preschool years is from the rating manual used in the study:

*Tendency to motoric hyperkinesis.* This variable assesses the degree to which *S*s motor behavior is described as impulsive, uninhibited, uncontrolled. At one extreme it is characterized by constant running, arm and leg movements, chronic motoric "fidgetiness" and restlessness; impulsive motor acts (e.g., dashing up and touching, pushing, or hugging the Fels visitor as she enters the house; running wildly around the Nursery School, etc.). At the other extreme it is characterized by slow, lethargic motor movements, lack of motor impulsivity with most children falling at Scale Points 3 or 4.

*Scale Points:* 1. *S* is generally lethargic and nonimpulsive in motor activity. 4. *S* shows some tendency to impulsive motor expression: some motoric restlessness. 7. *S* is markedly and chronically hyperkinetic; *S* is always motorically active; *S* is apt to flit from one activity to another with vigorous motor expression.

*Examples of the material upon which the ratings were made:* "He is rambunctious, active, into everything. *S* is small and very active — a runner, climber, explorer . . . he broke an ash tray, climbed on a table, turned out a couple of drawers." (at 1 yr.) or "Mother describes *S* as going through a 'jittery' stage — tearing through the house, making funny noises, jumping up and down. *S* didn't sit still, was 'on the go', running wherever she went" (6-10 yrs.).*

The findings indicated a marked lack of harmony in the early mother-child relationship. Hyperactive male infants were characterized by non-compliance toward adults and a lack of achievement striving in general, particularly on intellectual tasks. During the first 3 years of life the mothers of the hyperactive children were critical of them and showed a lack of affection; the maternal criticism and disapproval continued to be manifested in a variety of forms, including a low intensity of interaction, throughout the entire preschool and elementary school period.

These findings cannot be interpreted as indicating *direction* of effect. It is important to recognize *bidirectionality* of effect in the early mother-child relationship (Bell, 1968). A chronically difficult infant, such as the hyperactive infant, usually will elicit negative affect from his mother, and an indifferent or rejecting mother may produce a fretful, restless, or unresponsive infant. Once a pattern of hyperactivity is established, whatever its origin, both members of the dyad usually will contribute to the problem through an interactive process that maintains and exacerbates it. The main purpose of early intervention is to prevent the establishment of a pattern of negative interaction, or to interrupt this cycle if it is already in existence.

We wish to comment briefly here on the incorrect labelling of high active normal children as "hyperactive,"** a practice that implies a continuity between high activity levels and hyperactivity for which there is no convincing evidence. This misuse of terminology takes two forms: Findings on normal children with high activity scores are interpreted as being *applica-*

* Personal Communication, Battle, 1974.
** This criticism does not apply to Battle and Lacey's (1972) study. Their rating scale definition and the examples given strongly suggest that the term *hyperactive* accurately described some of the children in their study.

*ble to* hyperactive children, or they are interpreted as findings *on* hyperactive children. In both cases high active normal children and hyperactive children are incorrectly and naively viewed as identical. Even when an investigator carefully refrains from using the term *hyperactive* in connection with the high active normal children in his study, others are not deterred from quoting the findings as either applicable to or on hyperactive children. The result is that a fairly substantial body of information is built up in the literature on hyperactivity for which, in fact, there is absolutely no basis. A case in point is the study by Maccoby, Dowley, Hagen, and Begerman (1965) of activity level and intellectual functioning in normal preschool children. At no point in the study did these investigators use the term or imply that their subjects could be considered to be hyperactive, yet their findings are cited frequently as research on hyperactive children. For example, Forness (1975, p. 160) "interprets" the Maccoby et al. findings as:

. . . no differences were found between a group of hyperactive kindergarten children and their normal classmates when sheer level of motor activity was measured during free play.

Taken at its face value, this is the kind of statement that would then lead to hypotheses about optimal kindergarten programs for young children. In fact, the study on which it is based included neither hyperactive nor kindergarten children.

## PRESCHOOL

The preschool hyperactive child usually constitutes a far more serious management problem for his parents than he did as an infant because he is so much more mobile, is fearless, and does not learn from experience (Nichamin, 1972; Stewart & Olds, 1973). Evidence of the difficulty of managing the hyperactive preschool child is apparent from mothers' and clinicians' accounts. A mother of 2-year-old twins, one of whom, a boy, was clearly hyperactive although his twin sister was normal in activity level, reported that in the space of 1 week the boy had climbed out of a second-story window onto a tree, removed all of the books from a large bookcase and thrown a number of them out of the window, and uprooted a large number of new plants in the garden. When the twins ran to meet her husband each evening when he came home, the boy always dashed to the carpeted stairs to the main floor and unless restrained often hurtled down head first, but his sister, after her one and only fall on the stairs, grasped the railing firmly as she descended. In a report of early intervention with young hyperactive preschool children Drash (1975, p. 17) describes the following cases:

S1. John (C.A. 2 years, 6 months). This child was initially totally uncontrollable by either parent. He would not follow instructions, would engage in screaming temper tantrums which would last for at least a half hour, was cruel to animals, threw toys about the room and at his parents, would run away if left in the yard alone, used very little speech, and was so disruptive and uncontrollable that his parents had not taken him out to eat in more than a year.

. . . S4. Ryan (C.A. 2 years, 4 months). Ryan was "always on the go and into things." He was described as strong-willed, excessively demanding, and having a sharp temper. His typical behavior included turning on the iron, burning himself on the stove, climbing on top of an eight-foot bookcase, and covering the bathroom with soap powder. He slept only four or five hours per night and was generally non-compliant with both parents.

The child continues to show irregularity of movement, mood, and function as he did in infancy. He often seems very tense and then abruptly and with no intervention from others suddenly relaxes. He is still a light sleeper and often is the last one to go to sleep at night, but he also awakens early. Some hyperactive children go to sleep almost as soon as they touch the pillow, but they awaken suddenly during the night and are wide awake, alert, and usually noisy. The preschool child sometimes has violent fits of rage and temper tantrums that are well above average in frequency and intensity, and these reactions are heightened by a low tolerance for frustration. When frustrated he may cry for as long as an hour, although he is more likely to scream with rage. He may have a short attention span. He sometimes functions well in a one-to-one relationship and in strange situations may appear subdued, so that there may seem to be a real discrepancy between how his parents say he behaves and how others say he behaves. He generally does poorly in a group because he is sometimes aggressive and often destructive, thus evoking negative reactions from preschool teachers, other adults, and peers. Often he is excluded after a few sessions from one preschool after another and this series of failures and rejections helps to establish a basis for poor self-esteem, particularly if his siblings have had no such difficulties. He generally shows little concern for others' feelings and seems to be genuinely unaware when he has hurt another child. He often cannot meet parental and teacher demands and this failure, plus his difficulties in peer relations, lays the groundwork for the development of a poor self-concept. In order to gain some kind of recognition he may resort to negative-attention-getting behavior in the form of teasing, showing-off, name-calling, deliberate destruction of others' work, shouting, and blatant disobedience. At the same time he is typically quite unresponsive to discipline, discussion, or persuasion. His distracted caretakers regard him as accident-prone. In fact, Stewart, Thach, and Freidin (1970) have found that a significant proportion of preschool boys who were accidentally poisoned were diagnosed as hyperactive at a follow-up 6 years later. A history of accidental poisoning was significantly more common (*p* < .01) among hyperactive children of both sexes than among children in general. The association between instances of accidental poisoning and hyperactivity is a reasonable one: hyperactive children are more prone than normal children to get into things, so the probability that they will come into contact with a greater percentage of dangerous household items, including poisonous substances, is higher. The data of Stewart et al. suggest that one boy out of four brought to a hospital for accidental poisoning in the preschool years will be hyperactive when he is in grade school.

Hyperactive preschool children sometimes seem to be compelled to touch and handle, often with negative consequences. According to some clinicians and researchers, the inability in *any* child to inhibit touching is one result of slow or delayed speech development (Burns, 1972; Crowe, 1972). The hyperactive child is sometimes delayed in speech development (Creager & Van Riper, 1967) so that he may still be jabbering in his second year and saying only single words in his third year. Some hyperactive children do not say short sentences until their fourth year (Nichamin, 1972). This delay in overt speech has two consequences, both of which are likely to exacerbate the child's difficulties. One effect of his slower speech development is a concomitant slowness in the acquisition of covert speech skills, which are important because they enable the child to observe events in his environment and verbally code the events for later usage. The child who lacks the verbal repertoire needed to engage in such mediational activity is at a marked disadvantage in the acquisition of a variety of skills and cognitions that facilitate daily functioning. Typically, he is far behind his same-age peers long before the end of the preschool years. A second effect of his slower speech development is that the shift from tactual to visual dominance is delayed. The shift from constant touching to looking is dependent in part on naming, which serves as a substitute for the tactual feedback produced by touching. When a child lacks verbal ability, the shift to visual dominance is not accomplished as early or as easily as it normally would be. The child remains touch-dominated and this serves as an increasing source of difficulty not only in peer relations (children typically dislike being held or grasped while being spoken to or played with) but also in the increased probability of breakage of objects through handling. The verbal difficulty may be due in part to the early mother-child relationship: Kagan (1971) has reported that mothers of normal children typically engage in less social talk with infant boys than with girls, a predisposing factor in the verbal superiority of girls in the preschool years, and clinicians have noted that weary and exasperated mothers of hyperactive infants engage infrequently in social talk, thus partly setting the stage for the child's verbal deficit.

Usually the preschool hyperactive child's progress in physical growth and development is normal, although he may be slow in some aspects of motor development. He walks early and soon seems to run more often than he walks, and his running has a curious driven quality. He frequently shows unusual success (as a function of persistence) in getting into and out of locked and closed rooms, emptying drawers, and opening food and other supplies, so it is not surprising that he is often the victim of accidents and accidental poisoning (Manheimer & Mellinger, 1967; Stewart, Thach, & Freidin, 1970). At the toddler stage it is often almost impossible to monitor his behavior so he must be tethered in a way that protects him from harming himself with the tether cord or any other objects within reach (Stewart & Olds, 1937).

The following is a case study of a hyperactive child in a preschool setting (Ross, 1961):

Jerry was a four-year-old child whose mother stated that she had never noticed anything unusual about him until he was almost two years old. At that point he had a severe case of mumps and this illness seemed to be the turning point from a calm infancy to a disruptive preschool period. The abruptness of the change suggests that his mumps *may* have been a mumps encephalitis with subsequent brain damage, but there was no mention of this possibility in his pediatric history. His activity was characterized by a high speed coupled with an erratic quality. He rarely stood still: when he was not running, jumping, or climbing he jiggled up and down in place much as a boxer does while waiting for his opponent's next move. He lacked fine motor skill and some of his gross motor behavior was characterized by clumsiness and awkwardness. He spent a major part of each morning running, climbing, and swinging. If an adult offered to push him or help him with any project he sometimes accepted the help, but at other times he burst into screams of rage and often pounded the adult with his fists. When he went to the toy corner he would throw all the toys off the shelves until he found the one he wanted. If another child had the toy he wanted, he took it by force, then, when an adult intervened, he had a tantrum. He had a short attention span and was unable to sit in a group and listen to a short story.

His speech was somewhat delayed. Although his IQ on the Stanford-Binet was 120, he never seemed to learn from experience: he repeatedly tried to stand on the seat of his tricycle even though he had many nasty falls. He rarely cried on falling but he often sobbed disconsolately over minor frustrations and hurts. At times he seemed almost desperate for attention and would engage in what could best be described as daredevil and reckless behavior to get it. On one occasion he climbed a tall tree in the preschool yard and attracted a fascinated audience by his promises to "go down the chimney like Santa Claus." To reach the roof he had to make a difficult jump from the tree, which he did without any hesitation or overt evidence of fear, and was prevented from going down the chimney only because it was too small for him to enter. When he was brought down from the roof he exhibited only pleasure at his feat and at "having all the kids watch me like that." On another occasion he picked up some bottles of prescription pills that had been carelessly discarded in a trash can and set himself up as doctor outside the preschool, dispensing pills to children as they entered (many came by themselves from a nearby housing development). When he was severely reprimanded his only comment was that he liked having "every kid do what I tell them." His behavior in any one session had a Jekyll and Hyde quality, with periods of calm interspersed with frequent periods of intense upset. The other children generally feared him, so even his serene periods were never reinforced by positive peer attention. Although he appeared to enjoy the preschool he often tried to climb the fence and was successful on several occasions.

The hyperactive child generally is not referred for treatment until he reaches the point of school entry. Hyperactivity is more difficult to diagnose in the preschool than in the school years, partly because the symptoms are ones that differ only in degree from those of the normal preschool child. Also, the pediatrician often has only the mother's report to use as a basis for assessment of the child's behavior, whereas in the school years he also has the teacher's report, which describes the child in a structured setting. However, in recent years parents have become more aware of the symptomatology of hyperactivity as a result of a marked increase in articles in the mass media and have begun to seek help for their children in the preschool years, and researchers have shown increasing interest in early intervention with hyperactivity (see, for example, Drash, 1975; Jacob [Smithsonian Science Information Exchange, 1975]; and Schleifer, Weiss, Cohen, Elman, Cvejic, & Kruger, 1975). In the latter study Schleifer et al. obtained observations of nursery school behavior and administered tests of cognitive style and motor impulsivity to 28 3- and 4-year-old hyperactive preschool children (M = 25, F = 3) of normal intelligence and 26 (M = 23, F = 3) matched control children. The study is a model of good methodology. The purpose was to attempt to isolate behavioral descriptors and cognitive characteristics that could facilitate diagnosis of hyperactivity at the preschool level.

The children in the hyperactive group had all been referred with a major presenting complaint of chronic, sustained overactivity. This group was dichotomized into two subgroups, one of which contained 10 children (called true hyperactives) whose mothers' complaints of hyperactivity were confirmed by teachers' and psychiatrists' ratings; the other group consisted of 18 children (situational hyperactives) who were reported to be hyperactive at home but were not hyperactive in the nursery school setting. Each of the 54 children was placed in a group of 6 children (3 hyperactive and 3 controls) and participated in 2-hour nursery school sessions, once a week for 9 weeks, which were conducted by a teacher and a helper. The data used to compare the hyperactive and control groups consisted of observations of the children in free play and structured play activities, individual psychological tests, psychiatric interviews with the mothers, and home assessments by the psychiatrists. With the exception of one psychiatrist who assigned the children to groups, no other participant in the study, that is, no teacher, psychologist, or psychiatrist, was given any information about the children's experimental status or the purpose of the study.

None of the free-play observations differentiated true hyperactives from situational hyperactives, or either of these subgroups from the controls. Furthermore, the two psychologists who were doing blind ratings of the free play of the six-child groups were not able to identify the hyperactive children in each group at a level better than chance, a finding which suggests that in free play in a preschool setting similar behaviors occur in both hyperactive and normal children. This interesting finding suggests that for the most part the hyperactive children were indistinguishable from the controls not only in activity level but also in social behavior, a finding that is consistent with the Battle and Lacey (1972) report of good peer relationships and social behavior in the preschool years for children of both sexes. However, in the structured play period in which the children were required to remain seated and participate in activities introduced by the teacher, both subgroups of hyperactive children were out of their chairs, but not away from the table, more often than the controls ($p < .0001$), and were more aggressive ($p < .01$). The true hyperactive children more often left the table than the situational hyperactives ($p < .01$). Schleifer et al. noted a parallel between this finding and one reported with older children (Douglas, Weiss, & Minde, 1969; Sroufe, Sonies, West, & Wright, 1973) showing that school-aged hyperactive children differed from controls in exhibiting more irrelevant behavior and poor conduct in the classroom, but did not differ on measures of overactivity *per se*. In the present study the true hyperactive subgroup differed from the situational hyperactive subgroup on away-from-the-table behavior, which was essentially the ability to attend to the teacher in a structured situation, but not on the out-of-seat variable, which was actually a more pure measure of activity.

Psychological tests were conducted to determine if these preschool hyperactive children exhibited cognitive styles similar to those of school-age hyperactive children. The cognitive style dimensions assessed were reflection-impulsivity, field independence-dependence, and motor impulsivity. The status of these constructs is the center of a controversy, with Block and others (Block, Block, & Harrington, 1974, 1975; Weisz, O'Neill, & O'Neill, 1975) questioning their validity and applicability to different age-groups of children, and Kagan and Messer (1975) defending their use. Unpublished research from Douglas and her research group (personal communication, 1975) supports Kagan's position in the controversy. However, in following the discussions at points throughout this chapter on the use of these measures of cognitive style, keep in mind that their validity is presently being questioned. *Reflection-impulsivity* is important in situations that offer a choice among several alternatives and is measured by the time it takes a child to consider alternative solutions on a match-to-sample task. The impulsive child responds quickly, without thinking, and typically makes many more errors than does a reflective child. *Field independence-dependence* assesses the ability of the child to separate a figure from the field in which it is embedded. The field-independent child is able to isolate figure from ground; the field-dependent child responds globally to the most attention-directing features of the task. *Motor impulsivity* assesses the child's ability to control and restrain impulsive motor action when a task requires him to perform slowly. The results of these three sets of measures suggested that some of the cognitive styles that characterize school-age hyperactive children are already apparent in hyperactive children of pre-school age. The Early Childhood Familiar Figures Test, a test of reflection-impulsivity, distinguished the hyperactive group from the normal controls: the hyperactive children made fewer correct responses ($p < .0006$) and were more impulsive ($p < .00001$). The true hyperactives were more field-dependent than the situational hyperactives, as measured by the Early Childhood Embedded Figures Test ($p < .05$), and were less able to control and restrain impulsive action on the Draw-A-Line Slowly Test than the situational hyperactives ($p < .05$). Note that both sets of results could have resulted as easily from differences in motivation as from differences in cognitive style. The data from the psychiatric interviews showed that the mothers of all the hyperactive children saw them as more hyperactive ($p <$

.0001) and more aggressive ($p < .0002$) than did mothers of the controls. When the subgroups of hyperactives were compared, no differences occurred on either this measure or family ratings. The homes of all the hyperactive children were judged as more tense, with the mothers talking and playing less with their children than did the control mothers. Schleifer et al. concluded that hyperactivity in preschool children is a heterogeneous phenomenon that varies in its pervasiveness from one situation to the next, and that follow-up data would be needed to determine how many of the preschool hyperactive children would be hyperactive in grade school.

## MIDDLE CHILDHOOD

Clinical descriptions and research on the school-age child have shown that hyperactivity may affect all major facets of the child's life in the middle childhood years (Cantwell, 1975; Minde, 1971; Stewart & Olds, 1973; Wender, 1973; Werry, 1968).

### Home

In the home the child may become less of a problem than he was in the preschool years, because he spends substantially less time in the house. He may continue to be a hazard when he is there, particularly when there is some sort of special event and he tries to be helpful. Many of his attempts to help end in disaster, with his parents exasperated and the child upset. He is often still extremely active and his activity is usually of a precipitate nature with an underlying clumsiness. He may have difficulty sitting still and be unable to remain seated at the table throughout a meal (Wender, 1973). He tends not to persist with any activity and is easily discouraged. He may be disruptive, distractible, and may create many difficulties for his siblings. He is often a light sleeper, with sleep patterns that are qualitatively different from those of normal subjects (Luisada, 1969). The hyperactive children in Luisada's study spent less of their total sleep time dreaming, had fewer dreams per sleep period, and more frequently disrupted their dream periods by awakening. Just as in the previous age periods, he has a Jekyll and Hyde quality, with some days when, as one mother put it, "he acts like an ordinary child and we all enjoy a brief period of normal living."

Ament (1974) has noted that very few hyperactive children are free of psychiatric problems. In case studies the hyperactive child is often depicted as sad, unhappy, or depressed. Such feelings usually stem from a poor self-concept and feelings of hopelessness, which in turn may be linked to parental rejection of the child. In a discussion of the relationship between depression and hyperactivity Zrull, McDermott, and Poznanski (1970) hypothesize that depression may stem from the poor self-image that begins with parental, particularly maternal, rejection of the infant who manifests hyperactivity early in life. Such rejection may result from the mother's unwillingness to accept or recognize the problem of hyperactivity. These authors state that the child's negative feelings about himself are likely to be reinforced by his awareness early in the preschool years that he cannot control either his tendency to impulsivity or his motor behavior, and by his knowledge that he is unable to meet many of his parents' expectations concerning his performance. He may begin to hate his inability to perform, with the result that he directs aggressive feelings inwardly toward himself and outwardly in the form of accident-proneness and antisocial behavior, both of which elicit negative parental reactions that further contribute to his poor self-image.

The following case study (Zrull, McDermott, & Poznanski, 1970, pp. 36–37) is an example of the way in which hyperactivity present in infancy interacts with emotional components in the elementary school years to produce depression:

Tommy was a nine year old, who had a long history of hyperactivity, aggressive behavior, slowness in attaining developmental milestones, and learning difficulties. Tommy's hyperactivity was noted first when he was a toddler and it had become progressively worse. Along with this, his behavior had become increasingly aggressive as he had more contact with other children. His parents found him almost unmanageable and the school placed him in a classroom for emotionally disturbed children . . . In the clinical interview, his conviction that little could be changed in his life was striking. He recognized his mother's preferential treatment of the girls (two younger sisters) and was resentful of it. He also believed his father would never be able to spend more time with him. Tommy could not even guess at what he would like to be when he grew up because, as he put it, he was having a great deal of difficulty getting through his childhood . . . In the projective aspects of testing he consistently saw boys as being sad and dejected, he saw his parents as gone, with little hope for their return. In general, he was an unhappy boy, who felt separated from his family and expected little comfort or support from his parents. He recognized his own inability to cope with his feelings in the world around him.

## Neighborhood

In the neighborhood the hyperactive child may have poor peer relationships attributable almost completely to various aspects of his hyperactivity

(Stewart & Olds, 1973; Wender, 1973). His social skills are generally inadequate even for the relatively uncritical peer group. Patterson, Jones, Whittier, and Wright (1965) have suggested an interesting hypothesis that links hyperactivity to poor social skills. Figure 1 is derived from their suggestion that there is a curvilinear relationship between the activity level of the child and the acquisition of socially acceptable behavior. At both extremes along the activity axis the acquisition of socially acceptable behaviors is markedly reduced because these extremes of activity reduce the frequency of the child's positive interactions with peers and adults. At the low end of the activity axis the young, educable, mentally retarded child provides strong support for Patterson et al.'s hypothesis. This child typically is both inactive and significantly behind his chronological age group in level of social skill. He has an experiential deficit in interacting with others, particularly peers, that has a profound effect on the acquisition of socially acceptable behavior. He isolates himself from group play by choosing observer rather than participant roles even when he has the skills needed for the activity and the situation is a welcoming one (Ross, 1970). For the low activity child (whether retarded or not) the reduced interaction with others is of a neutral nature so that he tends to be overlooked by both peers and adults rather than either praised or punished by them for his inactivity.

Up to moderately high levels of activity the child's behavior will elicit an increasing number of presumably generally positive reactions from peers and adults so that he will have more opportunities for acquiring social skills and will acquire them at a faster rate. However, the extremely high rates of activity at the upper end of the axis are aversive to other people, so that in addition to limiting their interactions with the child they are also more punitive when they do interact with him. And they are often punitive *even*

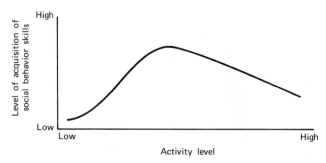

**Figure 1.** Curvilinear relationship between activity level and acquisition of socially acceptable behavior.

*when the child is displaying socially acceptable behaviors* such as friendliness and helpfulness. Punishment for these behaviors is highly confusing to the hyperactive child: it makes it difficult for him to master the rules of social interaction and contributes to his feelings of anger and resentment at the injustice of others' treatment of him. For the hyperactive child the higher ratio of punishment to reward results in a reduced rate of acquisition of social behavior skills.

The hyperactive child's poor social relations with his peers are sometimes exacerbated by two behaviors. One is his attempt to dominate his peers in an effort to inject some stability into his already shaky psychological environment, a behavior that is rarely tolerated by this age group; and the other is a tendency to engage in immature kinds of behavior, such as touching his peers when he talks to them, a habit that may make the peer group rather uneasy, particularly if the hyperactive child has aggressive tendencies (Wender, 1973). The touching behavior occurs because the hyperactive child has not made the shift from tactual to visual dominance that ordinarily is well-established at the point of school entry. Instead, he relies on tactual and kinesthetic cues far beyond the time when his peers have moved on to the predominant use of visual and auditory cues. The failure to shift dominance causes him to touch when it would be more appropriate for him to stand back and look.

He often has poor self-esteem and his esteem is further diminished by the fact that he is unable to play games properly and consequently disrupts them. His inability to play well is due to his clumsiness and also to his inability to sustain attention, which causes him to lose interest in a game long before his peers do. His tendency to be easily distracted, coupled with his poor emotional control, often results in his being labeled as a quitter, a crybaby, or a poor sport (Stewart & Olds, 1973).

## School

In school his teacher may complain that he cannot stay in his seat, finish his work in a reasonable period of time, keep his mind on his own work, stay at one task, refrain from calling out, and inhibit aggression. The hyperactive child is often very impulsive (Weithorn, 1970). He makes many errors in both oral and written work because he does not stop to think. He seldom follows oral directions accurately. His impulsivity is irritating to his teacher because he does not seem to care about his mistakes; his hand is often the first to be raised in answer to a question, and the answer is almost always incorrect. Teachers are seldom tolerant of this behavior and the peer group picks up the teacher's attitude and tends to make fun of the child when he impulsively blurts out a clearly incorrect answer. Sometimes the hyperactive child welcomes the attention, negative though it is, and makes a game of giving wrong answers. Once the teacher begins to doubt the child, her disbelief causes her to resent his interruptions and misbehavior, and this attitude is soon picked up by the other children in the class with the result that school becomes an intolerable experience for him (Brown, 1969). As his self-esteem continues its downward spiral, his performance worsens and he is subjected to a barrage of deficit-amplifying-feedback (Wender, 1971) that serves to exacerbate his difficulties. It is interesting that although a teacher may complain bitterly about him, she may also like the hyperactive child, as do many adults. Often, however, his peers, and particularly his schoolmates, dislike him.

Both the behavior and academic performance of the hyperactive child are very unpredictable, and this works to his disadvantage: A teacher who sees a child act like a disorganized tornado for the first 2 weeks of school and then suddenly switch to being obedient and industrious has a hard time believing that the child's behavior is out of his control. Furthermore, his grades often fluctuate from high to low, so that the teacher usually concludes that having done it once he could do it again if he wanted to. Stevens, Stover, and Backus (1970) did an interesting experiment designed to cast some light on the issue of motivation in the hyperactive child. They examined rapid finger-tapping performance of hyperactive and normal elementary school boys under three incentive conditions: free response, verbal urging, and monetary rewards. Under conditions of free response the hyperactive boys tapped faster than the normal boys, but when incentives were introduced the normal boys tapped faster. The hyperactive boys appeared to be unable to adjust to the changing incentive conditions. Stevens et al. attributed the inability to tap faster to defects in the brain structure regulating arousal and concentration. Their results indicated that the hyperactive group was slower than the normal group in their rapid tapping only when they were operating under specific instructions to tap as rapidly as possible. Basically, the hyperactive group had one response tempo, moderately fast, regardless of incentive condition; the normal group responded more appropriately by conserving energy when the situation did not call for sustained output, and by responding with considerably greater speed when called on to do their best. In an analogous situation in the classroom, we might expect that during free play or unstructured activities the hyperactive child would perform more rapidly than the average child, yet, when instructed to do his best on a task involving concentration and rapid intentional motor responses, would be far outstripped by his peers. The results of the Stevens et al. study suggest that the hyperactive child may *not* do better when he is trying his hardest and this idea is extremely hard for his teacher to understand and accept.

Much work is needed in this area, particularly research on how well the hyperactive child can perform under varying conditions of motivation. Freibergs and Douglas (1969) attribute the poorer performance of the hyperactive child to attentional and motivational factors rather than to central nervous system impairment. Their study involved a comparison of self-paced concept learning in hyperactive and normal children under different conditions of reinforcement. The two groups performed equally under a continuous reinforcement schedule, but a significant decrement occurred in the hyperactive group under a partial reinforcement schedule, and this difference still existed in retention testing done 2 months later. Further research from the McGill laboratories on the effect of different reinforcement parameters on performance in hyperactive children has suggested that these children "have rather unique reactions to reinforcement contingencies" (Douglas, 1975, p. 204). In one study (Parry & Douglas, in press) the use of positive reinforcement appeared to overexcite hyperactive children, with a consequent impairment of performance. In other studies partial reinforcement resulted in more distress in hyperactive subjects than in normal subjects, and performance on a variety of tasks deteriorated. Furthermore, there was evidence that termination of reinforcement sometimes resulted in a rapid deterioration of performance to prereinforcement baseline levels and at other times was associated with frustration and withdrawal (Douglas, 1975). However, mildly negative verbal feedback and negative reinforcement, used carefully, appeared to improve performance in part by reducing some of the hyperactive subjects' tendencies to respond impulsively (Douglas, 1975; Firestone, 1974). The implications of these findings for the use of reinforcement procedures in the school setting are discussed in Chapter 6.

## School Performance and Intelligence

One major focus of research on the hyperactive child centers around his performance at school, mainly in the areas of intelligence, academic achievement, and cognitive skills. Interest has centered on whether the hyperactive child has a lower IQ and/or a lower level of academic achievement than other children. One hypothesis is that the child exhibits a performance deficit, the implication being that his IQ is well above his actual level of achievement. Research in which one of the independent variables is the child's IQ test score is confounded by the effect on the IQ score of previous educational training, specifically, the hyperactive child's apparent inability to benefit from academic experiences in the way that other children do. IQ testing was originally developed to predict success in school, so the typical IQ test has a large component of school-learned tasks. For example, if a child has not learned to count he will fail a number of items on the Stanford-Binet regardless of his "innate" intelligence. The negative characteristics of the hyperactive child have a detrimental effect not only on the acquisition of academic skills but also on the demonstration of skill in the test situation. His short attention span, lack of confidence, and expectations of failure all lower the probability that his capabilities are being accurately assessed. Since it is quite possible to raise test performance in one subject area by providing training in test taking skills within the context of an *unrelated* subject area (Ross, 1969), the hyperactive child's performance on IQ tests almost certainly could be enhanced by working on the elimination or reduction of some of his negative characteristics. These qualifications concerning the accuracy of intelligence evaluations of hyperactive children should be kept in mind when considering the literature on this topic.

Findings from research on children in the early primary grades have shown that the mean IQ of hyperactive boys (Loney, 1974) and hyperactive girls (Prinz & Loney, 1974) in Grades 1 and 2 did not differ from that of the controls. However, in these studies the IQs of hyperactive children in Grades 5 and 6 were significantly lower than those of the controls. Although the sample size in both studies was small, the results do suggest that hyperactive children initially perform equally with other children on IQ tests but later do differ. These later differences are supported by the research that suggests that in the elementary grades the hyperactive child typically has a lower IQ score than that of his classmates. Palkes and Stewart (1972) compared 32 hyperactive elementary school children who had been referred to a psychiatry clinic with 34 controls having no known behavior problems in school, on IQ as measured by the Wechsler Intelligence Scale for Children (WISC), school achievement, and perceptual motor performance. They found that the hyperactive children were at a disadvantage in the school situation because, in addition to their behavior problems, their IQs were lower ($p < .001$) than those of the controls. The hyperactive children were learning at a rate normal for their IQs, and the gap between their school performance and that of their peers reflected the differences in IQ. Contrary to Douglas' findings (1974) in which hyperactive children were matched for WISC IQs with nonhyperactive controls, no evidence was found for the perceptual motor handicap that is commonly attributed to the hyperactive child. Further evidence for the tendency of the hyperactive child to have a lower IQ test score comes from the Miller,

Palkes, and Stewart (1973) study showing that hyperactive children in Grades 3 to 6 in a large suburban school population were significantly lower ($p < .001$) in IQ than were controls, and this was true for both sexes (M = 22, F = 3). These results are consistent with those of Wikler, Dixon, and Parker (1970) who reported significantly lower scores for their hyperactive group on the WISC Full Scale and Performance IQ. In most comparisons of this sort the variability in WISC performance of the hyperactive groups is significantly greater than that of the control groups. This greater variability supports the presence of an erratic quality in the hyperactive child's performance that is highly irritating to teachers and parents (Douglas, 1974).

Minde and his associates (Minde, Lewin, Weiss, Lavigueur, Douglas, & Sykes, 1971) selected a group of 37 elementary school children, with a mean age of 11 years, who had been diagnosed as hyperactive 4 to 6 years previously, and compared their academic performance with that of an equal number of nonhyperactive classmates. Their results showed that the hyperactive children generally did less well in school than their normal peers, having repeated more grades, scored lower on all the basic academic subjects and on behavior as evaluated with a conduct checklist, and scored lower on a group IQ test, the Henmon-Nelson Test of Mental Ability, with the nonhyperactive mean IQ being 112.0 as compared to the hyperactive mean IQ of 101.5. When matched for IQ with controls, the hyperactive children still repeated more grades and did less well on the basic academic subjects (a result that contradicts the Palkes and Stewart [1972] finding that hyperactive children learned at a rate that was normal for their IQs). The test results showed that many of the hyperactive children had uneven cognitive patterns and a preponderance of verbal difficulties of a magnitude that made satisfactory academic progress in a regular class setting unlikely. It is important to note that despite the relatively early identification of learning problems, only one of the hyperactive children had received extended help by age 11. Hyperactivity and associated problems had not disappeared in the later middle childhood years, as is often supposed. Instead, hyperactivity, a lack of concentration, and distractibility all persisted. In addition, problems not primarily associated with hyperactivity, for example, day-dreaming and delinquent behavior, also occurred. One possible reason for the onset of antisocial behavior is that after years of academic and social failure the acting-out behavior elicits peer recognition. Minde and his associates found that poor school performance persisted far beyond the latency period, a finding that is consistent with those of Weiss, Minde, and Werry (1971) and Mendelson, Johnson, and Stewart (1971). Many of the children had a sense of failure and a lack of motivation that was heightened, in some cases, by the presence of specific learning disabilities. These investigators concluded that hyperactivity profoundly affected the personal and academic life of the individual child, and that long-term psychological, academic, and remedial assistance would be required if these effects were to be avoided.

Further evidence that hyperactive children do not learn at the rate that would be expected on the basis of their intelligence test scores is provided by Cantwell (1975), who compared hyperactive children with matched normal public school children to determine whether they were functioning at a level appropriate to their chronological age and IQ scores. Significantly more of the hyperactive children were educationally retarded in reading, spelling, and arithmetic, and their level of retardation was below that of the subgroup of normal children, who also were performing below their expected grade level.

Overall, the studies reviewed here suggest a downward spiral in the academic facets of the hyperactive child's school performance. This is probably the result of an *interaction* between his defects in attention and cognitive functioning (Douglas, 1972) on the one hand, and his sense of failure and lack of motivation on the other. It is clear that early remediation within a context of meaningful success experiences is of critical importance for these children.

## Cognitive Skills and Styles

Douglas and her associates at McGill University have suggested that the problems of attention and impulse control, which they consider to be reciprocal aspects of the same process, are major determinants of the inability of the school-age hyperactive child to function effectively on a variety of cognitive tasks and in a number of learning and social situations. Their work is notable for the systematic approach they have used in describing attention in the hyperactive child. Their basic research strategy has been to study the performance of hyperactive and normal children on a wide range of tasks in which the role of attention and the kind of attention required varies. With this approach it is possible to manipulate task and testing parameters, and to specify the amount and kind of attention required by each task. Such an analysis allows the investigator to specify strengths and weaknesses in attention and thus avoids the tendency to attribute a generalized attention deficit to the hyperactive child. The picture that emerges from this systematic study of attention in the hyperactive child is indeed complex. It suggests that his attentional problems constitute a heterogeneous group of strengths and weaknesses: the child performs as well as his normal peers when he is helped to focus his attention prior to the presentation of the test stimulus and when he is allowed to work at his own rate; he shows evidence of a costly impulsivity of response, and his behavior is characterized by lapses of attention; but he is not more easily distracted from normal children on *some* tasks. The picture is further complicated by the finding that the hyperactive child often performs better on individual rather than group tests, and has difficulty with some tasks even when he is performing in a sound-deadened room with a minimum of distracting stimuli present (Douglas, 1972, 1974). The latter finding raises serious questions about the efficacy of the minimal stimulation classroom advocated by Cruickshank, Bentzen, Ratzeburg, and Tannhauser (1961). Douglas et al. have also attributed some of the hyperactive child's difficulties with school tasks to his inefficient cognitive styles, that is, to his general approach to problems rather than to his intelligence or specific cognitive abilities. Their research has focused on four cognitive styles: reflection-impulsivity, field independence-dependence, constricted-flexible control, and strong versus weak automatization. (The first two styles have been defined in the section on the preschool child.) *Constricted-flexible control* is the ability to focus on relevant aspects of the task and to inhibit incorrect verbal responses. The flexible child is able to ignore distractions and inhibit verbal response to them. *Strong versus weak automatization* is the ability to respond rapidly to simple repetitive tasks, particularly the ability to overlearn routine material.

When previous research data and clinical descriptions of the hyperactive child are viewed in terms of cognitive style, one would expect that the hyperactive child would be more impulsive and field-dependent, would display more constricted control of attention, and would be a weaker automatizer than normal, same-age, equally intelligent control children. For the most part these predictions have been confirmed experimentally. In a study of hyperactive children of grade-school age, Campbell, Douglas, and Morgenstern (1971) found that hyperactive children approached cognitive tasks quite differently from normal children, and typically utilized less efficient problem-solving strategies. When the task required the hyperactive child to select one of several alternative answers to a multiple-choice type problem, he tended to respond impulsively, and often incorrectly, because he did not take time to critically evaluate the alternatives. The hyperactive children had difficulty focusing on the relevant parts of a task and excluding any irrelevant information. On tasks where success depended on isolating a stimulus, such as an embedded figure from a confusing background, the focus of the hyperactive child was easily drawn away by attention-directing cues in other parts of the field. Furthermore, the children were slower than normal children on tasks that required rapid response rates and on rote memory-type tasks requiring the ability to sustain concentration. These and other hyperactive-normal comparisons by this group of investigators (Campbell, 1973; Douglas, 1972) suggest that much of the school difficulty of the hyperactive child may be attributed to his inefficient cognitive styles.

Of particular relevance to the clinical description of the hyperactive child in middle childhood is the study by Battle and Lacey (1972). Observational data collected in infancy and childhood, and interview data collected in adolescence and young adulthood from the Fels Longitudinal Study, were used to identify some of the behavioral and environmental correlates of high levels of motor activity in a normal, nonclinical population of 74 white middle-class children (M = 43, F = 31) of normal intelligence. All available data were divided into five age periods: birth to 3 years, 3 to 6 years, 6 to 10 years, the adolescent period of 13 to 17 years, and the young adult period of 18 to 26 years. The data were then rated by age period. Hyperactivity was rated separately for each of the three earliest age periods, and ratings of hyperactivity for a given age period were correlated with child and maternal variables during the same and subsequent age periods. A comparison of the mean hyperactivity scores of boys with girls at each of the first three age levels shows that the difference was significant only at the 6 to 10 year period. Hyperactivity was relatively stable for boys across these three periods, but fluctuated from one period to the next for girls. The overall picture that emerges of the hyperactive boy in this study is remarkably consistent with the clinical descriptions of other observers. Hyperactive boys showed a general lack of achievement striving and intellectual withdrawal in the earliest age periods, estimated their intelligence to be low during adolescence, and expressed anxiety about their intellectual competence during adulthood. They showed early and continued evidence of physical boldness and aggression, and exhibited persistence and effort in mastering physical tasks, possibly because the boys were capable of excelling in this area, and it may have been the only area in which they could attain satisfaction in their own performance and positive recognition from their peers. During the first two age periods they were noncompliant toward adults, but in middle childhood they sought attention from adults and peers, tried to dominate them, and were physically aggressive to same-sex peers. During the preschool years the hyperactive boys were socially active in a positive way; in the early school years this positive tendency was replaced by a pattern of undesirable attention and control seeking in peer interaction. During the infancy period the mothers were critical and disapproving and in the preschool and school years added to these reactions a lack of protectiveness and affection, severe penalties for disobedience, a low intensity of interaction and an absence of involvement with their sons, and a tendency to underestimate the boys' level of intelligence.

The composite picture for the hyperactive girls in the Battle and Lacey study suggests that the hyperactive girl generally fared much better. She showed a marked lack of concern about physical harm in infancy and was generally achievement striving in the preschool years, tending to choose achievement tasks suitable for older children and to attack these tasks vigorously and with persistence. In the preschool years the hyperactive girl was highly sociable, quite aggressive to her peers, attempted to dominate them, but was clearly accepted by them. This same pattern persisted in the school years when, for the first time, the hyperactive girl was noncompliant with adults while also trying to dominate them. It is interesting that, in contrast to boys, girls who were hyperactive as infants placed a high estimate on their own intelligence in adolescence. The fact that hyperactivity in infancy was predictive of a positive estimate of one's own intelligence in adolescence for girls, and a negative estimate for boys, may be partly due to the differences in maternal attitudes. Whereas the boys' mothers were critical, disapproving, noninvolved, and tended to place a low evaluation on their sons' intelligence, the girls' mothers exhibited none of these behaviors and, in fact, attempted to accelerate the girls' development during the early school years.

## ADOLESCENCE

It is our opinion that adolescence is a more difficult period for the hyperactive child than are the middle childhood years, since there are now two distinct sets of problems which interact with one another. One set of problems is the result of hyperactivity and may include poor school performance despite an adequate intellect; a poor self-image; difficulties in the home, particularly rejection by parents and siblings; a lack of social skills, particularly social game skills; a difficult personality; and more than the usual tendency to be nonconforming and to engage in antisocial behaviors. The other set of problems includes those that normally beset adolescents in our culture, for example, concern about one's identity and future, peer acceptance, physiological changes, and heterosexual adjustment. In regard to the identity crisis, the hyperactive child who is taking medication until adolescence and then has the medication discontinued, suddenly has a whole new post-drug personality to contend with, for which neither he nor his family are prepared (Stewart, 1973).

In the 1950s and 1960s much of the clinical literature presented a positive prognosis by supporting the view that hyperactivity disappears or diminishes sharply in adolescence. In a discussion of the management of the hyperactive child, Eisenberg (1966, p. 593) stated that:

. . . typically hyperkinesis follows a developmental course, diminishing in later childhood and usually disappearing by adolescence. In this it resembles the activity pattern of normal children but displaced chronologically to the right by four to six years.

Bradley (1957) reported a marked decrease in hyperactivity with maturation in 500 hyperactive children whom he had observed over the long term. Laufer and Denhoff (1957) reported that hyperactivity tended to wane spontaneously and disappear between the ages of 8 and 18, and did not persist in the adolescents that they followed into adult life. Support for these reports is provided by other investigators (Bakwin & Bakwin, 1966; Laufer, Denhoff, & Solomons, 1959; Lytton & Knobel, 1958) as well as by the fact that a reduction in activity level does occur in children in general as a function of increasing chronological age (Cromwell, Baumeister, & Hawkins, 1963), and that hyperactivity is a symptom characteristic of younger age groups (Werry, 1968).

Equating the reduction of activity level to a positive prognosis for the hyperactive child, however, is a gross oversimplification of the problem. Although there is general agreement that the high activity levels associated with hyperactivity decrease in adolescence, clinicians who have had extensive experience with the hyperactive child agree that elimination of the activity problem does not alleviate the remaining major problems, particularly those in the areas of educational achievement and social and emotional adjustment. Laufer (1962) reported a variety of psychopathological symptoms and consistently poor school performance, despite adequate intelligence, in a group of 20 adolescents who had been diagnosed as hyperactive in childhood. Anderson and Plymate (1962), on the basis of extensive clinical experience, reported that hyperactive children are frequently characterized by serious problems in adolescence.

Prior to 1970 the foregoing kind of clinical experience was the sole basis for concern about the prognosis for the hyperactive child in adolescence. No systematic attempts to follow the progress of the hyperactive child during his adolescent years were reported. In 1935, Bond and Smith did a long-term study, but it was on children who had physically recovered from encephalitis. Their discouraging findings were that the children's behavior at home and at school was characterized by marked restlessness, disobedience, aggressiveness, and difficulties in interpersonal relations well into late adolescence, with only 25 percent of the 85 children returning to normal functioning. There are several reasons for the lack of long-term empirical investigations of hyperactivity. Awareness of the disorder was relatively new, therefore, clinicians and researchers focused first on diagnosis, assessment, and treatment. In the late 1950s and the 1960s the effect of drugs on hyperactive behavior was so dramatic in many cases that there was a tendency on the part of pediatricians, parents, and teachers to consider the problem of hyperactivity solved because the activity level was controlled. Also, extremely high levels of activity often diminish sharply or disappear in adolescence, so that the adolescent is no longer characterized by a specific and conspicuous dissorder. He usually has a residue of behavioral and emotional problems, but these problems are very similar to those of others in his age group who are experiencing difficulty in adolescence. Consequently, the formerly hyperactive child is no longer a member of a clearly defined group.

Since 1970 there has been an increasing awareness among clinical researchers and educators of the need for more information concerning the outcome for the hyperactive child in adolescence. This interest reflects growing concern about the high prevalence of hyperactivity in our society and also about emerging evidence (Cantwell, 1972; Morrison & Stewart, 1971, 1973) of an association between hyperactivity in childhood and specific psychiatric disorders in adulthood. The result of this concern has been two excellent follow-up studies, one by Weiss and her associates at McGill University, and the other by Stewart and his associates at Washington University, and several less extensive studies.

Weiss, Minde, and Werry (1971) did a 5-year follow-up study of 64 hyperactive children (M = 60, F = 4) who were characterized by long-term and sustained hyperactivity. The children ranged in age from 10 to 18 years with a mean of 13 years, and in IQ from 85 to 134 on the WISC. The criteria for inclusion in the study were that a child had to have been seen at least 4 years previously, have no demonstrable brain damage or dysfunction, have no psychosis, and be living at home with at least one parent. Hyperactivity had been the chief complaint on referral, but 5 years later 70 percent of the mothers complained about other problems, such as aggression, distractibility, emotional immaturity, and poor academic functioning. Eighty percent of the children had repeated at least one grade, 10 percent were in special classes, and 5 percent had been expelled. Only 5 percent were doing above average work. Data from rating scales and classroom observations suggested that the children did not outgrow their hyperactivity but merely expressed it in less gross and disturbing ways; and they were still rated as having more behavioral problems than a control group matched for age, sex, and intelligence. Weiss and her colleagues concluded that the high activity diminished but that other major problems, particularly disorders of attention and chronic underachievement despite normal intelligence, remained. These adolescents exhibited a tendency toward psychopathology, being characterized by emotional immaturity, inability to attain goals, feelings of hopelessness, and poor self-image; nearly one-third had no close same-age friends. Of particular relevance to the question of prognosis were the findings that one-quarter of the hyperactive group were characterized by greater restlessness, aggression, and antisocial behavior at follow-up, and that poor mother-child relationships, parents described as "in poor mental health," and punitive child rearing practices were the factors distinguishing this antisocial subgroup from the remainder of the group at the time of the initial evaluation. Conrad and Insel (1967) have reported that the children of parents who were rated as grossly deviant or socially incompetent tended to respond less well to pharmaceutical intervention regardless of other factors. These findings suggest that the prognosis is even less encouraging for the hyperactive child or adolescent with a parent who has psychiatric difficulties than it is for hyperactive children in general.

Mendelson, Johnson, and Stewart (1971) reported a follow-up study on 83 children (M = 75, F = 8) who had been diagnosed as hyperactive 2 to 5 years earlier. They ranged in age from 12 to 16, with a mean of 13.4 years, and in IQ from 60 to 120, with a mean of 96. These investigators interviewed mothers in their homes, using a systematic structured interview consisting of an open-ended evaluation of the child, questions about specific behavioral symptoms, and questions about school, family, police record, and effectiveness of treatment. About half of the children were markedly improved, one-quarter remained unchanged, and the remaining quarter lay in between. Sixty-five percent were attending regular school and 25 percent were in special schools or classes. They were less active, distractible, impulsive, and excitable than they were in elementary school, although these symptoms were still troublesome. The children were disobedient and rebellious at home and at school, however, and were still having serious difficulties with their school work. A high percentage were characterized by low self-esteem. Forty percent of the parents had seriously considered having their hyperactive child live away from home. A significant minority of the hyperactive children, perhaps 25 percent, were involved in enough antisocial behavior to make Mendelson and his colleagues pessimistic about their future.

In an attempt to identify some of the academic skills contributing to the consistent retardation in school performance that is characteristic of the hyperactive adolescent, Hoy, Weiss, Minde, and Cohen (1972) compared the test performance of adolescents previously diagnosed as hyperactive with that of nonhyperactives similar in age, IQ, and socioeconomic status. The test battery measured specific academic skills, such as oral reading, comprehension, vocabulary, and spelling. Although the hyperactive group had failed more grades, they differed from the nonhyperactive group only on spelling. Even on a difficult auditory continuous performance task with both meaningful and nonsense distractors, no differences were found. This finding does not mean that hyperactive adolescents are as resistant to distraction as their normal peers, nor do the overall findings suggest that the hyperactive group were as able academically as the normal group. The findings do show that the two groups were similar in *competence*, which is the demonstration of proficiency under ideal testing conditions. However, in terms of *performance*, that is, the ability to use skills appropriately and consistently in everyday situations, the hyperactive group were far less able. Well-documented clinical and research evidence supports this distinction. The hyperactive adolescent possesses the requisite skills for effective classroom performance but does not make consistent use of them, resulting in a marked discrepancy between his overall classroom performance and the level predicted on the basis of his IQ. This discrepancy has been attributed in part to a *generalized motivational deficit*. However, it is our opinion that a more specific contributing influence is a *cognitive energy deficit*, an *inability*, rather than an *unwillingness*, to continuously mobilize the intellectual forces needed to perform routine classroom tasks. This hypothesis is consistent with the findings that the hyperactive adolescent generally performs effectively in one-to-one situations and attends closely to television programs for relatively long periods. In both situations his cognitive energy is to a great extent being mobilized for him: in one case by a compelling adult in a novel situation and in the other by an attention-directing presentation. This explanation differs markedly from the motivational deficit explanation in its implications for classroom management. It follows that approaches to remediation based on these two constructs would be quite different.

Further evidence that all is not well in adolescence is provided by a long-term follow-up of hyperactive children (Huessy, Metoyer, & Townsend, 1974) in which many formerly hyperactive children continued to have difficulties in adolescence, including school problems, unsatisfactory family and peer relations, and trouble with the law. In this follow-up the number that had been hospitalized for psychiatric reasons was substantially greater than the expected rate of psychiatric hospitalization for the adolescent age group. These findings confirm those of Quitkin and Klein (1969) and Hartocollis (1968), who reported specific serious psychiatric difficulties in previously diagnosed hyperactive children whom they studied in adolescence and young adulthood. Tec (1971, 1973) has suggested that some hyperactive children who do not receive proper treatment in childhood become bitter and disillusioned and search for relief from drugs during adolescence. As adolescents they manifest clinical symptoms that Tec calls the *Staccato syndrome*: their behavior has a disjointed, staccato quality and is appropriate at some times and bizarre at others. The symptoms resemble schizophrenia to some extent, but the hyperactive adolescents maintain good peer relationships.

The results of the foregoing studies suggest that the tendency to discontinue various forms of intervention in early adolescence is an error that has potentially serious implications for the adolescent's development and success as an adult. What is needed is increased intervention of a kind differing markedly from that used with the hyperactive child in his middle childhood years. Hyperactivity does not disappear in adolescence. Instead, it diminishes, but the adolescent is still noticeably more restless, distractible, impulsive, and emotionally labile than his peers. Underachievement, attentional difficulties, poor self-esteem, and depression remain major problems. Some of the predominant problems change, for example, for the first time antisocial behavior becomes a major problem and leads to police contact and court referral in a significant number of the hyperactive group. The spectrum of hyperactivity-related problems interact with the stresses normally associated with adolescence in our culture. The result is a period of great difficulty that the adolescent is ill-prepared to handle.

## ADULTHOOD

There is little information about what happens to the hyperactive child in adulthood. On the basis of a series of clinical studies Anderson and Plymate (1962) concluded that hyperactive children do not outgrow their problems in adulthood but instead may develop a variety of serious personality disorders. These investigators used the term "associate deficit pathology," which appears to assume brain damage.

The earliest relevant empirical data come from a follow-up study by Menkes, Rowe, and Menkes (1967) on 14 adults (M = 11, F = 3) who had been seen 25 years earlier in an outpatient psychiatric clinic. The diagnosis of hyperactivity was made *retrospectively* on the basis of the fact that, as children of ages ranging from 2 to 15 years with IQs from 71 to 128, they had been characterized by hyperactivity, learning disorders, and one or more of the following symptoms: impaired or delayed speech, clumsiness on fine motor tasks, and visual-motor deficits. One purpose of the study was to determine the level of social functioning in adulthood, and to identify factors that could serve as indices of prognosis. At the time of follow-up four were hospitalized as psychotics, two were mentally retarded and were supported by their families, and eight were self-supporting. Of these eight, four were from seriously inadequate homes and had spent some time in institutions, and three still complained at age 30 of restlessness, and reported that they had a hard time settling down to anything, even a TV program, and changed jobs frequently. In the remaining 11 subjects signs and symptoms associated with hyperactivity had disappeared during early adolescence in the majority and during early adulthood in a few. A major prognostic factor was the IQ obtained during the initial evaluation; almost all of the subjects who were self-supporting had an IQ score over 90. In this study the investigators noted a number of methodological weaknesses, such as incomplete records. In addition, home conditions for some subjects were so inadequate that they could have been the prime reason for difficulties in adulthood.

The possibility that the hyperactive behavior pattern might be a childhood prologue to psychiatric disorders in adulthood has been suggested by the results of several recent investigations. Morrison and Minkoff (1975) have presented three case reports that suggest that an explosive personality in adulthood may be one of the sequelae of hyperactivity in childhood. Morrison and Stewart (1971) interviewed the parents of 59 hyperactive and 41 control children and found a significantly higher prevalence of psychiatric illness, particularly alcoholism, in the parents of the hyperactive children. In 21 of the 59 families of hyperactive children, at least one parent was alcoholic, hysteric, or sociopathic compared to only four of the 41 control families. Twelve parents of hyperactive children (M = 9, F = 3) were retrospectively diagnosed as having been hyperactive children, as compared to two parents of control children; and of these 14 parents, 11 qualified for a psychiatric diagnosis. These data indicate the association of hyperactivity in children with specific psychiatric disorders in their parents, and suggest that hyperactivity may be etiologically related to alcoholism, hysteria, and sociopathy. The finding of a higher prevalence of psychiatric disorder in parents of hyperactive children has been confirmed by Cantwell (1972), who also reported a high prevalence of reported alcoholism, hysteria, and sociopathy in second-degree relatives of the hyperactive children. Cantwell found that 10 of the 100 parents of the children ($n = 50$) in his study had been hyperactive children themselves, and *all* of these 10 parents were psychiatrically ill, which suggests that hyperactivity may be a precursor of specific psychiatric disorders. Neither study provides more than suggestive evidence for whether this association is the result of genetic or environmental influences. However, a second study by Morrison and Stewart (1973) found a high prevalence of psychiatric disorder in the *biologic* parents of hyperactive children, but not in the *adoptive* parents, a finding that is consistent with the genetic transmission of hyperactivity.

The foregoing data provide support for speculations by Huessy (1974), on the basis of extrapolations from existing epidemiological data (Robins, 1966), that one-third of adults diagnosed in early childhood as hyperactive will have serious problems in adulthood, ranging from total psychiatric disablement to acute handicaps. Huessy's comments were made in connection with his finding in a therapeutic community setting, that a number of young adults who had been diagnosed as schizophrenic showed little evidence of the primary symptoms of schizophrenia, but in each case had been diagnosed as hyperactive in childhood. The Morrison and Stewart (1971, 1973) and Cantwell (1972) data receive some support from the results of a follow-up study by Huessy and his associates (Huessy, Metoyer, & Townsend, 1974) on a group of 84 hyperactive children who had been placed on medication 8 to 10 years previously. Their ages at the time of follow-up ranged from 9 to 24 years. The follow-up data showed the hyperactive child to be seriously at risk for academic, emotional, and social problems in later life. The school dropout rate was five times higher than expected. Of those who were employed ($n = 37$), one-third had a poor work record and many were in trouble with the law, their families, or peers. Ten of the total group of 84 had required hospitalization for psychiatric treatment, and 18 had been institutionalized, a rate that was 20 times the expected rate.

Preliminary findings from a questionnaire follow-up of hyperactive children ($n = 100$) who ranged in age from 3 to 13 years at initial evaluation, and from 15 to 26 years with a mean of 20 at follow-up, have been reported by Laufer (1971) and Denhoff (1973). Of the patients ($n = 66$) who returned the questionnaire, two-thirds were still hyperactive, more than one-third had required psychiatric help, 9 percent were continuing to have psychiatric help, and 5 percent had been hospitalized. A substantial number had had difficulty with the law, but none had been jailed. Academically the group had done quite well: 75 percent had had special education, 47 percent were either enrolled in or had completed high school, and almost one-third were attending or had graduated from college. Although these results are encouraging they may not apply to hyperactive individuals in general, since they may partially result from the fact that the respondents had been treated in private practice and were presumably in a socioeconomic group that could afford private schools and other services. Also, the accuracy of the questionnaire data could not be checked, one-third of the sample failed to respond, and of those who did return the questionnaire, each did not answer all the questions.

The most optimistic report of hyperactivity in adulthood has been presented by Shelley and Riester (1972), and concerns 16 cases (M = 14, F = 2) of previously undiagnosed minimal brain damage located as a result of psychiatric referral because of difficulty in coping with the basic tasks of military training at an Air Force base. A careful evaluation of the subjects included psychological testing with the Wechsler Adult Intelligence Scale (WAIS), Bender-Gestalt, and Rorschach; a psychiatric evaluation; a neurological evaluation including an EEG; and a Child Development Questionnaire completed by the subjects' parents. Some of their test results were consistent with a minimal brain damage diagnosis; the subjects were within the normal range in intelligence, most did better on the verbal tests on the WAIS, and many scored in the dull-normal range. Many subjects had difficulty on the Bender-Gestalt with tasks that generally are done poorly by patients with neurological dysfunction. The neurological evaluation failed to reveal any "hard signs," but all 16 manifested two or more "soft signs." The term *hard signs* describes unequivocal evidence of neurological damage, whereas *soft signs* refers to borderline equivocal neurological signs, such as awkwardness, clumsiness, mixed laterality, speech defect, short attention span, and poor fine motor coordination (Clements & Peters, 1962). Both the psychiatric examination and the parents' responses to the questionnaire were consistent with a retrospective diagnosis of hyperactivity in childhood. Most of the group had had problems in school, but all had been able to complete high school and some had finished college prior to enlisting in the Air Force. The results of the evaluation of these 16 young adults suggested that their hyperactivity was of a relatively mild type; that the problem was handled well in childhood by their families, who combined helpfulness with the children's motoric problems with firm demands for achievement; and that the subjects themselves were reasonably intelligent, motivated to do well, and astute at avoiding areas in which they performed badly. Apparently this combination of attitudes and behaviors carried them along until they entered the Air Force and were thrust into a situation that demanded precise and effective visual-motor skills, one of this group's weakest performance areas.

Further evidence of a good prognosis is contained in preliminary data from an ongoing 10-year follow-up study (Weiss, 1975a) of previously hyperactive children ($n = 80$) and matched controls ($n = 50$). Although the extensive measures of educational achievement, intellectual ability, cognitive style, work achievement, psychiatric status, and assessment of these young adults by their families had not been completed, Weiss (1975a, p. 234) noted:

It is our impression to date that the previously hyperactive young adults have adjusted surprisingly well once they have left those environmental circumstances with which they could not cope (for most this included secondary school, and for some it included rejecting homes). It seems that young adult life offers a wider range of life-styles, including varieties of continuing education (more choices of course in pre-university and university studies), large choice of jobs, and so on. It is possible, of course, that maturation itself has also played a large part in what seemed to indicate a narrowing of the gap between the experimental and the control subjects. So far we have seen no evidence of psychosis or severe depression in any of the subjects, although some have personality disturbances.

Few of the subjects in this study are married. We will continue to follow the two groups into an older age period in order to be able to assess their ability as husbands and fathers (only a few are female), their final work adjustment, and the presence or absence of psychosis or criminal behavior. Our clinical impression is that in young adulthood the adjustment of the previously hyperactive child is considerably closer to the normal than it was in the primary-school and secondary-school years.

Experienced clinicians say that with judicious use of medication, manipulation of home and school conditions, and psychotherapy, and with continued careful follow-up and adjustments in the treatment regimen, the hyperactive child can develop into a productive adult. Without this level of care the emerging evidence suggests an unrelenting downhill course (O'Malley & Eisenberg, 1973). Stewart and Olds (1973), who stress educational and therapeutic measures for the hyperactive child, are optimistic because on the one hand the high level of activity tends to diminish in adolescence, and on the other hand the demands of adult life are more flexible. Also, some of the characteristics of hyperactivity can facilitate performance in certain jobs. They have noted that adults who were hyperactive as children are often restless, lively, energetic extroverts as adults, and are frequently very successful in their careers despite poor school performance. Jobs requiring endless energy, an outgoing manner, quick decisions, physical risk, and allowing some flexibility and individual freedom, are well suited to individuals with a hyperactive temperament. The fact that adult life offers the hyperactive person alternatives that suit his temperament and allow him to function effectively supports the contention that many of the problems of the hyperactive child would diminish if schools were modified to meet the requirements of some of his behaviors.

The ability of the hyperactive adult to function effectively in the right job is highlighted by the performance of a stewardess observed by one of the authors on a crowded cross-country flight. From the moment she burst into the cabin she made the other three stewardesses, all of whom were quite industrious, look as though they were standing still. Before the plane departed she sped down the aisle checking seatbelts in approximately half the time that it took another stewardess to accomplish the same task. Although one of the other stewardesses had pronounced the compartment for storing carry-on luggage full and advised passengers to store their cases in the overhead compartment, this stewardess picked up extra cases, forced the hangers into position, and flung herself repeatedly against the crowded compartment, emitting aggressive comments as she did so, until she forced all the cases in and closed the compartment. Throughout the flight she moved about rapidly, responding to passenger requests with astonishing promptness, talking and joking with the passengers and other stewardesses, all of whom appeared to find her very congenial. On one occasion, as she was waiting to load a tray in the kitchen area, she ran in place while keeping up a lively conversation; on another, when a small boy asked for a comic book, she rushed into the storage compartment, returned with a stack of miscellaneous papers and magazines, flung them down on the floor, threw herself down beside them, and sorted them with a frenetic haste until she found a comic book, then moved rapidly up and down the aisle dispensing the other magazines. It was the author's impression that she never stood still during the entire flight and took only one very short break. When a passenger, obviously impressed with her unlimited energy, asked if she found the job tiring, she replied cheerfully that she had always been one to be "on the run," and that in grade school her teachers had recognized this and had often given her "all the good monitor jobs." When another passenger commented on the fact that she had not had a lunch break, she assured him that all she needed for lunch was coffee and chocolate bars. The fact that this nutritional routine was satisfying to her could be explained in terms of the efficacy of continuing doses of central nervous system stimulants in the form of caffeine (see Schnackenberg, 1973, in Chapter 4).

Although isolated observations and anecdotal and retrospective accounts of the hyperactive child in adulthood are of interest, comprehensive long-term investigations are needed to determine the prognosis for the hyperactive child in adulthood, and this research has not yet been done. Nor has there been any research demonstrating unequivocally that singly or in combination pharmaceutical, psychotherapeutic, and educational forms of intervention do effectively modify the long-term outcome for the hyperactive child. In the studies reviewed here most of the hyperactive children were on medication for various periods of time and some were receiving psychological treatment or counseling and remedial educational help, but the descriptive data are sparse as to the extent, quality, and regularity of the intervention provided. None of the studies provide evidence that any systematic intervention programs were provided for the hyperactive subjects in the period between the initial evaluation and the point at which follow-up measures were obtained. For definitive statements about prognosis, prospective studies on a large population of hyperactive infants and children, similar to the Terman gifted child series (Terman & Merrill, 1926; Terman & Oden, 1947; Terman & Oden, 1959), are needed. These could follow children from the onset of hyperactivity through adulthood, with periodic assessments of performance and personality. For optimum information such a population should be divided into diagnostic subgroups on the basis of etiological factors. Thus some kind of prognostic index could be formulated for children with known etiological agents, such as lead poisoning, and for those in which factors such as genetic determinants seem to be of major importance. The assumption here is that the basis for such an index would include factors such as IQ (Menkes, Rowe, & Menkes, 1967), paternal behavioral and academic history (Mendelson, Johnson, & Stewart, 1971), parent-child relationships and general adequacy of home environment (Weiss, Minde, & Werry, 1971), behavioral adjustment other than hyperactivity (Minde, Lewin, Weiss, Lavigueur, Douglas, & Sykes, 1971), as well as duration of time on medication, duration of symptoms, and time of onset of symptoms. Such an index would have considerable value for planning a treatment strategy as well as for determining prognosis.

# CHAPTER 3

# *Etiological Factors*

The earliest scientific descriptions of hyperactive children (Still, 1902) established the fact of etiological subgroups, and a variety of medical and psychological conditions characterized by hyperactivity have since been identified (McMahon, Deem, & Greenberg, 1970). However, it is apparent from the literature that *most* of the clinical descriptions and experimental studies from the turn of the century to 1970 have treated hyperactivity as a homogeneous phenomenon. There have been frequent acknowledgments that etiological subgroups do exist and strong recommendations that they be identified and studied, but there has been little evidence of action. Interest that focused on etiological classification prior to 1970 tended to emphasize an organic-nonorganic dichotomy (Cruickshank, Bentzen, Ratzeburg, & Tannhauser, 1961). One of the few exceptions was Bender's (1953) categories of organic, constitutional, and environmental hyperactivity. That there was a paucity of clinical and research interest in the etiology of hyperactivity until the end of the 1960s is evident from the comprehensive review articles of Werry (1968) and Werry and Sprague (1970). In both articles the authors carefully considered the supportive evidence for the genetic, organic, and psychogenic etiologic factors and concluded that there was insufficient empirical support for these hypotheses. In the years that have elapsed since the publication of their articles, considerable evidence has accumulated for the importance of genetic and psychogenic factors in the etiology of hyperactivity and also for several other factors that, prior to 1970, had not entered into etiologic discussions. The support comes from two sources: experienced clinicians and experimental investigations. Several clinicians have rejected the unitary concept of hyperactivity and, on the nonexperimental basis of extensive experience with hyperactive children, have identified subgroups of these children. Although experimental evidence for these classifications is lacking, the value of clinical observations should not be discounted, particularly when detailed and supportive case history data are provided. Nor should it be forgotten that many productive hypotheses have evolved as a direct result of astute clinical observation.

Howell, Rever, Scholl, Trowbridge, and Rutledge (1972) have suggested a treatment-oriented classification for assigning excessively active children to two classes: *primary hyperactivity,* in which the excessive movement is the root of the child's difficulty, so that the child is best treated by focusing on the activity itself; and *secondary hyperactivity,* in which the high level of activity is a symptom of a more basic problem, or a reaction to it, so that therapeutic efforts should be directed to the underlying cause. Marwit and Stenner (1972) have also identified two patterns of hyperactivity. In the first of these the child consistently exhibits a high level of activity that is often inappropriate. He is clumsy, often has perceptual and learning deficits, is unable to stay with tasks, and has poor peer relationships. The etiological factors that this pattern is often associated with are organic brain damage and maturational lag, but the pattern can also occur as a normal variant of temperament. The second pattern represents a learned response and is essentially a life style developed by the child as a means of coping with his environment. The child who is characterized by this pattern is clearly capable and does not have the basic learning and behavioral deficits of the first pattern, although he may be emotionally disturbed or anxiety-ridden as a result of precipitating social and nonsocial environmental factors. Ney (1974) has used clinical histories and test results from a large group of referrals ($n = 263$) to designate four types of hyperactivity: *genetic hyperactivity* includes children who have been hyperactive from early infancy and whose prenatal and perinatal histories were normal; *behavioral hyperactivity* refers to children whose hyperactivity was conditioned by parental handling; *minimal brain dysfunction* describes children with early continuous hyperactivity and histories of abnormal pregnancies or perinatal events; and *reactive hyperactivity* occurs in children from chaotic home environments. Although the labels are different, Howell et al.'s secondary hyperactivity, Marwit and Stenner's learned response pattern, and Ney's reactive and behavioral categories are all somewhat similar, which attests to the reasonableness of these groupings. Doubros and Daniels (1966) have conceptualized hyperactivity as a class of heterogeneous inappropriate responses maintained by an unspecified number of social and nonsocial environmental factors. Thomas, Chess, and Birch (1968) consider a high level of activity accompanied by other difficult behaviors to be a normal variant of temperament that can become a behavior problem if it results in conflict with the child's environment. Bender (1953) has designated three kinds of hyperactivity: *constitutional,* which is similar to Thomas, Chess, and Birch's normal variant of temperament; *organic,* a brain-damage syndrome; and *environmental,* which is learned. Other categorizations of hyperactive children that are based on a number of medical and environmental factors include those of Lesser (1970), who has suggested seven etiological groups; McMahon, Deem, and Greenberg

(1970), who have listed 12 etiologic considerations; and Bax (1972), who considers genuine hyperactivity to be rare, but has described a variety of social and cultural factors that can elicit overactive behavior.

In addition to these nonexperimental but potentially valuable descriptions of subgroups of hyperactive children, four major categories of etiological influence have been investigated: genetic, organic, psychogenic, and nonsocial environmental factors. The relevant theoretical formulations and the available direct and indirect empirical support for them are discussed here. Although most of these formulations are of a fragmentary nature, with varying amounts of supportive evidence due in some cases to their comparative recency, some have already generated hypotheses that represent interesting new directions in the search for knowledge and understanding of hyperactivity, particularly in the areas of effective prevention and treatment methods. It is important to note that although the available empirical data are not adequate to establish an unequivocal cause-effect relationship, the evidence to date for some of the factors, and the potential importance of others, qualifies them for serious consideration as having an etiological relationship to hyperactivity. Furthermore, some of the environmental factors to be discussed here had not actively been considered prior to the 1970s and are particularly worthy of etiological consideration since the prevalence of hyperactivity appears to have increased sharply over the last 25 years. One explanation for such an increase could be the presence of new environmental causative agents; another could be that a heterogeneous set of misbehaviors has become defined as hyperactivity. Conrad and Teele (Smithsonian Science Information Exchange, 1975) are currently studying factors that were involved in the purported increase in the identification, diagnosis, and treatment of hyperactive children during the period from 1953 to 1973.

## GENETIC FACTORS

The present decade has been notable for attempts to evaluate the relative roles of genetic and environmental factors in this behavior problem. Omenn (1973) has noted that this task has been made difficult by the fact that the clinical phenotypes in behavior disorders are highly variable and far removed from the direct effects of single genes. Furthermore, a specific analysis of the interaction of a genetic predisposition and some environmental stresses may be impossible.

Although no studies have directly established that genetic factors are important determinants of hyperactivity, several sets of well-documented findings have suggested that such a relationship may exist. There has been unequivocal evidence since the early part of this century that animals could be selectively bred for high or low activity level (McClearn, 1970); human twin studies have suggested a genetic component to activity level (Scarr, 1966); many parents of hyperactive children remember themselves as hyperactive (Stewart & Olds, 1973); and a significant parent-child resemblance in activity level exists when parents of children within the normal range of activity level are asked to report on their own childhood activity levels (Willerman & Plomin, 1973). None of the foregoing data can be regarded as conclusive, but they have important implications for the etiology of the hyperactivity problem.

Following are several epidemiological methodologies that have been used to study the role of genetic factors in the transmission of hyperactivity.

## First Degree Relatives

In this method first degree relatives (parents, siblings, and children) of hyperactive children are studied to determine whether they have a higher risk of being or becoming hyperactive than do control groups of comparable individuals from the general population. Morrison and Stewart (1971) interviewed the parents of 59 hyperactive and 41 control children to determine whether the parents or any of the second-degree relatives (aunts, uncles, cousins) had been hyperactive as children, and found a trend toward an association between hyperactivity in parent and child. Twenty percent of the hyperactive children had a parent (M = 9, F = 3) who had been hyperactive, compared to 5 percent of the parents (M = 1, F = 1) of the control children. When the findings for first- and second-degree relatives were combined, hyperactivity occurred significantly more often in the families of hyperactive children ($p < .001$). These families also had a higher prevalence of psychiatric disorder, with one-third having some psychiatric diagnosis as compared to one-sixth of the control group parents ($p < .025$). The major differences were the greater prevalence of alcoholism, sociopathy, and hysteria (p < .01). The fact that in 21 of the 59 families of hyperactive children at least one parent was alcoholic, sociopathic, or hysteric, whereas only 4 of the 41 control families were so affected ($p < .025$), suggests that these three adult disorders may all bear a familial relationship to hyperactivity (Morrison & Stewart, 1971). Agreement with these findings was reported by Cantwell (1972), who interviewed the parents of 50 hyperactive children and 50 matched control children seen in a pediatric clinic in a military setting. Ten percent of the parents (M = 8, F = 2) of the hyperactive children were diagnosed as having been hyperactive themselves as children, and 45 percent had some psychiatric diagnosis (alcoholism, sociopathy, hysteria, and probable hysteria). In the control families only 2 percent of the parents were diagnosed as having been hyperactive as children; this figure is probably spuriously low, however, because the pediatrician who located the control group was asked to recommend families who were not known to have hyperactive members. Eighteen percent of the control parents had some psychiatric diagnosis. The results of these two studies confirm the common clinical finding that hyperactivity passes from one generation to the next, and that there is an increased prevalence of psychiatric disorder in the families of hyperactive children. They do *not* distinguish between genetic and environmental modes of transmission of the hyperactivity, and they do not specify the nature of the relationship between the hyperactivity and the adult psychiatric disorders.

## Twin Studies

This method compares identical monozygotic (MZ) twins with fraternal dizygotic (DZ) same-sex twins. If *genetic factors* are important in the transmission of hyperactivity, one would expect to find that when one MZ twin is hyperactive the probability would be high that the co-twin would also be hyperactive, that is, a *concordant* relationship would exist. However, the rate of concordance in DZ twins would be significantly lower, resembling that for same-sex singleton siblings. If *environmental factors* are important the rate of concordance in MZ twins should not differ significantly from that in DZ twins, except that MZ twins are treated more similarly than are DZ twins. The only twin study with children diagnosed as hyperactive was one by Lopez (1965) in which methodological weaknesses rendered the findings invalid. However, there have been several studies of activity in normal twins. Willerman (1973) asked the mothers of 93 sets of same-sex twins to complete questionnaires on the activity level and zygosity of their twins. The adjusted score intraclass correlation ($r = .92$) for activity level in MZ twins was significantly higher ($p < .001$) than that ($r = .60$) for DZ twins; but this similarity could be attributed in part to the fact that parents who believe that their twins are identical would be more likely to give them identical ratings. Estimates of *heritability,* the proportion of variance accounted for by genetic factors, were also computed. The results showed a heritability of .82 for males and .58 for females. Among twin sets in which at least one member of the pair scored in the top 20 percent on the Activity Level Questionnaire (Werry & Sprague, 1970), MZ twins ($n = 8$ sets) showed a high correlation ($r = .70$) for activity level, and DZ twins ($n = 16$ sets) showed a zero correlation, apparently due to the restricted range of scores in the hyperactivity sample (top 20 percent of the scores). Taken together these results suggest a substantial genetic component to *activity level* but not necessarily to *hyperactivity*. Willerman arbitrarily designated scores in the top 20 percent on the Activity Level Questionnaire as *hyperactive* without obtaining confirmation of hyperactivity in these subjects from other sources. If such scores are indicative of hyperactivity, then the results of this study are consistent with the view that genetic factors are important in hyperactivity. It is essential that researchers distinguish between the most active in a subject population and the truly hyperactive. There is a regrettable tendency to treat a high level of activity as synonymous with hyperactivity, and as we have already pointed out, hyperactivity is *qualitatively* different from a high level of activity. Further evidence of a genetic basis for activity level in normal children is provided by a study in which Vandenberg (1962) administered the Thurstone Temperament Schedule to adolescent twins and found a heritability of .67 for activity. Also, Scarr (1966) reported a significant hereditary component to activity level in a study in which twin girls of elementary school age were measured on a variety of procedures related to activity level. These findings suggest that genetic influences are involved in activity level, but it is also clear that the findings cannot sustain a purely genetic mode of transmission.

The basic assumption in the twin study method of investigating the genetic contribution for a specific characteristic is that differences between MZ twins are a result of environmental factors, whereas those in DZ twins reflect both genetic and environmental factors. Therefore, the greater the resemblance of MZ twins, and the smaller the resemblance of DZ twins for that characteristic, the stronger the assumption of a genetic contribution. This assumption is subject to two criticisms that would be difficult for even a methodologically sound study to cope with: MZ and DZ same-sex twins may differ in homogeneity of treatment by others, with MZ twins having more similar experiences, which could reduce interpair differences in MZ twins and thus provide spurious support for a genetic hypothesis. Also, MZ twins are more at risk than DZ twins for some of the prenatal and perinatal problems that appear to be etiologically related to hyperactivity, and these *environmental factors* could spuriously increase the concordance rate for hyperactivity in MZ twins (World Health Organization, 1966).

## Adopted Children

One method here is to study adopted or foster children and their biological and adoptive parents. Children in these studies preferably have been reared from infancy by adults who are not their biological parents. Morrison and Stewart (1973) interviewed the legal adoptive but not the biological parents of 35 hyperactive children (M = 31, F = 4) who had had no contact since birth with their biological parents, and who had been permanently placed by the age of 2.5 years. The results of the interviews were then compared with previously reported groups of the biological parents of other hyperactive children and control parents (Morrison & Stewart, 1971). In this study and in a similar one by Cantwell (1972), the biological parents used for comparison purposes unfortunately were not the parents of the hyperactive children in the study, but were the biological parents of *another group* of clinically diagnosed hyperactive children. Consequently the results of both studies are considerably weakened by the fact that the biologic and adoptive parents did not share the same offspring. However, two findings provided support for the role of genetic transmission in the development of hyperactivity. The biological first- and second-degree relatives reported a significantly higher prevalence of childhood hyperactivity than did the adoptive relatives or controls (who did not differ on this measure). This finding clearly favors a genetic transmission hypothesis. Second, hyperactivity was more often associated with the adult personality disorders of sociopathy, hysteria, and alcoholism in the biological group than in the adoptive group. There is considerable evidence to suggest that these three personality disorders have a genetic basis, and the fact that hyperactivity has been shown to be linked with them in these studies supports a genetic mode of transmission for hyperactivity.

Another type of adoption study involves comparisons between twins, siblings, or half siblings who have been reared apart. Safer (1973) reviewed the medical histories and social service charts of the full siblings (*n* = 19) and half siblings (*n* = 22) of 17 index children with minimal brain dysfunction, all of whom had been assigned to foster homes at an early age. The major difference in group description was that the full siblings had the same fathers as did the index minimal brain dysfunction children, but the half siblings did not. The data were consistent with the genetic transmission of hyperactivity: there was a significantly higher incidence of the major signs of minimal brain dysfunction in the full siblings than in the half siblings; 10 of the 19 full siblings were classified as having minimal brain dysfunction as compared with 2 of the 22 half siblings.

These studies suggest the existence of a hereditary factor in the transmission of hyperactivity that operates in combination with environmental factors. The question of which model of genetic transmission could account for such a factor has been pursued by Morrison and Stewart (1973, 1974). They point out that the well-established excess of affected males argues against a *single autosomal dominant gene pattern*, because for this pattern there should be no sex differences in prevalence. Also, with this pattern no generations should be skipped and one parent should have been hyperactive, and there is considerable clinical evidence that these events do not occur with any consistency. It should be noted that if a *reduced penetrance explanation* is invoked, generations could be skipped with a single autosomal dominant gene pattern. With a *single autosomal recessive gene* both parents would be carriers but neither should have been affected, and approximately one-quarter of the siblings of the hyperactive child should be hyperactive. The number of affected parents in the Morrison and Stewart (1971) and Cantwell (1972) studies, coupled with the lack of evidence of the prevalence rate in siblings, excludes this mechanism of transmission. The well-documented evidence of apparent transmission of hyperactivity from father to son (Cantwell, 1972; Omenn, 1973) is inconsistent with a *sex-linked mode of transmission*. In the only chromosome study of hyperactive children in the literature, Warren, Karduck, Bussaratid, Stewart, and Sly (1971) reported no evidence of any *chromosome aberrations*. Morrison and Stewart (1973) conclude that the high ratio of males to females afflicted with this syndrome suggests some sort of *polyfactorial transmission* in which a sizable number of different hereditary and environmental influences interact to produce the behavior, with the hereditary component being polygenic, that is, reflecting the activity of many genes rather than of a single major gene. Wender (1971) considered the fact that minimal brain dysfunction did not "breed true" to be support for a theory of polygenetic transmission.

Polyfactorial transmission implies a genetic predisposition to hyperactivity that puts the individual at risk so that the extent to which he is affected by hyperactivity, if he is affected at all, is determined by various environmental influences that operate on the substrate of the genetic predisposition. A polyfactorial hypothesis would be consistent with the sex differences in hyperactivity as well as with its variability. To test the hypothesis of polygenetic transmission Morrison and Stewart (1973) reexamined the data of a previous study (Morrison & Stewart, 1971) that had demonstrated an association between hyperactivity and the adult psychiatric disorders of alcoholism, hysteria, and sociopathy. Two aspects of the polygenetic hypothesis were tested, the first being that the greater the number of individuals in a family who are hyperactive, the higher the risk component for related conditions in that family. Thus if hyperactivity is linked with alcoholism, families with several cases of hyperactivity in the immediate or extended families of the proband would be expected to have a higher incidence of alcoholics than families with no secondary cases of hyperactivity. This hypothesis was supported: the incidence of alcoholism in first- and second-degree relatives was nearly twice as high in families with secondary cases of hyperactivity as in families with no secondary cases. According to the polygenetic theory, if a proband has a first-degree relative who is hyperactive, that family probably has a higher dose of the genes responsible, and hence would be more likely to have more remote relatives affected than would a family in which only the proband is hyperactive. This hypothesis was also confirmed. Of the families ($n = 15$) with an affected first-degree relative, seven had an extended relative with hyperactivity and eight had none. Of the families ($n = 44$) with no affected first-degree relatives, eight had an extended relative with hyperactivity and 36 had none. Although these data do not rule out other modes of genetic or social transmission, they do support the polygenetic transmission model. In a second study Morrison and Stewart (1973a) used Slater's method (1966) to distinguish between polygenetic transmission and dominant gene transmission with reduced penetrance. With this method family histories are analyzed to determine whether secondary cases occur almost exclusively on one side of the family, as would be expected with a single dominant gene, or whether a significant number of affected persons have *both* paternal and maternal ascendant relatives so affected, which would support polygenetic transmission. When the family histories of 12 hyperactive children were examined, relatives affected with hyperactivity or adult psychiatric disorders were found on both sides of the families, a finding congruent with a polygenetic mode of transmission. For an excellent discussion of this mode of genetic transmission see Carter (1969).

Although the results of this rather diverse group of studies suggest a genetic mechanism of transmission, they have not proven it. The crucial genetic study of hyperactivity or any trait, condition, or disorder must specify the precise genetic mechanism involved. The only procedures that can precisely define a genetic mechanism are *segregation studies,* which could only be done with humans under very unusual circumstances, and *linkage studies,* which would require the identification of the genetic marker associated with hyperactivity (Cantwell, 1975b). One difficulty in conducting such genetic studies is the possibility that different etiological subgroups may be represented in the subject population and their characteristics could confound the findings. Researchers in this area would do well to locate children whose hyperactivity began in the neonatal or prenatal stage, with no identifiable cause (see, for example, the 1972 study of David, Clark, and Voeller discussed in the section on lead poisoning in this chapter). Since there is ample evidence to suggest that hyperactive children are an etiologically heterogeneous group, it is time for researchers to treat this heterogeneity as a significant variable in research on hyperactivity.

## ORGANIC FACTORS

The earliest descriptions of hyperactivity (Still, 1902; Ebaugh, 1923) usually attributed the condition to *brain damage* that had occurred as a result of traumatic events, such as severe illness, injury, and prenatal and perinatal problems. The assumption that brain damage caused hyperactivity was strengthened by a report (Strauss & Lehtinen, 1947) citing hyperactivity as one of the primary behaviors of the brain-injured, mentally retarded child. Although hyperactivity does occur in children with severe and demonstrable brain damage, there is little empirical evidence to support the view of brain damage as a major etiological factor in hyperactivity. Stewart and Olds (1973) estimate that less than 10 percent of the referrals for hyperactivity have histories suggesting brain injury, and point out that the frequency of birth process complications is no greater among the hyperactive than the general population; even when such complications do occur they are not necessarily significant. Evidence from the Kauai pregnancy study (Werner, Bierman, French, Simonian, Connor, Smith, & Campbell, 1968) showed little relationship between severe perinatal stress and later performance. Werry and Sprague (1970) state that when the criteria for subject selection are either *demonstrable* brain damage or brain damage *inferred* from noxious events, such as severe perinatal anoxia that carry a high probability of causing significant damage, the research produces little evidence that brain damage causes hyperactivity. However, when the criterion for subject selection is *hyperactivity,* there is a higher incidence of minor abnormalities in the experimental group than is usually the case for the normal control children. The neurological significance of minor EEG, perceptual, and sensorimotor abnormalities is a matter of dispute, with some investigators (Werry, Weiss, & Douglas, 1964) reporting that hyperactive children have slightly more than the usual number of events in their histories that might have caused brain damage. Others (Stewart, Pitts, Craig, & Dieruf, 1966) have found no differences between hyperactive and normal groups on this variable. Although there is evidence from animal studies (Cromwell, Baumeister, & Hawkins, 1963) and clinical psychopharmacology (Werry & Sprague, 1970) consistent with the hypothesis that interference with cerebral function can result in hyperactivity, Werry's (1968) conclusion that there is no firm evidence for the organic etiologic hypothesis still stands.

## Brain Dysfunction

There is increasing theoretical and empirical interest in the role of brain dysfunction in hyperactivity. As noted earlier, we do not dispute the possibility that minimal degrees of brain dysfunction, which are exceedingly difficult but not impossible to demonstrate (Towbin, 1971), may be etiologically related to hyperactivity. Our objection concerns the *designa-*

*tion* of brain damage purely on the basis of certain behavioral symptoms or obstetrical complications. For example, one group of clinicians considers that a combination of hyperactivity, other behavior symptoms, and cerebral anoxia in the delivery process *automatically* justifies a diagnosis of minimal brain dysfunction. Many clinicians agree with Handford's (1975) hypothesis that infants who suffer brain hypoxia prenatally, perinatally, or immediately postnatally constitute a population at risk for minimal brain dysfunction. Empirical evidence against such a conclusion has been provided by the methodologically sophisticated prospective study by Graham, Ernhart, Thurston, and Craft (1962) of development 3 years after perinatal anoxia and other potentially damaging neonatal experiences. Their results showed an increased number of adverse cognitive and neurological effects as a function of these early traumatic experiences, but there was no evidence that the obstetrical complications were associated with hyperactivity or any specific behavior disorder.

Several theoretical formulations of brain dysfunction as an etiological factor in hyperactivity are based on models that emphasize the interaction of excitatory and inhibitory systems within the central nervous system. The most comprehensive of these theories is that of Wender (1971, p. 186). There is relatively little empirical support for this theory, and some of its assumptions about high arousal level and defective reward mechanisms in the hyperactive child have been questioned or contradicted by recent empirical evidence (Sroufe, 1975). It is presented here because it is the most comprehensive theoretical attempt thus far to integrate data on hyperactivity and to relate hyperactivity to brain dysfunction (Sroufe, 1975). As such, it should generate a strong body of research in this area. According to the interpretation of this theory offered by Sroufe (1975), the increased arousal and activity, and the diminished capacity for positive and negative affect in the hyperactive child, can be attributed to an abnormality in the metabolism of the monoamines (serotonin, noradrenaline, and dopamine), specifically, to a low cortical noradrenaline level with a consequent deficiency in the inhibitory system. In this theory activity level is assumed to be a function of the comparative levels of the inhibitory and excitatory systems and both systems are assumed to be monoaminergic so that both respond to amphetamine. If the excitatory system is at a higher level of activity (as mediated by the monoamines), the child is more active; if the inhibitory system is at a higher level, the child is more controlled. The activity level of the normal child represents a balance between the two systems. The low noradrenaline level that Wender has postulated in the hyperactive child decreases activity in the inhibitory system and thus results in a high level of activity in the child. Because the amphetamines are chemically similar to noradrenaline, they can substitute for it and thus modify the low cortical noradrenaline level, with a consequent calming effect in the hyperactive child. Although the amphetamines act on *both* the inhibitory and excitatory systems, the effect of the usual therapeutic dose of amphetamine on the hyperactive child is a calming one because, according to Wender, the curvilinear inhibitory function is more steeply sloped near the zero point. Consequently, the *net effect* of amphetamine on a child with a low noradrenaline level is an increase in the activity of the inhibitory system (see Figure 2). In considering this *ad hoc* explanation it is important to keep in mind that the validity of the assumption of a paradoxical drug effect (that is, that over-aroused children become quieter and normal children become over-aroused with a subsequent deterioration in performance as a function of moderate doses of stimulant medication) is crucial to Wender's explanation: it also is important to note that there is no evidence that moderate doses of stimulant medication impair performance in normal

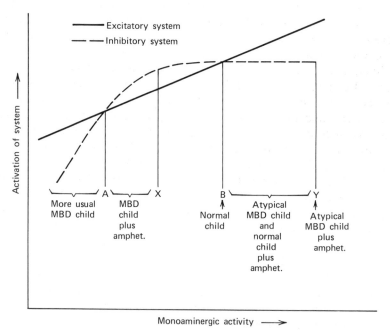

Figure 2. Level of arousal and monoaminergic activity. (Reprinted, by permission, from Wender, P. H. *Minimal brain dysfunction in children.* New York: Wiley-Interscience, 1971, p. 187.)

children (Sroufe, 1975). Indeed, the evidence from studies on adults would suggest that many types of performance might *improve* as a function of the amphetamines (Weiss & Laties, 1962). Wender (1971) cites as support for his theoretical position research with rats that demonstrated a progressive increase in the monoamines with age. If we can assume that the same changes in the monoamine system occur with maturation in humans, this research finding suggests an explanation for the fact that activity level decreases with age in the hyperactive child. Also, another study cited by Wender (1971) showed that testosterone administration increased the level of the monoamines in rats. Since increased androgenic activity normally occurs at puberty and thus could increase the level of the monoamines, this finding would also provide an explanation for the fact that hyperactive behavior often decreases at puberty.

Several other less explicitly formulated attempts have been made to explain hyperactivity as a result of some dysfunction in the central nervous system. Gellner (1959) suggested that damage to the midbrain structures, specifically the superior colliculi, may result in an inability to respond meaningfully to visual arrays which, in turn, causes a child to seek compensation by obtaining an increased amount of kinesthetic, tactual, and proprioceptive stimulation. In the process of seeking such stimulation the child exhibits a high level of activity. Zaporozhets (1957) also emphasized the role of tactual stimulation in the explanation of hyperactivity. According to his explanation, early motor activity provides a primal basis of motor-touch associations with the young child's world. This set of tactual associations provides a basis for the development of visual associations, which in turn mediate the acquisition of word and sensory associations. Neurological impairment could cause the child to be fixated at the tactual stage and thus continue to react to external stimuli with motor-touch activity. In the early childhood years such a response pattern might not cause any problems, but in the preschool and early school years it would appear as hyperactivity. Laufer and Denhoff (1957) have postulated a diencephalon disorder to explain hyperactivity; their explanation and the related research is discussed in Chapter 4.

## Delayed Maturation as an Alternative to Brain Dysfunction

Some investigators (Abrams, 1968; Bax & MacKeith, 1963; Laufer, Denhoff, & Solomons, 1957) have emphasized the role of of maturational factors in hyperactivity and have discounted the role of brain dysfunction. There is both physiological and psychological support for a subgroup of hyperactive children characterized by delayed and/or irregular maturation.

In a carefully conducted study Oettinger, Majovski, Limbeck, and Gauch (1974) demonstrated that elementary school children ($n = 53$) diagnosed as having minimal brain dysfunction were significantly retarded ($p < .01$) in bone age as compared to standard norms, with two-thirds of the subjects falling below the norms. Oettinger et al. concluded that the concept of physiological immaturity should be considered in school and home planning for such children. Peters, Romine, and Dykman (1975) reported that although younger children with minimal brain dysfunction showed significantly more lags or deficits at the highest levels of central nervous system functioning than did control children, many of these signs diminished or disappeared with age, so that older children with minimal brain dysfunction were more like the control children. On psychological measures of impulsivity Weithorn (1970) found greater similarity of performance between older hyperactive and younger nonhyperactive boys than between same-age hyperactive and nonhyperactive boys. These differences were more clearly defined in comparisons between first and fourth grade groups than they were between fourth and sixth grade groups, a finding that is consistent with a delayed development hypothesis. Further support for a maturational lag is provided by Butter and Lapierre (1974), who compared 6- to 12-year-old hyperactive children with normal matched controls on the Illinois Test of Psycholinguistic Abilities and found that the hyperactive group were from 18 to 24 months less mature than the controls. Note that the possibility of a maturational lag does not mean that treatment should be postponed, instead it suggests the direction that some aspects of the management program should take.

## PSYCHOGENIC FACTORS

### Child Rearing

One explanation of the etiology of hyperactivity centers around the traditional view that the mother's behavior with her child is primarily a function of her attitudes, motives, and philosophy of child rearing, and as such, is relatively independent of the infant's characteristics. Bettelheim (1973) has proposed that there are children who are *predisposed* to hyperactivity because of constitutional factors, and who then react with hyperactivity when they are stressed with environmental pressures that exceed their tolerance. According to this diasthesis-stress formulation many potentially normal infants become restless and cranky because their mothers are impatient or resentful of the trouble the infant causes them; presumably a mother with an unusual capacity for calming, or considerable tolerance for restlessness, would not react to the infant in a way that would exacerbate his difficult temperament. Often the unhappy dyadic relationship deteriorates into a continuing battle, with the infant fighting back through restlessness and resistance as he finds himself unable to cope with his mother's demands for quiet compliant behavior. As he moves chaotically through the preschool years his performance elicits increasing maternal disapproval with a consequent deterioration in his behavior. As his mother becomes increasingly anxious about his ability to adjust to school, she conveys her anxiety and disapproval to him explicitly and implicitly; the child thus sees himself as more and more of a problem, and his already battered self-concept deteriorates further. The demands in the school situation for conformity and compliance, particularly inhibition of motor movement, are often far beyond the child's capacity and soon his teacher and peers label him as a failure.

According to Bettelheim, the inability to learn that so often characterizes the hyperactive child is partly a function of his low self-esteem and restlessness, but is primarily the child's way of defending himself against an environment that has been characterized since his infancy by rejecting agents of socialization. The increasing demands to perform lead to an inability to perform at the level expected on the basis of the child's intelligence, or to an inability to perform at all. Bettelheim portrays the child as driven into a state of hyperactivity and advocates more warmth, acceptance, and flexibility on the part of women in the child's environment, the implication being that the same child would probably be able to maintain an acceptable pattern of behavior if the environmental stresses were modified.

Of relevance to the latter point is a study by Gelfand (1973) in which the task performance of children with minimal brain dysfunction was compared under two sets of conditions. In one condition the child was required to perform the experimental task in the presence of his mother; in the other he performed the task in the presence of an experimenter whom he knew well, and who created an interpersonal climate that was as different as possible from that of the child with his mother. The maternal climates were more nonresponsive and generally more negative than those of the experimenter. The hypothesis that the children would perform better with the experimenter was confirmed. They showed greater absorption in the task and more exuberance with the experimenter, whereas their behavior with their mothers was more distractible, angry, and anxious. These results are consistent with Bettelheim's view that the child's behavior and performance are not isolated variables; instead, they covary with the general behavior and affect of socialization agents within specific interpersonal situations.

There is other support in the clinical and research literature for the etiological explanation proposed by Bettelheim. Henderson and his associates (Henderson, Dahlin, Partridge, & Engelsing, 1973, 1974) believe that the mother can be the source of the child's difficulty, thus supporting Bettelheim's position; they also think that the infant can trigger off the difficult relationship. They regard the etiology of hyperactivity as a chain of events in which one primary factor is an overreactivity to touch and handling that manifests itself in an avoidance response pattern evoking negative responses from the caretakers in early infancy. As a function of the infant's fussiness and difficult behaviors the mother may become tense, guilt-ridden, and anxious, with the result that the early mother-child interaction spirals into an increasingly tense and difficult dyadic relationship. Henderson et al. note that such difficulties may also originate with the mother: inadequate maternal handling may result in an originally calm infant becoming a problem. The infant and young child who has experienced these difficulties is ill-equipped to cope with school stresses, and one outcome may be the pattern of school performance and social relationships similar to that described by Bettelheim (1973). To modify the early avoidance response pattern Henderson et al. recommend an increase in the usual amount of physical contact. In a pilot study they have demonstrated successful use of this procedure with both infants and elementary school children (Dahlin, Engelsing, & Henderson, 1975).

Battle and Lacey (1972) have reported the correlates of hyperactivity in boys who participated in the Fels Longitudinal Study. The mothers of hyperactive male infants were critical of their difficult babies during infancy and showed a lack of affection for them, continued to be disapproving during the later preschool years and tended to pressure the child to be independent, tended to use severe penalties for disobedience during the primary school years, and assessed their sons' intelligence as lower than did mothers of boys with a moderate level of activity. Hyperactive boys were characterized from early infancy by an absence of compliance with adults and also of achievement striving. Thomas, Chess, Birch, and Hertzig (1960) have identified a pattern of behavior characterized by high activity level, irregularity, nonadaptability, high intensity, and negative mood that is discernible early in the first year of life and continues to be characteristic of the preschool child. This temperament pattern is similar to Bettelheim's description of these infants' behavior. Chess, Thomas, Rutter, and Birch (1963, p. 145), in studying children with the temperament pattern that they describe as difficult, provide impressive evidence of the differences in behavior and adaptation to the school environment that occur as a result of differential parental practices in child management. For example:

The first pair of children, a girl and a boy, both showed the characteristics of irregularity, non-adaptability, negative mood and intense reactivity in the infancy period. Both were what are often called "difficult infants" to manage, with irregular sleep patterns, constipation and painful evacuations at times, slow acceptance of new foods, prolonged adjustment periods to new routines, and frequent and loud periods of crying. Adaptation to nursery school in the 4th year was also a problem for both children.

In terms of parental attitudes and practices, however, the children differed greatly. The girl's father was unusually angry with her, in speaking of her gave the impression of dislike of the youngster, was punitive, and spent little or no recreational time with her. The mother was more concerned for the child, more understanding, and more permissive, but quite inconsistent. There were only two areas in which there was firm but quiet parental consistency, namely safety rules and choice of clothing.

The boy's parents, on the other hand, were unusually tolerant and consistent. The child's lengthy adjustment periods were taken in stride and his strident altercations with his younger sibling were dealt with good-humoredly. They waited out his negative moods without getting angry. They tended to be very permissive but set safety limits and consistently pointed out the needs of his peers at play.

By the age of five and one-half years these two children, whose initial characteristics had been so similar, showed qualitative behavioral differences. The boy's initial difficulties in nursery school had disappeared, he was a constructive member of his class, had a group of friends with whom he exchanged visits and functioned smoothly in the major routine areas of daily living. The girl, by contrast, had over the previous few years developed a number of symptoms of increasing severity. These included explosive angers, negativism, fear of the dark, encopresis, thumb-sucking, insatiable demands for toys and sweets, poor peer relationships, and protective lying. It is of interest that there was a lack of any symptomatology or negativism in the two areas where parental practice had been firmly and quietly consistent, i.e., safety rules and choice of clothing.*

The *existence* of the temperament pattern described by Bettelheim and supported by others is unquestioned. Many children fit this description. Disagreement arises concerning the *source* or eliciting stimuli for the mother's immediate behavior to her infant. Research in the last two decades suggests that the *unidirectional* effect proposed by Bettelheim (1973) and other traditionalists is quite inaccurate (Bell, 1968): in fact, the direction of effect is *bidirectional*. The environment is not an autonomous force as Bettelheim would have it, but instead is caused just as the behavior is caused (Bandura, 1974). Temperamental differences among neonates have

* Reprinted, by permission, from Chess, S., Thomas, A., Rutter, M., & Birch, H.G. Interaction of temperament and environment in the production of behavioral disturbances in children. *American Journal of Psychiatry,* 1963, Vol. 120, pp. 142–148, Copyright 1963, the American Psychiatric Association.

been clearly identified in research projects, but because of the chasm between research reports and their application to socialization practices, the findings and their effect on the early dyadic relationship are often not considered. There is firm evidence that the infant, with his pattern of difficult response, partly determines his social environment. Although the mother's behavior to the infant is guided by her beliefs and attitudes, it is also controlled to a substantial degree by the infant's behavior, just as the infant's behavior can be determined to a great extent by the mother's behavior. The mother may by her negative and rejecting attitude *cause* her infant to behave in a difficult manner, or she may become impatient, critical, and rejecting as a *result* of her infant's behavior. Unfortunately, her behavior and response patterns then serve to heighten and maintain the infant's negative behaviors. In discussing the resultant strained and tense relationship between the child and the mother, Huessy (1967, p. 131) writes:

It is our feeling that it is not the poor relationship which has brought about the child's problem, but that the child's problem has brought about this strained relationship.

Acceptance of the bidirectional view as a philosophical base for determining the specific content of the intervention program will result in a program markedly different from that based on a unidirectional view of the child's problem.

## Learning

There is both theoretical and empirical support for the early acquisition of hyperactivity as a function of direct reinforcement or through observational learning processes.

### Direct Reinforcement

Consider first the case for the development of a hyperactive behavior pattern either through early direct reinforcement of physiological needs or as a coping response that is strengthened through social reinforcement. Clinical reports strongly support a wide range of fetal activity during pregnancy, and mothers of hyperactive children have often commented on the unusually active nature of these children during the latter part of the pregnancy. These recollections can often be verified from the obstetrical histories. Let us suppose that the high level of prenatal activity reported in children, some of whom were subsequently diagnosed as hyperactive, represents an attempt by a fetus characterized by a high level of arousal to maintain an optimal level of stimulation (Berlyne, 1960; Leuba, 1955).* As Wender (1971) has theorized, such a state of overarousal could result from a deficient inhibitory system which might cause the fetus, and later the infant, to strive to reduce his level of arousal by seeking stimulation. The activity response would be strengthened initially by self-reinforcement, that is, as a result of the reinforcing value of the fetal activity a *tendency* toward high motility could be acquired prenatally. In the postnatal period optimal stimulation would continue to be maintained through physical activity, and as long as this behavior was not also accompanied by irritability or any other difficult attributes it is likely that the infant would receive considerable positive attention for this response pattern. That neonates do differ widely in motility in the early days of life is well-documented (Kessen, Hendry, & Leutzendorff, 1961). There are several possible explanations for a high level of activity; the instigating factor could be that the optimal level of stimulation for a particular infant is one that requires considerable activity. Since high motility in an infant elicits attention from adults more often than does passivity, the behavior pattern is likely to be strengthened in the infancy period; and in the preschool years both adults and peers tend to react favorably to the lively child. Another pattern of response likely to occur in such a child is one of marked absorption in watching television, accompanied by an attenuation of his high level of activity. The same phenomenon occurs when he is a passenger in a moving vehicle, apparently because the quality of audio-visual stimulation in the television situation and the tactual-kinesthetic stimulation provided by the moving vehicle are sufficient to induce inhibition of activity. Although parents often point with relief to the fact that their overactive child can sit still for hours in front of the television set, in fact, it may be a cause for concern. When it occurs with the hyperactivity pattern some clinicians would consider it to be a diagnostic index (Zuk, 1963).

Often the first difficulties occur at the point of school entry when a high level of motility is unacceptable and likely to elicit considerable teacher disapproval and, at this point in the school cycle when the desire to conform is high, peer disapproval. The high active child is not equipped to

---

* After this manuscript had been submitted for publication, a theoretical paper by Zentall (1975) appeared proposing a similar explanation, namely, that hyperactive behavior may function to optimize stimulation rather than being a consequence of too much stimulation. The Zentall paper provided a comprehensive review of research suggesting that hyperactive behavior may result from a homeostatic mechanism that functions to increase stimulation for a child experiencing insufficient sensory stimulation. Zentall also presented evidence that the efficacy of drug intervention and behavior therapy in hyperactivity are consistent with a theory of a homeostatic mechanism that attempts to optimize sensory input.

cope with this situation; the pattern of high motility is well up on his hierarchy of responses, and often he becomes even more active in a desperate bid for the social reinforcement that in the past has always been forthcoming for such behavior. Unfortunately, he is likely to get the most attention in the school setting when he is hyperactive, and even though the quality of the attention is negative, it may serve to further strengthen the behavior. Thus the level and kind of activity that the child manifests may be gradually shaped by the social reaction of others into a pattern of behavior that elicits concern and remedial action.

In some children hyperactivity is a response to demands in the school situation that far exceed their capacity to respond. Several years ago, one of the authors observed a girl in kindergarten who after 3 months had become so restless and difficult to contain in the school setting that her teacher had labeled her as hyperactive. In fact, this particular kindergarten was highly academically-oriented and the child, whose IQ on the Stanford-Binet was 84, was seldom able to perform most of the tasks that were presented to her. However, she was also very achievement-oriented, and in order to avoid failure she had learned to move from one activity to another to avoid aversive consequences. Her teacher frequently worked quite intensively with her in an effort to improve her performance, and these interactions produced a generalized anxiety reaction which increased when she persisted with a task because she had apparently recognized that the longer she stayed at a task, the higher the probability of failure. Terminating the task and moving to another for a period that was too short to result in failure reduced the anxiety and thus reinforced the high rate of motility. In this child hyperactivity was not a disturbance in motility, instead it could more accurately be regarded as perpetual avoidance behavior. It was recommended that she be moved to a less achievement-oriented kindergarten, and that she be given special tutoring on readiness tasks with the provision that, at least in the early stages, the tutoring situation offer a very high proportion of success experiences. Because her solution for avoiding failure at a task was at a higher level of problem solving than one would expect of a child with an IQ of 84, it was also recommended that she be tested again after a period of time in the new setting. With these changes, hyperactivity disappeared in a few weeks and a subsequent follow-up revealed that she was quite successful in the first grade, and her IQ now measured 98.

## Observational Learning

Of relevance to the influence of observational learning on the development of a hyperactive behavior pattern are the findings from genetic investigations of hyperactivity (Cantwell, 1972; Morrison & Stewart, 1971), long-term drug studies (Gross & Wilson, 1974), and individual case studies (Daniels, 1973) which have consistently shown that the parents of hyperactive children were often hyperactive as children themselves. This finding is consistent with a social as well as a genetic mode of transmission. The possibility that activity level could be transmitted through modeling processes receives extensive support from observational learning research. A diverse body of research (Bandura, Ross, & Ross, 1961, 1963; Kaspar & Lowenstein, 1971) has demonstrated that children of preschool and elementary school age who were exposed to active models showed an increase in activity level, and that those who observed more passive models exhibited a more sedate form of response. If a single, brief exposure to a live or symbolic model can result in the transmission of a particular level of activity, it is reasonable to expect that daily exposure to a highly active parent could result in the acquisition of an unusually active *personal tempo* (Rimoldi, 1951) or characteristic way of responding. Several factors would serve to enhance the probability of observational learning of activity level from the parent (Bandura, 1969). The parent possesses characteristics known to elicit imitative behavior: he is typically powerful, competent, attractive, and of high status. Conversely, the child has characteristics that increase the probability of observational learning: he is incompetent, generally low in self-esteem, and, in the preschool years, often high dependent. Furthermore, in parent-child interactions the child would be rewarded for keeping pace with the parental tempo. In view of the prevalence of hyperactivity, it is surprising that there has been no research on the observational learning of this behavior, although Daniels (1973) has reported the successful modification of hyperactive behavior in a 6-year-old boy through operant conditioning combined with modeling. In this study the child's parents were overactive: the mother, who never sat down to relax, was constantly engaged in housework and was described by her husband (who was also very active) as "jumpy, nervous, high strung, and on the run all day." The maternal grandmother was also characterized as constantly running back and forth at household tasks, and was considered by Daniels to have been the original model for the hyperactive behavior in both the mother and grandson. Part of the modification procedure required the parents to curtail their overactivity drastically.

## ENVIRONMENTAL FACTORS

### Lead Poisoning

Lead is a trace element that has no known essential role in the human body, but it occurs so widely in the environment, particularly the urban environment, that exposure to it is almost inevitable, even for fetuses (Lin-Fu, 1972). Its toxic significance has been recognized for centuries. Pliny warned of the dangers of using lead pots in wine-making (Gilfillan, 1965), and in the latter half of the 18th century Baker traced the cause of colic among cider drinkers in Devonshire to lead poisoning that developed as a result of the cider being transported in leaden pipes (Needleman, 1973). Although lead poisoning has long been recognized as an industrial disease, lead poisoning in children was not described until the 20th century when Aub, Fairhall, Minot, and Resnikoff (1926) published a monograph on the diagnosis and treatment of this syndrome.

In the United States lead poisoning in children is sufficiently widespread that it has been referred to as a silent epidemic (Needleman, 1973; Oberle, 1969). Most cases of lead poisoning in this country are associated with the eating of lead-pigment paints in deteriorating urban housing areas by pre-school children characterized by *pica*, the tendency to ingest nonedible materials. Although lead-based paints have not been used since World War II, there are many deteriorating inner-city urban housing areas where peeling paint still contains lead pigment. A chip of paint the size of a penny can contain between 50 and 100 mg. of lead, and the repeated ingestion of a few chips a day over a 3-month period can lead to clinical symptoms and eventually to the absorption of a potentially lethal body burden of lead (Chisolm, 1971). Another major source of lead is high octane gasoline. In the United States almost all of the 200,000 tons of lead emitted into the atmosphere each year results from the combustion of gasoline containing lead. Inner-city and suburban children may inhale lead from this source or may ingest it by eating roadway dust or snow on busy city streets (Environmental Protection Agency Report, 1972). When lead poisoning does occur the onset is insidious and, because the symptoms of fatigue, pallor, irritability, anorexia, and nausea are not distinctive, a child with lead poisoning might easily be incorrectly diagnosed and treated unless the pediatrician is alert to the possibility of lead poisoning. Treatment is with a compound known as a *chelating agent*, which removes lead atoms from the body tissues for excretion through the kidneys and liver. Even high lead levels can be rapidly reduced to levels approaching normal with chelating agents (Chisolm, 1971).

The effects of lead are relevant to the topic of hyperactivity in two conditions: children with *confirmed lead poisoning* often sustain severe neurological and psychological sequelae, one of the latter being a behavioral pattern of hyperactivity, short attention span, and impulsivity (Byers & Lord, 1943; Wiener, 1970). Recent research (David, Clark, & Voeller, 1972) has established that children with *elevated body-lead burdens* below the level needed to produce overt symptoms of toxicity also exhibit hyperactive patterns of behavior. It is not known whether the involvement of lead in the hyperactivity is primary, contributory, or incidental. Although there is no evidence yet that the association between elevated but not toxic body-lead concentrations and hyperactivity is a causal one, the research findings to date are highly suggestive of such a relationship.

David, Clark, and Voeller (1972) have presented epidemiological evidence for the association of hyperactivity with a history of lead exposure in children, and for the fact that significant numbers of hyperactive children live in housing with a high probability of lead-painted surfaces. In their study children were designated as hyperactive on the basis of one or more of the following: a doctor's diagnosis, a teacher's rating scale, and a parent questionnaire. The hyperactive children were then assigned to the following groups: *pure hyperactive,* with no evidence of any event known to be associated with the hyperactivity; *highly probable cause of hyperactivity,* such as prenatal or perinatal complications; *possible cause,* in which there was a history of an event that could have resulted in hyperactivity; and a *history of lead poisoning* that had been treated. In addition to these hyperactive subgroups, there was a control group of nonhyperactive children. Overall, the hyperactive children had significantly higher values than the controls on two measures that reflected the presence of body lead and on a lead exposure questionnaire, thus supporting the hypothesis of a relationship between hyperactivity and a concomitant condition of increased body lead stores. Since these findings suggested that many of the hyperactive children had probably had *increased,* but not toxic, lead stores for some time and that one consequence of such a long-term minimal poisonous assault might be hyperactivity, David and his colleagues examined the subgroup results for support for the assumption that lead poisoning might cause hyperactivity and found two comparisons supporting this possibility. First, the *highly probable cause group* did not differ in lead values from the controls, a finding that would be expected since there was a likely cause of the hyperactivity in this group and it was not lead poisoning. Second, the *pure hyperactives* (no known cause but no reason why it could not be lead-associated) showed raised lead levels ($p < .01$) as compared to the controls. A sobering finding about the *lead poisoning* group ($n = 8$), all but one of whom had had chelation therapy 5 years previously, was that they all had elevated blood and urine levels, indicating either that the chelation therapy and follow-up procedures had been inadequate, or that the children had subsequently been reexposed to lead. The investigators have suggested that it might also mean that hyperactivity may not be an after-effect of lead poisoning, instead it might be a condition that is dependent upon continuing, nontoxic elevations of body lead.

In an ongoing 3-year study of the relationship between hyperactivity and body lead levels in children, David and his colleagues (Smithsonian Science Information Exchange, 1975) are comparing lead chelating and non-chelating (methylphenidate) treatments in hyperactive children. Data are also being collected on the relative efficacy of different procedures for determining body lead level and for identifying the source of lead in children with elevated body lead levels. Preliminary data (David, personal communication, 1975) have substantiated the earlier finding (David, Clark, & Voeller, 1972) of an association between lead and hyperactivity. Increased body lead levels have been demonstrated in approximately 50 percent of their hyperactive population; this lead presence occurs significantly more often in children with no other etiologic reason for their hyperactivity than in those who do have a good reason for it. Hyperactive children with elevated levels differ markedly in psychological test scores from those with normal levels. There is not yet evidence of a causal relationship between lead and hyperactivity, but David et al. expect that within 2 years an unequivocal statement on the existence or nonexistence of such a relationship will be forthcoming.

Two animal studies by Silbergeld and Goldberg (1973, 1974) provide support for a causal relationship between lead and a high level of activity. In the first of these, one group of mice was given one of three concentrations of lead in their drinking water from birth, and a second group was given sodium acetate. Activity level was measured for 4 consecutive days when the mice were between 40 and 60 days old. Mice who had ingested lead were more than three times as active as the controls ($p < .001$). Sauerhoff and Michaelson (1973) reported similar findings with rats. Silbergeld and Goldberg (1973) consider this finding to be conclusive evidence of a causal relationship between chronic ingestion of lead and a high level of activity in mice. The fact that the lead-induced hyperactivity was not dose-related, at least in the range of doses used, coupled with the fact that there were no deaths in the experimental group, suggests that increases in motor activity may be a symptom that occurs early in the period of exposure to lead, while the body level is increased but not toxic. Also, increases in the amount of lead given to the mice produced other sequelae of lead intoxication, such as peripheral ataxia and splayed gait. In a second study, Silbergeld and Goldberg (1974) replicated the causal relationship between lead ingestion and hyperactivity in mice and then administered to the lead-treated and control mice the stimulant drugs that are used in the treatment of hyperactivity: dextroamphetamine, levoamphetamine, and methylphenidate, and also chloral hydrate and phenobarbital, which is contraindicated in hyperactive children because it exacerbates their hyperactivity. Lead-treated mice responded with decreased hyperactivity to the three stimulant medications and with increased levels of activity to the phenobarbital. Controls showed an increase in activity with the amphetamines and a decrease with phenobarbital. Chloral hydrate effected an equal decrease in activity level in the experimental and control groups. Related work by Sobotka and Cook (1974), in which rats were subjected to early lead exposure, has demonstrated a reduction of motor activity and an alleviation of a performance deficit on a two-way shuttle task with amphetamine treatment. These investigators concurred with Silbergeld and Goldberg (1974) that perinatal lead exposure might be etiologically related to some forms of minimal brain dysfunction. The parallels between this animal model of hyperactivity and the clinical description of hyperactivity are impressive and strongly suggest that lead may be an etiological agent in the hyperactivity of children in urban areas. The fact that Silbergeld and Goldberg (1973, 1974) have produced and replicated a lead-induced animal model of hyperactivity, and demonstrated a striking parallel between the efficacy of stimulant medication at the infrahuman level and at the human level, represents a potentially major contribution to knowledge about the etiology and treatment of hyperactivity. What is urgently needed now is an extension of their animal model of hyperactivity to determine if the toxic effects, particularly the hyperactivity, are reversible with chelation therapy, and if this reversal, once accomplished, is maintained as long as there is no further exposure to toxic levels of lead.

## Radiation Stress

A Florida photobiologist, John Ott, has suggested that hyperactivity may be a radiation stress condition that occurs as a result of exposure to conventional fluorescent lighting and to certain conditions of television viewing. Ott believes that the conventional fluorescent lighting typically used in schools and offices is harmful because it gives off soft X-rays through the cathode ray guns at the ends of all fluorescent tubes, and inadequate because it lacks certain of the long ultraviolet wavelengths of the natural light spectrum that are essential to humans/Ott believes that harmful and inadequate fluorescent lighting and unshielded TV cathode tubes may result in sufficient radiation exposure to directly cause hyperactivity, or may serve as environmental stressors that alter the body so that hyperactivity results (Ott, 1974). His premise that these sources of radiation might directly or indirectly cause hyperactivity is based on research by Frey (1965) who found that animals experienced behavioral changes and transient changes in the central nervous system following repeated exposure to radio and television frequencies.

Evidence that the X-rays given off by the cathode ray gun used in fluorescent lights and television picture tubes may trigger hyperactive behavior and prove detrimental to health comes from a study by Hartley (1974). Rats who were placed in front of a color television set with standard (unshielded) cathode tubes became hyperactive within 3 to 10 days, remained hyperactive until the 30th day of radiation exposure, and then became lethargic and died. Rats exposed to the same conditions with lead-shielded cathode tubes showed no change in behavior or physical wellbeing. These findings were replicated in two subsequent studies in the same laboratory.

Further support for an association between radiation and hyperactivity comes from a case study (Hartley, 1974) in which an exceedingly hyperactive girl was found to be exposed for long periods to the radiation leak from a television set that was placed against a living room wall so that the set was separated from the head of her bed by the wall between the adjacent rooms. When lead shields were put on the television tubes the girl's behavior began to calm down and eventually returned to normal.

Similar findings were obtained in replications, leading Ott to investigate the effects of shielded versus standard unshielded fluorescent lights on established cases of hyperactivity in children. Ott conducted a 90-day experiment with primary school children that allowed a comparison of the effects of conventional and improved fluorescent lighting (Mayron, Ott, Nations, & Mayron, 1974). Four windowless first-grade classrooms were used. Two were illuminated with standard cool white fluorescent lights and two with fluorescent lighting having three special features: long ultraviolet wavelengths present in sunlight, lead foil shields over their cathode ends to keep X-rays from escaping, and a wire grid screen over their entirety to ground radio frequencies. In all four classes there were some hyperactive children who were about to be transferred to special classes because they were unable to function in the regular class setting. Time-lapse pictures taken while the four classes were in session and teacher reports showed that the disruptive behavior, irritability, and poor attention spans of the hyperactive children working in full spectrum, shielded fluorescent lighting diminished so sharply that special class placement was not required. No change occurred in the behavior of the hyperactive children in the two classes with conventional fluorescent lighting. Analyses of the time-lapse photographs, disciplinary referrals, absenteeism, and other factors relevant to the findings suggested that the improvements that occurred could be attributed to the lighting variable rather than to other environmental or social factors, such as difference in teacher efficiency.

Ott's research may prove to have enormously important implications for hyperactive children. If hyperactivity proves to be a radiation stress condition, this causative factor could be eliminated simply by installing lead shielded lighting that contains the missing ultraviolet rays and does not leak X-rays. Ott's research on television radiation exposure raises critical questions about the adequacy of the safety standards of the 1968 Radiation Control Act. How many of the apparently increasing number of hyperactive children are victims of continuous exposure to radiation through fluorescent lights at school and long hours of television viewing close to the set at home?

## Food Additives

During the past 50 years numerous reports have appeared linking hyperactivity, irritability, and other nervous system reactions to allergic conditions, particularly to food allergies (see, for example, Baldwin, Kittler, & Ramsay, 1968; Moyer, 1975; Randolph, 1947; Shannon, 1922). The underlying physiological cause of the behavioral reaction has not yet been established, but one possibility (Moyer, 1975) is that the allergens directly affect the central nervous system by causing a noninflammatory swelling of the brain in areas that contain the neural connections controlling aggression, with a resultant increase in sensitivity of these areas to stimulation. A second possibility suggested by Moyer (1975) is that of a disinhibitory effect on areas of the brain that normally control aggressive tendencies. Kittler (Taub, 1975) noted that inhalation, elimination, and diet restrictions not only improved the behavior and learning performance of 20 children (M = 15, F = 5), but even led to correction of abnormal electroencephalograms. Recently Feingold (1973) has suggested that chemicals that add color and flavor to food may be a causative factor in some cases of hyperactivity and learning disabilities. His interest in food additives stemmed from the case of a woman who was referred to him for allergic problems while she was also under psychiatric care for compulsively frenetic behavior. Feingold decided that the patient might be sensitive to aspirin and other salicylate compounds and he prescribed a diet free of those chemicals. The results were dramatic: both the allergic symptoms and her frenzied behavior disappeared within a few weeks. Feingold concluded that the allergic symptoms of the patient, and others who responded equally well to a salicylate-free diet, did not constitute an allergy in the classic immunological sense but instead seemed to be symptoms provoked in some way by an unexplained biochemical mechanism that interfered with the central nervous system. The mechanism by which the salicylates cause the adverse reaction has not been identified. Feingold then began to consider the prevalence in food additives of salicylates, and other chemicals similar to salicylates but unrelated to them, and found that the compounds were in 34 food colors and 1610 synthetic food colorings, all of which have been classified as safe by the Food and Drug Administration. When hyperactive children ($n$ = 194) were put on diets free of these compounds, 58 children showed a level of response that Feingold (1975) termed "dramatic" and 35 responded favorably. Approximately half of the children were able to discontinue stimulants and other medications within 10 days. The degree and rapidity of response to the Feingold diet appears to be a function of age, the younger the child, the more rapid and complete the improvement. Three- to 5-year-old children show a marked cessation of symptoms within a few days (Feingold, 1975); those in the middle childhood years require 2 to 3 weeks before they manifest complete improvement; and adolescents require still longer and even then often do not show clearcut improvement. A recent study by Hawley and Buckley (1974) has provided support for the efficacy of a salicylate-free diet for some hyperactive children. The diets are difficult to follow in that most of the prepared foods and some fresh fruits and vegetables must be eliminated, but it is essential to follow them because even a minor lapse precipitates a return of the hyperactive symptoms.

Although these preliminary clinical reports are impressive, Feingold has not yet conducted a controlled study of his hypothesis. Although there is some evidence from case studies (Crook, 1974; Moyer, 1975), and confirmation from clinical reports (Havard, 1973), there is no firm empirical support for the Feingold theory from other sources. The prospect of any workable alternative to drug intervention merits consideration and further investigation. A major study under the direction of Conners (Goyette, 1975) is currently underway in Pittsburgh to test the Feingold hypothesis. The study is set up as a double-blind crossover experiment in which each patient is placed on either the Feingold elimination diet or a control diet from which randomly selected food items have been eliminated. Following initial selection of the hyperactive subjects the parents maintain the child for 2 weeks without medication. During this period and throughout the experiment the parents are expected to keep a careful diet diary. Subjects are randomly assigned to condition and the dependent variables are weekly parent and teacher ratings, and global ratings based on parent interviews by the principal investigator under double-blind conditions. Although the final data on this study are not yet available, Feingold (1975) has reported that preliminary observations on a pilot group of 12 boys validate the relationship of artificial food colors and flavorings to behavioral disturbances.

Conners' test of Feingold's theory depends on strict adherence to the Feingold dietary requirements. A major weakness in the experimental procedure concerns the total dependence on the parents for the manipulation of the major independent variable, that is, strict adherence to the diet. Even though the investigators are requiring the parents to keep a written account of the food given to the children, and are meeting with them on a weekly basis throughout the experiment, they will not know with *absolute certainty* that the diet is being followed. As Feingold himself has said (Petit, 1974, p. 2):

Some parents just give up my diet as too much trouble. They'd rather have their doctors prescribe drugs for their kids than spend all that time cooking up recipes from raw foods.

There is ample evidence that parents of hyperactive children are notably unreliable in following simple medication instructions even when apparently highly motivated to do so (Conrad & Insel, 1967). In Conners' study the effort needed to prepare the Feingold diet is considerably greater than that usually expended on family food preparation, and in addition, the children's medication will be halted 2 weeks prior to the introduction of the new diet, an essential requirement but also a further source of stress for the parents. Altogether, it would appear that a real test of the Feingold approach would require a live-in test period, perhaps in a summer-camp setting, but the ingenuity of Feingold's hypothesis and its potential impact would certainly justify the expenditures involved. Confirmation of the hypothesis would represent a major contribution in that it would simultaneously identify an etiological factor in hyperactivity and a method of treatment. The question is also of practical concern to educators not just because of the prevalence of hyperactivity in the schools, but because the school lunches that many districts supply contain a high percentage of food additives.

## Maternal Smoking and Drinking

It is an established fact that heavy maternal smoking during pregnancy is associated with an increased incidence of *obstetrical complications*. Some of these complications are of a severity sufficient to produce fetal anoxia and consequent brain damage. The possibility that heavy maternal smoking might be associated with hyperactivity has been explored by Denson, Nanson, and McWatters (1975). They describe the mechanism through which such an association might occur as follows: The supply of oxygen to fetal tissues often falls to a critical level during delivery. If the lack of oxygen (anoxia) falls sufficiently, permanent damage may be done to the brain, with one possible manifestation of such damage being hyperactivity.

One factor that can compromise oxygenation during delivery is the presence of an increased amount of carbon monoxide in the fetal bloodstream. Such an accumulation may occur when a woman smokes heavily during pregnancy. If it is high enough it could result in cerebral anoxia in an apparently normal delivery. Another factor that can sharply reduce oxygenation is a difficult or prolonged delivery, a phenomenon that commonly occurs in the woman giving birth to her first child. It follows that if an association does exist between heavy maternal smoking and hyperactivity, ordinal position might also be linked to hyperactivity. If ordinal position is involved, an increased proportion of hyperactive children having the above set of pregnancy factors should be firstborn. To investigate the possibility of an association between heavy maternal smoking and hyperactivity, Denson et al. conducted a carefully controlled study using three groups of 20 subjects each and matched for sex (M = 18, F = 2), age (5 to 15 years), and social class. The children in the first group had been diagnosed as hyperactive by accepted criteria. Dyslexic children formed the second group and normal controls the third group. Each of the 60 mothers was interviewed to determine her own and her spouse's smoking habits and to obtain information about her child, including birth weight and ordinal position. The results showed that there were more firstborn among the hyperactive group than in either of the other two groups ($p < .01$), and the mothers of the hyperactive group smoked an average of 14.3 cigarettes daily during pregnancy as compared to mothers of the dyslexic (Mean = 6.0) and control (Mean = 6.3) groups. Mothers of the hyperactive children had continued to smoke heavily and their maximum daily consumption at the time of the study far exceeded ($p < .01$) that of the other two groups. Although these findings do not establish a causal connection between heavy maternal smoking during pregnancy and hyperactivity, they clearly justify further investigation of this possibility. The investigators make an interesting point, that the prevalence of cigarette smoking in young women has increased markedly in the past 30 years, and the incidence of hyperactivity in children also appears to have increased.

A recent series of reports by Jones and his colleagues (see, for example, Jones, Smith, Streissguth, & Myrianthopoulos, 1974) has identified heavy drinking during pregnancy as another maternal behavior that may be etiologically linked to hyperactivity. As yet there is no evidence to implicate moderate drinking, but research on this possibility is in progress. These investigators have estimated that one-third of the children of women who drink heavily throughout pregnancy will suffer some kind of damage, much of which will be irreversible. The kinds of damage that may be sustained include brain damage, mild facial deformities, and heart disorders. The magnitude of the problem is evident from the fact that experts regard the results of this fetal alcohol syndrome as more serious than those of Thalidomide. The mechanism through which the damage occurs has not yet been identified but Jones et al. state that the fetal brain is especially susceptible to damage from this source. It follows that infants who are afflicted with this fetal alcohol syndrome could be hyperactive.

## Environmental Constraints

The possibility that hyperactivity can develop from environmental constraints has been suggested by McNamara (1972) and Thomas, Chess, Sillen, and Mendez (1974). In the first paper, McNamara described the environmental conditions, demands, and stresses that he viewed as causative factors in the onset of hyperactivity in lower-class Puerto Rican children in New York City. The picture that he presented was a bleak one of high density slums, overcrowded schools, a lack of green space, virtually no recreational outlets, and a high crime and accident rate. In this setting parents were, with reason, fearful for the safety of their children. The combination of this fear and the nonavailability of recreational services caused them to keep the children indoors as much as possible, thereby imposing a major restriction on physical activity. According to McNamara a typical day in the life of one of these children consisted of going to school, trying to learn in an overcrowded classroom from a teacher who often was not bilingual, returning home, doing homework, and watching television. Many children responded to this general curtailment of their physical activity with a pattern of behavior, particularly in school, that was characterized by hyperactivity, attention problems, lethargy, and indifference, and that resulted in a referral for neurological evaluation and subsequent drug intervention. In fact, McNamara concluded that the only remedy needed for this apartment-bound hyperactivity was the obvious one of adequate and safe outlets for the normal physical activity of childhood. Unfortunately, there is no empirical evidence of the efficacy of such a solution.

In the second paper, Thomas, Chess, Sillen, and Mendez (1974) reported a cross-cultural comparison, also in New York City, of the behavior patterns of Puerto Rican working-class children ($n = 31$) and non-Puerto Rican middle-class children ($n = 42$). Although the economic, social, and cultural backgrounds of the two groups presented a sharp contrast, there were some striking similarities, with both groups being characterized by a relatively high degree of family stability, living in two-parent homes in which geographic and economic stability prevailed, and not differing in the incidence of prenatal and perinatal complications. Like their middle-class counterparts, the Puerto Rican parents were clearly concerned about the wellbeing of their children, but they were more demanding about compliance to rules, less child-problem oriented, and less prone to pressure their children for early achievement and independence, particularly in the preschool years. Of relevance here is the finding that in the Puerto Rican sample there was a significantly higher incidence ($p < .001$) of parental complaints about excessive and uncontrollable motor activity than in the middle-class group; 53 percent of the Puerto Ricans under 9 years presented problems in activity level, as compared to only one child in the other group who was brain damaged. Thomas and his colleagues attributed the hyperactivity to the fact that these East Harlem parents coped with the dangers of the street by keeping their children in and expecting them to restrain their physical activity. This restrictive method of coping and its resultant hyperactivity effects are precisely those described by McNamara (1972) in his Puerto Rican group. The problem was exacerbated by the fact that children who *temperamentally* had high activity levels (Thomas, Chess, & Birch, 1970) were even more likely to be restricted to the home because their parents were already aware that they were more accident-prone (Stewart, Thach, & Freidin, 1970) and, therefore, in greater potential danger on the streets than their less active siblings. The children typically reacted to parental demands for restraint with disobedience, eliciting physical punishment and further disobedience, and setting up a cycle that led to the children whose activity level presented a problem also being described as disciplinary problems. Thomas and his colleagues pointed out that the number of complaints about hyperactivity would almost certainly have been sharply diminished if these children had been in an environment with more space for physical activities and fewer hazards. Note that the primary problem here was a lack of safe physical space for physical activity, rather than social crowding. As evidence for the effect of a lack of physical space, Thomas et al. noted that one Puerto Rican boy who had been described as "uncontrollably active" at school and "a whirling dervish" at home improved markedly when the family moved to a house with a small yard. Their conclusion concerning the sample was that (Thomas, Chess, Sillen, & Mendez, 1974, p. 63):

It is likely that this high motility did not represent pathological hyperactivity as such but, rather, the normal temperamental characteristic of high activity level which became exacerbated and the basis for a behavior problem development because of environmental constraints.

All of the preceding etiological factors have been discussed singly. An additional possibility that should be considered is that a multifactor etiology is operative. In such cases no single factor would be sufficient to cause the hyperactivity, but the cumulative effect of several factors would result in the behavior problem. For example, a child could be born with a temperament that predisposes him to hyperactivity, but is not expressed as hyperactivity unless he is also exposed to a variety of lesser environmental stressors whose combined effect is powerful enough to cause hyperactivity. In this example, which is essentially a diasthesis-multistress model, the mode of multifactor action is *interactive:* factors within the child interact with environmental stressors. The mode of multifactor action may instead be *unidirectional:* here the combined force of stressors in the environment is sufficient to cause hyperactivity even though the child himself is characterized by physiological and psychological integrity. In clinical reports hyperactivity is often diagnosed with the qualification of "no known cause." Yet when the clinical description is carefully considered a number of possible causes may exist, which taken together could constitute a powerful etiological effect. In one hyperactive child that we knew there was a history of obstetrical difficulty but no demonstrable brain damage; the child had a raised blood-lead level which did not approach toxicity; he lived in a crowded ghetto area with few opportunities for activity, but so did his siblings who were not hyperactive; he was in great difficulty academically and behaviorally at school, as were a number of his nonhyperactive peers; and he and his siblings had poor relationships with their parents. It seems reasonable that this complex of probable and possible etiological factors could combine to cause hyperactivity.

It would be interesting to locate a group of hyperactive children with no known cause of their hyperactive behavior, as David, Clark, and Voeller (1972) did, and for each child to compile a score indicating his status on all known etiological factors. A raised blood-lead level or parent-child difficulties would be assigned higher scores than a normal lead level or harmonious home relationships, so that the higher the total score, the greater the number of nonoptimal factors in the child's total environment. If these children's scores were then compared to those for a group of children with identifiable causes for their hyperactivity, we would predict that the no-known-cause group would have high scores, indicating a conglomerate of contributory factors, whereas the known-cause group would have low scores, indicating only one or two etiological factors. This scoring system, which is analogous to the *optimality score* developed by Kalverboer, Touwen, and Prechtl (1973) to provide a global measure of the integrity of the nervous functions in the newborn, would have important implications for the prevention and management of hyperactivity.

In this chapter we have discussed a number of factors that appear to be etiologically related to hyperactivity and have classified them on the basis of various parameters, such as epidemiological causes and biological and psychological mechanisms. It is important to remember that these factors are *labels*. To say that certain groups of children are hyperactive because they are being exposed to an identifiable environmental stressor is not, in itself, of value to the children, their parents, or society. It is only the first step in the management of the problem. The remainder of this book is concerned with the problems and procedures of the treatment, prevention, and management of hyperactivity.

# CHAPTER 4

# *Drug Treatment*

I have never prescribed stimulants for these patients, and I never will . . . Stimulants merely mask the symptoms without curing the disease . . . I have found that the hyperactive child's problem can almost always be identified and treated if the physician is willing to take the time and trouble . . . (Walker, 1974, p. 43.)

If after this time (three to six months) things seem just as bad as ever . . . no matter how they (the parents) have changed the pressures at home or at school, no matter how they have rewarded their child's efforts to improve, no matter how they have dealt with the school and with professional consultants . . . then it may be time to think about medication. (Stewart & Olds, 1973, p. 246.)

The basic flaw of drug treatment is that it cannot teach a child anything, and it is not yet established that drug treatment makes the child more accessible to other intervention techniques. (Sroufe & Stewart, 1973, p. 411.)

It is difficult to assess the deleterious effects of psychotherapy and other forms of behavior modification . . . All who have practiced medicine, however, have seen patients who have become worse with counseling or other behavior therapies. In attempting to evaluate all the factors pertaining to the use of drugs, as compared to no therapy or to other forms of therapy, it would seem that the hazard from drugs is no greater and may in fact be less dangerous, since drug effects can be rapidly terminated. (Oettinger, 1971, p. 164.)

To those who have seen the results of such treatment (stimulant medication) in minimal brain dysfunction children, many of whom had failed to improve or had worsened with traditional therapies, the present limited use of drug therapy is as upsetting as it is unbelievable . . . It would not be hard to argue that in many instances psychotherapy of children with this syndrome virtually constitutes malpractice — a harmful withholding of useful treatment from a child . . . Barring the future disclosure of chronic toxic consequences of stimulant drug therapy for such children, one must argue that it is the treatment of choice, and that withholding it represents an injury to the patient and his family. (Wender, 1971, p. 130.)

The foregoing comments are representative of the spectrum of dissent concerning the use of stimulant medications in the treatment of hyperactive children. The lack of consensus concerning the extent to which drug

**95**

intervention constitutes appropriate treatment for the hyperactive child has contributed to, and is also a result of, inadequate and unsystematic research with conflicting results due to methodological weaknesses. Since criteria for acceptable research procedures are well established, the presence of major methodological weaknesses in many drug studies can only be the result of indifference, ignorance, or bias on the part of the researchers. Whatever the reason, the effect is to render the findings of these studies virtually worthless. One result is that many practitioners are prescribing drug intervention in the absence of a firm empirical basis for their decisions. At the present time the majority seem to favor drug intervention alone, despite a substantial body of criticism and evidence contraindicating this approach. The ease and time-saving aspects of drug intervention, coupled with a lack of awareness or acceptance of the potential efficacy of other available forms of intervention, appear to outweigh the contradictory evidence in the decision process. As a result, opinions based on inadequate clinical observations and personal preference have largely determined what treatment approach has been used in hyperactivity and what directions drug research has taken. To advance the state of the art the reverse should be the case: research results should form opinions and guide treatment.

The use of drugs to quiet restless children is not a recent phenomenon; drugs have been used for this purpose for hundreds of years. The last of the great Greek physicians, Galen, prescribed opium for restless, colicky infants; medicinal blends containing substantial amounts of alcohol have been used for centuries to sedate irritable infants; and bromides and barbiturates were used extensively for chronic restlessness in the late 19th century (Goodman & Gilman, 1970). However, the central nervous system stimulants are a product of 20th century technology. They were first introduced for use with children having behavioral and learning problems in the 1930s (Bradley, 1937; Molitch & Eccles, 1937), but reports of their efficacy attracted little clinical and research attention. It was not until the late 1950s that they were widely used with hyperactive children. By the middle 1960s one group of respected clinicians and researchers considered them the treatment of choice, and a second group expressed strong dissent in the form of critiques that demonstrated serious methodological flaws in much of the research on the use of stimulant medication. This controversy became a public issue in 1970, when the *Washington Post* reported that between 5 and 10 percent of the school children in Omaha, Nebraska, were being given central nervous system stimulants to improve their classroom behavior (Maynard, 1970). Although this statement proved to be erroneous (the figures represented the estimated incidence of learning disabilities in the elementary school population of Omaha), the rash of publicity that followed disclosed that the use of stimulant medication was indeed wide-spread in schools throughout the nation. The effect of this information was catalytic. Panels were convened by professional organizations (American Academy of Pediatrics, 1970) and government agencies (Office of Child Development, 1971) to investigate the use of stimulant medication, and the results were disquieting: Nothing was known about the long-term effects of stimulant drugs, the only evidence being a single follow-up study involving 67 children (Gallagher, 1970). Between 150,000 and 200,000 children were being treated with stimulant drugs and the National Institute of Mental Health estimated (Hunsinger, 1970) that approximately 4,000,000 hyperactive children in the United States could benefit from drugs, which suggested that the trend could be expected to increase. Educators (Yanow, 1973) estimated the incidence of hyperactivity at 15 to 20 percent of the elementary school population in contrast to the 5 to 10 percent figure set by those in other disciplines (Huessy, 1967; Stewart & Olds, 1973), and the enthusiastic endorsement by educators of the stimulant medications had resulted in alarming proportions of children in some school districts being treated with drugs (Miller, 1970). Respected clinicians charged that stimulant medications were being prescribed indiscriminately, with the prescription often depending primarily upon a report of a child's behavior provided by his teacher or parents (Denhoff, 1971). There was unequivocal evidence that the drug industry was exerting every effort to extend the use of the stimulants (Hentoff, 1972; Lennard, Epstein, Bernstein & Ransom, 1971).

In the 5 years that have elapsed since the Omaha incident the amount of real progress in this area of psychopharmacology has not been encouraging. A number of methodologically sound experiments have demonstrated beneficial effects of a short-term nature on behavior and performance; but there has been relatively little concern shown with the long-term side effects of drug treatment, although the sparse information that we do have indicates that these effects are generally mild (Weiss, Minde, Douglas, Werry, & Sykes, 1971; Werry, 1968; Werry & Sprague, 1970). There is well-documented evidence that stimulants are being prescribed without real justification for prolonged periods and without adequate supervision (Solomons, 1973). There is little reliable information about the possible detrimental behavioral effects and physical consequences of long-term drug treatment despite the fact that many children are on stimulant medications for years.

The purpose of this chapter is to discuss the current status of the drug treatment of hyperactive children, with the primary emphasis being on the clinical facts, empirical findings, and practical considerations relevant to the use of the central nervous system stimulants because there has been more clinical experience and research reported with these drugs than with other categories of psychoactive drugs. No attempt is made to provide an exhaustive review of the voluminous literature on the drug treatment of hyperactive children. For the reader who is interested in such comprehensive coverage, several summaries of different aspects of drug treatment are available (Conners, 1972; Eisenberg, 1968; Eisenberg & Conners, 1971; Erenberg, 1972; Freeman, 1966; Grant, 1962; Sprague & Werry, 1971). Sroufe (1975) has written a critical review of the drug treatment of hyperactive children that is the best statement in the literature and, as such, should be required reading for anyone seriously interested in the psychopharmacotherapeutic and research aspects of hyperactivity.

## CENTRAL NERVOUS SYSTEM STIMULANTS

The central nervous system stimulants that have been most extensively used with hyperactive children are dextroamphetamine (Dexedrine) and methylphenidate (Ritalin). The amphetamines were used by Bradley in 1937 but methylphenidate was not introduced until the late 1950s (Zimmerman & Burgemeister, 1958). Although reports in the mass media (Hentoff, 1972; Maynard, 1970) have suggested that between 5 and 10 percent of all elementary school children are being given medication for behavior disorders and learning difficulties, the results of two recent surveys indicate that these figures may be exaggerated. Stephen (Sprague & Sleator, 1973) conducted a questionnaire survey of 700 Chicago physicians who were asked to *estimate* the dose and frequency of psychoactive medication that they prescribed for school-age children. The major findings were that in 1970–1971 approximately two percent of elementary school children received medication for hyperactivity; the stimulants were clearly the preferred medication with methylphenidate being the stimulant of choice; the average dosage of methylphenidate was 17 mg per day as compared to 11 mg per day of dextroamphetamine; and the average period of medication was 9 months. In 1971 and 1973 Krager and Safer (1974) asked school nurses in a large suburban Maryland area to list children known to be on medication and provide details about the medication. The data from this survey were generally consistent with the Chicago data. In 1971, 1.07 percent of elementary school children received medication for hyperactivity and in 1973 this figure had increased to 1.73 percent. Stimulants were the medication of choice and methylphenidate was clearly the preferred stimulant with twice as many children ($n = 672$) using it as were using dextroamphetamine ($n = 333$). Although the Krager and Safer data could have been spuriously low because some children had been told not to discuss their medication at school or were reluctant to admit that they were on medication (Kline, 1975), and the Stephen data (Sprague & Sleator, 1973) involved estimates rather than factual data, the results of these two surveys suggest that the mass media reports may be overestimating the prevalence of the use of medication with hyperactive children.

The Krager and Safer (1974) finding that methylphenidate was the treatment of choice is consistent with contemporary medical opinion concerning the greater efficacy of methylphenidate as compared to dextroamphetamine. The widespread clinical acceptance of methylphenidate is surprising since there is very little empirical basis for its supposed superiority. In one of the few *direct* comparisons of the two stimulants, Nichamin and Comly (1964) reported a 70 percent improvement rate for both drugs, the criterion for improvement being a rise in letter grade for classroom conduct. Comparative data from the long-term clinical study by Gross and Wilson (1974) showed that fewer severe side effects occurred with methylphenidate than with dextroamphetamine, but there was no evidence that target behaviors improved more with one drug than with the other. The widespread belief in the superiority of methylphenidate appears to stem from comparisons reported by Millichap and Fowler (1967), who averaged the percentages of children reported to have shown improvement in separate studies by different investigators, all of whom used different dosages and criteria for improvement. The methodological flaws in Millichap and Fowler's approach are obvious, but what is less obvious is the way in which their report of 83 percent improvement with methylphenidate versus 69 percent improvement with dextroamphetamine has shifted from the status of a carefully qualified finding in the 1967 paper to an unqualified and established fact in later publications by Millichap (1968, 1972). The extent to which this kind of loose treatment of the data has contributed to methylphenidate becoming the preferred stimulant medication is not known. For a thoughtful discussion of this topic see Arnold and Knopp (1973).

**Therapeutic Regimen**

The appropriate dosage procedure for the central nervous system stimulants is a matter of contention, with dosage being based on personal opinion rather than on established empirical fact. There has been a disappointing and potentially costly lack of research interest in the empirical determination of appropriate dosage level. What is needed is the delineation of *dose-response curves* for general activity level and for specific problems that often occur concomitantly with hyperactivity, such as impulsivity and short attention span. The dose-response curve refers to the fact that changes may occur in the target behavior with alterations in the amount of drug administered. As the dose is increased there is a greater effect on different response systems to a point of maximal response, and after that point is reached for a specific response system, further increases in the amount of drug ingested have no positive effect and, in fact, may cause the response to diminish in efficacy. An example of this phenomenon occurred in a study (Sprague, Werry, & Davis, 1969) using a memory recognition test in which the child's task was to identify from a series of pictures those that he had previously been shown. Figure 3 shows two different dose-response curves: the *reaction time curve* was linearly related to dosage level, but the *accuracy of responding curve* was greatest at 0.20 and 0.30 mg per kg of methylphenidate with a marked diminution of accuracy at 0.40 mg per kg. The only research on the general behavioral effect in hyperactive children of parametrical manipulation of medication (Sprague & Werry, 1971; Werry & Sprague, 1974) has shown that for methylphenidate no increase in drug effectiveness occurred beyond a dosage of 0.30 mg per kg, which for an average 9-year-old boy would be approximately 10 mg per day, a dosage that is substantially lower than dosages commonly used in clinical practice.

A closely related problem concerns the relative efficacy of *standardized* versus *individually titrated dosages.* Many clinicians (Gross & Wilson, 1974; Pincus & Glaser, 1966; Solomons, 1971; Wender, 1971) prefer the

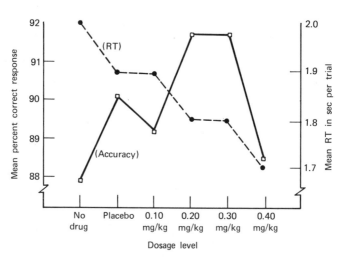

**Figure 3.** Dose-response curves of methylphenidate for speed and accuracy of responding. (Reprinted, by permission, from Sprague, R. L., Werry, J., & Davis, K. Psychotropic drug effects on learning and activity level of children. Paper presented at the Gatlinburg Conference on Research and Theory in Mental Retardation, 1969.)

standardized or average dose. However, Sprague and Sleator (1973) are opposed to it, contending that dosage should be titrated individually, beginning with small doses and gradually increasing them until a satisfactory reduction occurs in the hyperactivity, or side effects appear that are of sufficient severity to warrant no further increase in medication. It is our opinion that individual titration of the stimulants should be mandatory in view of the wide range of minimum effective dosage in hyperactive children (Knopp, Arnold, Andras, & Smeltzer, 1973; Schain & Reynard, 1975).

*Dextroamphetamine* may be administered in tablet form or in a sustained-release capsule with a duration of action of 6 to 18 hours. Tablets have the advantage of allowing greater flexibility and accuracy in maintaining optimum dosage, but have two disadvantages: a precipitous drop-off effect occurs when the medication wears off, and the child is more aware of being on medication particularly if the tablets must be administered by school personnel. The sustained-release capsule has a less precipitous drop-off effect and usually only a single daily dose is required. Wender (1971) suggests a beginning dose of 5 mg of dextroamphetamine before breakfast, at lunch, and again after school if necessary, but emphasizes, as does Solomons (1971), that many hyperactive children can tolerate much higher dosages, with 20 mg per day being considered the median effective dose. Other clinicians (Gross & Wilson, 1974; Pincus & Glaser, 1966) have advocated lower standardized doses of this drug.

*Methylphenidate* is less potent than the amphetamines, with *potency* defined as the amount of a drug that must be administered to obtain a particular response. Although it is often prescribed as if it were approximately half as potent as dextroamphetamine on a weight basis, a direct comparison (Sprague & Sleator, 1975) of the effects of the two stimulants on a laboratory test of learning showed that methylphenidate was more than half as potent as dextroamphetamine. Wender (1971) recommends a daily dosage range of from 20 to 100 mg of methylphenidate, whereas Lytton and Knobel (1958) have used up to 200 mg per day with some hyperactive children. Schain and Reynard (1975) have reported drug success with dosages ranging from 5 to 60 mg per day for elementary school children, with single doses being used for many of the children. An interesting finding in their study was that overweight children did not respond well to methylphenidate even though the milligram per kilogram dosage was equivalent to that in children who were categorized as drug successes. Gross and Wilson (1974) state that the dosage requirement can be reduced by half if liquid methylphenidate is used.

It is generally believed that only a few children can be satisfactorily maintained on a single morning dose of methylphenidate, with most children requiring a dose in the morning and again at noon. However, in a comparison of single and multiple doses of methylphenidate and dex-troamphetamine, Safer and Allen (1973a) found a single standardized morning dose of 20 mg of methylphenidate to be as effective for school day use as multiple dosage forms of dextroamphetamine. A single dose has the advantage of an appreciable reduction in the cost of medication; more important, the child is spared the embarrassment of being singled out for medication by school personnel. That being on medication can be a source of embarrassment is illustrated by the following excerpt from the response of an 8-year-old boy to the question, What would you like most?

Just one thing. I would like to only take these medications at home where no other kids know. I am calling them medications because ever since last year when we all had to write poems about real-life things I hate the word Pill. Last year my teacher was always saying, "Did you take your pill, David?" and pretty soon the other kids started saying it and then that dumb Susan Neilson wrote her poem on me and this is the poem. I heard it a million times already:

> David Hill
> Did you take the pill
> That makes you work
> And keeps you still?
> Take your pill, Hill.

And in baseball when I swing out and I almost always do the kids all yelled it. Sometimes I wish I could go to another school and start over. And once I wished that Susan Neilson would have to take pills and then she was away with some sickness and when she came back she did have to take pills and she had them in a little pink thing like my mother has powder in and all the girls thought it was cute and darling and no one ever said mean jokes about *her* taking her pill. I was real mad when everyone was just sort of interested in her pills.

The dosage levels reported above for dextroamphetamine and methyl-phenidate all refer to school-age children. Another point of contention in drug treatment is concerned with how early in the life cycle stimulant medications can be safely used. Some physicians are already using these medications with infants and young children (McMahon, Deem, & Green-berg, 1970; Nichamin, 1972) despite the fact that their use in the preschool years has not been approved by the Food and Drug Administration. Wen-der (1971) considers the amphetamines to be much less effective in pre-school children, and sets the trial dosage for these children at 2.5 mg twice a day. The treatment schedule reported by Gross and Wilson was 2.5 mg per day up to age four. The results of the following three in-vestigations question the efficacy of stimulant drugs for the preschool hyperactive child. In a comparison of the effects of methylphenidate and placebo on the psychological, motor, and cognitive test performance of preschool hyperactive children, and on ratings of them by teachers and pediatricians, Conners (1973) concluded that the children's overt behavior showed considerably less response to drug treatment than that which typically occurs in school-age children. On a mean dosage of 11.8 mg of methylphenidate per day the side effects were minimal, with no differences between groups. Schleifer, Weiss, Cohen, Elman, Cvejic, and Kruger (1975), using individually titrated dosages, also reported methylphenidate to be relatively ineffective with the preschool child. Although it reduced the level of activity exhibited by 3- and 4-year-old children at home, there was no evidence of improvement in their nursery school behavior or psychometric test performance. Significant overall improvement, that is, improvement in behavior plus an absence of side effects or only minimal side effects, occurred in only 3 of the 28 children in the drug treatment condition. A mean dose of 5 mg of methylphenidate in the morning and at noon often had a negative effect on mood, resulted in solitary play and poor peer relationships, and was associated with insomnia and anorexia. Zara (1973) reported that 4-year-olds who were on medication and who had shown a positive response to it were less competent verbally in an experimental learning situation than the same-age hyperactive controls who had never been on medication. In addition, those on medication were characterized by a cognitive inflexibility that was not exhibited by the control children.

**Prediction of Response to Medication**

To date no basis exists for predicting whether a specific hyperactive child will benefit from drug intervention, or for determining which medication will be most effective and what the minimum effective dosage is for him (Sroufe, 1975). The fact that there is no known method for predicting response to medication has attracted considerable clinical and research attention. Barcai (1971) was able to differentiate with a high degree of accuracy between stimulant responders and nonresponders on the basis of the child's history, teacher information, a clinical interview, and a finger-twitch test. Although the procedure is described in considerable detail and the finger-twitch test is simple to administer, the method has limited application because the only norms available are for 10- to 12-year-old boys. Unfortunately, there has been no attempt to cross-validate this procedure, and this limitation applies to all of the procedures described in this section.

*Environmental Social Factors*

One group of investigations has centered around environmental social factors. Conrad and Insel (1967) reported a negative relationship between drug response and psychologically turbulent households. Hoffman, Engelhardt, Margolis, Polizos, Waizer, and Rosenfeld (1974) found that hyperactive children who manifested consistent improvement as a function of stimulant medication were viewed as less of a problem by their parents than were children with a more variable response to medication. Knobel (1962) has emphasized the differential effects of medication-accepting and medication-rejecting households and research by Paxton (1972) and Weiss, Minde, Douglas, Werry, and Sykes (1971) suggests that the mother-child relationship is one determinant of drug response. The marked placebo effect that occurred in the Knights and Hinton (1969) study was undoubtedly one reason for their suggestion that the attitude of the parents and child toward drug therapy might have predictive value for response to medication. However, to date there has been no *systematic* study or research on any of these stimulus parameters.

## Neurobiochemical Measures

A second group of studies has focused on the relationship between neurobiochemical measures and drug response. Rapoport, Lott, and Alexander (1970) studied the level of excretion of adrenaline and noradrenaline in hyperactive elementary school boys and reported an inverse relationship between urinary noradrenaline and behavioral improvement as a function of stimulant medication. Of particular importance was the finding that noradrenaline levels prior to drug treatment predicted the decrease in playroom activity that occurred with stimulant medication. These findings suggest that biochemical measures may have predictive value for identifying children who may respond to medication. Epstein, Lasagna, Conners, and Rodriguez (1968) correlated dextroamphetamine excretion and drug response and concluded that organics with higher excretion rates responded best to amphetamine. In a brief discussion of this finding Knopp, Arnold, Andras, and Smeltzer (1973) noted that unpublished pilot studies by Corson with hyperkinetic dogs showed that following ingestion of amphetamine, good responders showed no increase in excretion of catecholamines, whereas poor responders showed increased excretion. Knopp et al. regard the Corson findings as at variance with the Epstein results. Despite the scarcity of studies in this area, and the conflicting results, the search for a biochemical index of potential drug response appears to have considerable merit and should be intensively pursued.

## Neurological and EEG Indices

In a major body of research on the prediction of drug response, subjects have either been categorized on an organic-nonorganic basis or their drug response has been correlated with their neurological and EEG findings. In some studies the stimulant medications have not proven to be differentially effective with either of these data treatments (Knights & Hinton, 1969; Millichap & Boldrey, 1967; Werry & Sprague, 1970). However, in other investigations neurological and EEG findings have been used with some success to predict drug response (Buchsbaum & Wender, 1973), or have demonstrated an association between the variables. For example, Satterfield, Cantwell, Saul, Lesser, and Podosin (1973) found that hyperactive elementary school boys with minor neurological abnormalities in four or more categories, such as gait, equilibrium disorder, dysarthria, and ambidexterity, responded with more improvement to methylphenidate than did boys without such abnormalities; boys with EEG abnormalities improved more than those with normal EEG's; and the degree of evidence of brain dysfunction correlated significantly with the probability of a good clinical response. A 30 percent improvement on the post-treatment versus the pre-treatment teacher rating of classroom behavior was considered to be evidence of a good response to medication. Callaway (Smithsonian Science Information Exchange, 1975) reported that increased EEG variability appeared to be a predictor of improvement with methylphenidate. In his study hyperactive children who showed the greatest improvement with methylphenidate had significantly more variable average evoked potentials in their EEG's than those who did not improve. A replication of this study is in progress. Conrad and Insel (1967) identified several factors that were associated with positive drug response, one of these being an organic background. They hypothesized that children with organically based or congenital hyperactive behavior would respond more favorably to the amphetamines than those with hyperactive behavior that was anxiety-based or emotional in origin. A retrospective review of charts of hyperactive children, combined with interviews concerning the current status of the children, indicated that the most positive response to stimulant medication was associated with an organic background, positive parent-child relationship, and the absence of severe psychiatric problems in the parents. Although several investigators (Cohen & Douglas, 1972; Dykman, Ackerman, Clements, & Peters, 1971; Spring, Greenberg, Scott, & Hopwood, 1974) have reported that hyperactive children who are not on medication do not differ from normal children in central nervous system arousal level as assessed by such measures as skin conductance level, EEG with the child at rest, and the sensory evoked cortical response, Satterfield and his associates have reported differences in all but one study (Satterfield, Atoian, Brashears, Burleigh, & Dawson, 1974). Their findings suggest the intriguing possibility that low central nervous system arousal is indicative of a good response to stimulus medication. In a series of studies with homogeneous groups selected on the basis of one set of criteria, Satterfield, Cantwell, & Satterfield (1974) identified a subgroup of hyperactive children all of whom had low central nervous system arousal and responded well to methylphenidate. In this subgroup they found that the lower the arousal level prior to treatment the greater the behavioral problem. For this group the stimulus medication functioned in a way similar to a stimulant (i.e., not paradoxically) in that it increased the arousal level, and the amount of increase in arousal level was positively correlated with clinical response as measured by teacher rating scales. Satterfield et al. note that the small numbers of subjects in some of the comparisons and the low, but significant, levels for the correlational data call for caution in interpreting their findings. This admonition is commendable, but the basic issue concerns the implications of their discrepant findings on arousal level.

Many discussions of the arousal issue assume that only two alternatives are involved, that is, that hyperactive children are either uniformly similar or dissimilar to normal children in central nervous system arousal level. This dichotomy is consistent with the opinion that hyperactive children are a homogeneous group. However Satterfield et al.'s (1974) discrepant finding can be interpreted as evidence for the existence of definable subgroups within the hyperactive population and, as such, supports the view that hyperactive children are a heterogeneous group. The fact that hyperactive children benefit from stimulant medication regardless of their arousal level may indicate that a higher optimal level of stimulation is characteristic of hyperactive children in general, and that those with normal arousal levels require a smaller daily dose than those with below-normal arousal levels. Research findings reported by Knopp, Arnold, Andras, and Smeltzer (1973) are consistent with reported variations in arousal level within the hyperactive population. In their sample of hyperactive children ($n = 22$), changes in the extent of pupillary contraction were measured by electronic pupillography before and after a test dose of amphetamine. The changes correlated with independent parent and clinician ratings of subsequent behavioral improvement as a result of stimulant medication. The findings were consistent with the hypothesis that the more a hyperactive child's light-reactive pupillary contraction deviated from the normal mean in *either* direction before medication, and the more nearly that contraction approached the norm after a test dose, the more likely the child's behavior would improve after medication. Prior to the test-dose administration there was marked variation in pupillary contraction above and below the normal mean, a finding that is consistent with Satterfield's findings concerning high and low arousal levels in hyperactive children.

There are several possible interpretations of the variations in level of arousal reported here, one being that in some subgroups of hyperactive children the high level of activity represents a physiological attempt to reduce the disequilibrium created by a low arousal level. This interpretation represents pure speculation at this point in empirical knowledge of hyperactivity; if true, however, it is possible that the *hypoactive* or lethargic children described by Nichamin and Comly (1964) and Wender (1971) are coping with high arousal levels through inactivity.

Although several of the foregoing clinical observations and research findings *appear* to have considerable potential as drug response indices, apparent potential should not be confused with proven value. Sroufe's conclusion (1975) remains unchallenged: No index of neurological status or battery of neurological indices has yet been shown through cross validation to have predictive utility, and physiological and psychological indices of drug response based on clinical experience are also empirically unsubstantiated.

## Response to Medication

There is a wide range in the literature in estimates of frequency of positive response to stimulants. Conrad and Insel (1967) have noted that researchers' claims of positive response center around the 70 percent level, whereas those of clinicians are around 30 percent. Many clinicians estimate positive drug response at around 70 percent with the qualification that allowance is made for *idiosyncratic specificity,* that is, the fact that many children will respond well, but not to the first stimulant or psychoactive drug administered (Knopp, Arnold, Andras, & Smeltzer, 1973; Weiss, 1975). There is also a wide range reported in the type of response in children who are given a trial of stimulant medication. It is estimated that from one-third to one-half of children experience an immediate and dramatic *positive response* (Fish, 1971; Office of Child Development, 1971); and with these children the omission of a single dose of medication results in a reappearance of the behavior problems in full force. Fish (1971) describes the positive response as dramatic and "very rapid when it works," so that children need only be kept on medication for a very short time to determine whether the drug will be effective.

An example of the immediate, dramatic, and very positive response to methylphenidate that Fish (1975) has described is contained in the following report (Fowlie, 1973, p. 354) by a mother of the response of her 5-year-old son:

When my son received his first half-tablet, the first thing he did was to get a rather complex jigsaw puzzle out of his toy closet. It was a puzzle that he had never been able to complete and that had particularly frustrated him. It had always angered him that his sister could do it without much difficulty. He worked at it for a whole hour, methodically fitting each piece or discarding it without evidence of temper or frustration. His concentration was deep, his patience unusual (for him) the ordinary distractions that always had interfered with his completing a task did not appear to disturb him. The change was extremely noticeable. It surprised me because never before had he been able to devote more than ten minutes to one activity. The repeated failure that he experienced every day had taken a toll on his self-esteem. We were both elated by the boost he got from his new success with the puzzle. Shortly after he finished the puzzle we held our first sensible two-way conversation. At five years old his interest in the sounds of words had seemed to distract him almost to the point of his ignoring their meaning.

However, Wender (1971) states that a positive response to medication is sometimes delayed, therefore a 2-week trial period should be allowed before deciding whether to continue with the medication or terminate it. Wender (1971) has suggested that the delayed positive response may be due to the occurrence of a metabolic change during the period between initial administration of the medication and onset of a positive response. One possible explanation offered (Wender, 1971, p. 101) for the mechanism of drug action in the delayed positive response is that of:

. . . drug-induced production of a false neurotransmitter. The theoretical model . . . is that the chronic administration of amphetamine might result in the production of a neurohormone(s) which does not normally occur, which in turn would interfere with or react with the neurotransmitters customarily present in the particular child.

*Moderate improvement* occurs in 10 to 20 percent of the children, a neutral response with no reaction other than minimal side effects occurs in some children, and in about 10 percent of the children three kinds of *negative responses* occur: The symptoms are exacerbated and this effect does not diminish with increased or reduced dosage but disappears gradually over a 48-hour period when the medication is discontinued; or the child becomes withdrawn and silent with a marked deterioration in his social relations; or he develops an acute psychotic reaction, which generally disappears with the withdrawal of medication. Fish (1975) has noted that some children manifest overt psychotic symptoms as a function of medication even though they were not apparently psychotic prior to medication. In her experience (Fish, 1971) these children were borderline psychotics whose symptoms were sharply exacerbated with medication. Occasionally a child exhibits immediate and dramatic improvement only to develop a rapid tolerance, a phenomenon called *tachyplaxis*. In this condition the child responds only temporarily to increased dosage and usually must be withdrawn from medication, although sometimes a different medication proves satisfactory (Gross & Wilson, 1974).

The foregoing categories of positive and moderate improvement refer to a generalized, overall improvement in cognitive and behavioral symptoms. The possibility that the response to stimulant medication may be hierarchical in nature has been suggested by a recent study from the Sprague laboratory. These data (Porges, Walter, Korb, & Sprague, 1975, p. 732) suggest that:

. . . although attention and behavioral hyperactivity may be influenced by methylphenidate the response affected may be a function of the individual's deficit . . . Influences on attentional behavior may precede influences on social behavior; or, if attention is adequate, social behavior may be influenced.

Reports of psychoactive drug action generally have relied on behavioral observations of children under naturalistic conditions or on standardized test performance of children under laboratory conditions. Arnold, Strobl, and Weisenberg (1972) have provided a subjective account of adult response to dextroamphetamine by a 22 year-old male university student who had clearly been hyperactive as a child, although his hyperactivity had not been treated, and who had continued to be hyperactive in adulthood. The subject stated that sometimes he needed to move so badly that he got up and walked around the classroom for no specific reason and friends confirmed that he was chronically nervous and restless. The subject had started taking dextroamphetamine in adulthood under a doctor's supervision, reported a definite calming effect, and stated that dextroamphetamine allowed him to concentrate, sit still, and study better. Arnold et al. obtained a subjective account of drug effect by having the subject do self-ratings of mood variables (concentration, anxiety, depression, and self-esteem) over 8 hour periods after double-blind administration of dextroamphetamine and placebo on 2 different days. Compared to placebo, dextroamphetamine increased concentration and depression, decreased anxiety, and had no effect on self-esteem. The investigators noted that this subjective evaluation is consistent with observations of drug effect on hyperactive children and differs markedly from those on normal adults, who typically react to amphetamines with a decrease in depression and a marked increase in anxiety and self-esteem. The subject's assessment of drug effect under controlled conditions is consistent with the informal reports of hyperactive adults who requested drug treatment after they had observed the marked improvement that occurred in their children's behavior with drug intervention (Gross & Wilson, 1974).

## Side Effects

Side effects are actions or effects of drugs other than those intended. They can be categorized in terms of *desirability* as positive or negative, with some of the negative effects being of a severity that justifies discontinuation of the medication, and in terms of *duration,* as short-term or long-term. Side effects do not occur in all children. When they do occur they generally increase proportionately with an increase in dosage (Sprague & Sleator, 1973).

### Short-Term Side Effects

The most frequent short-term side effects of the stimulants are *anorexia* and *insomnia,* both of which are usually of short duration and occur more frequently with the amphetamines than with methylphenidate. A common side effect that is particularly distressing to parents is the *"amphetamine look,"* a sunken-cheeked, sallow, dark shadows under the eyes look that Solomons (1971) calls the "panda effect." It is not considered to be of any physiological importance; however, it may do some psychological harm, as evidenced by the following statement from a 6-year-old boy with a marked amphetamine look:

I would like not to take those pills. I do not think those pills are good. Ladies say to my mom, "Why is he so *pale?* Doesn't he get enough sleep?" and my mom hates that and she says, "He's on medication," and they all look like I'm a new animal in the zoo and then real quick they start talking about some other things but they all keep looking at me in a real funny way and I don't feel good when they do.

Other short-term side effects of the stimulants that are less often reported include sadness, depression, fearfulness, social withdrawal, sleepiness, headaches, nail biting, stomach upset, and weight loss. It should be noted that weight loss often seems to be unrelated to appetite since slowing of weight growth has been reported when no anorexia was present (Gross & Wilson, 1974; Safer & Allen, 1973).

The few empirical investigations that have been conducted on the *sleep effects* of stimulants all suggest that these drugs have little effect other than insomnia. In an investigation of the effects of stimulants on rapid eye movement (REM) in children Feinberg, Hibi, Braun, Cavness, Westerman, and Small (1974) reported that dosages of amphetamine sufficient to produce clinical improvement did not substantially reduce the percentage of REM in spite of some increase in the amount of sleep preceding the first REM period (REM latency). Nor was there any elevation (REM rebound) in the percentage of REM on withdrawal of the drug even though REM onset occurred earlier. Furthermore, research by Haig, Schroeder, and Schroeder (1974) has shown that methylphenidate has little effect on the quality of sleep even with large dosages and with administration close to bedtime. Sleep latency and REM latency were the only measures affected and both were well below the levels indicative of sleep pathology.

Often the stimulant medications are given only in the morning and afternoon, the rationale for this procedure being that this dosage schedule will prevent sleep disturbances, particularly insomnia. Kinsbourne (1973) has questioned this procedure on the grounds that insomnia is not a stimulant effect but is a stimulant *withdrawal* effect. His argument is that by evening the medication effects have long since worn off, the child has returned to his hyperactive base state, and because of the rebound accentuation of his hyperactivity may be in a worse state than before medication, particularly if he is on amphetamines, which have a more marked rebound effect than methylphenidate. Kinsbourne reasons that the child should therefore find it easier to go to sleep if given a stimulant late enough in the day so that its period of effect overlaps bedtime; if he awakens during the night, giving him a stimulant should help him to go back to sleep.

## Long-Term Side Effects

There is little empirical evidence of the long-term risks of stimulant medication. However, two long-term studies are in progress, one by Satterfield and his colleagues and the other by Sprague (Smithsonian Science Information Exchange, 1975), and these may provide some information on this topic. The two major long-term side effects that have been identified are *increased heart rate* (Aman & Werry, 1975; Cohen, Douglas, & Morgenstern, 1971; Knights & Hinton, 1969; Sprague, 1972), the implications of which are not clear because the consequences of a chronic increased load on the child's heart are difficult to assess, and *growth suppression*. The latter was first reported by Safer and Allen (1973), who noted a mean loss of expected height of 5 percentile points in 20 children using dosages of more than 20 mg per kg of methylphenidate for an average of 3 years. This possibility created some anxiety among clinicians (Eisenberg, 1973). However, a subsequent study by Safer, Allen, and Barr (1975) showed a gain in the growth rate following the termination of drug intervention: the growth not only returned to normal, it also exceeded the expected level, a phenomenon which Safer et al. interpret as a growth rebound. Also, the reports of other investigators (Beck, Langford, MacKay, & Sum, 1975; Gross & Wilson, 1974), and preliminary reports from an ongoing study (Huessy, 1975), have suggested that although there may be an immediate period of growth suppression, over a longer period of observation the loss of expected growth is made up. Thus the data at the present time support a *delay* in growth rather than a suppression of it.

In 1971 Wender noted that there were no reports of *blood dyscrasias* occurring as a function of long-term amphetamine administration. However, a recent case-control study (Newell & Henderson, 1973) has demonstrated a possible link between Hodgkin's disease and the use of amphetamines. When the responses to an interview questionnaire of 100 patients with existing diagnosed Hodgkin's disease were compared with those of an equal number of controls matched for age, sex, race, and socioeconomic status, 19 of the 100 Hodgkin's disease patients had taken amphetamines for at least 2 months within 2 years of the onset of their Hodgkin's disease, as compared to 3 among the 100 controls (relative risk $= 6.33, p < .01$). Newell and Henderson emphasize that this finding is a preliminary one and must be replicated; nevertheless, the possibility of such a link suggests the need for investigations of bone-marrow changes, and particularly the importance of long-term follow-up studies.

It is generally believed that neither the amphetamines nor methylphenidate is characterized by a high incidence of severe side effects. Evidence of the low incidence of such effects comes from a long-term study of minimal brain dysfunction in 1056 children in which the mean duration of contact was 2-½ years (Gross & Wilson, 1974). Only four instances of side effects severe enough to warrant discontinuation of the medication occurred in the children treated with methylphenidate ($n = 377$), and only 16 instances in those treated with dextroamphetamine ($n = 371$). However, there has been an increasing number of reports in the literature of problems such as drug-associated psychosis (Ney, 1967), hallucinosis (Lucas & Weiss, 1971), and grand mal seizure (Chamberlain, 1974). Golden (1974) has written a case report of a 9-year-old boy who developed Gilles de la Tourette's Syndrome following methylphenidate administration. The explanation offered (Golden, 1974, p. 78) was that "methylphenidate stimulated an increase in dopamine turnover and brought about the onset of Tourette's Syndrome in a vulnerable patient." Greenberg, McMahon, and Deem (1974) have described significant personality deterioration in 5 of 26 children treated with relatively low dosages of dextroamphetamine. Although the symptoms subsided with discontinuation of the drug, the cases presented emphasize the need for careful observation for such reactions.

The possibility exists on both a theoretical and practical level that pharmacotherapeutic intervention for hyperactivity in childhood or early adolescence could result in an increased tendency to drug use in adolescence or adulthood. Clinical opinion based on clinical observation generally does not attach importance to this possibility, even though a definitive basis for accepting or rejecting it has not been established. Some clinicians (for example, Gross & Wilson, 1974, p. 108) state unequivocally that "the risk of addiction is zero," others (for example, MacKay, Beck, & Taylor, 1973) take a more cautious position by stating that they have never seen any evidence of it. Several investigations have failed to demonstrate an association between drug intervention in middle childhood and later drug abuse (Bradley, 1950; Office of Child Development, 1971). Beck, Langford, MacKay, and Sum (1975) compared 30 adolescents with histories of minimal brain dysfunction who had been treated with methylphenidate for at least 6 months with a control group comparable in age, sex, and socioeconomic background, but who had no history of drug intervention or psychiatric problems. The age range in both groups was 14 to 19 years. Following individual interviews these investigators concluded that (Beck, Langford, MacKay, & Sum, 1975, p. 437):

. . . adolescents who received methylphenidate during childhood are no more susceptible to later drug use than adolescents in the general population.

Indeed, it was stated that they might even be *less* susceptible:

Children who are receiving methylphenidate are eager to terminate the treatment in spite of their recognition of its positive effects. The experience of being controlled by medication apparently leads to later distaste of such restraint. Thus, contrary to general belief, early chemotherapy with methylphenidate appears to inadvertently offer a deterrent to the abusive use of drugs in late adolescence.

In this study at least two major independent variables were operating, minimal brain dysfunction and length of time on medication. To control for minimal brain dysfunction a third group of adolescents with this history but no medication history should have been included. In respect to the second variable additional information should have been provided, including statistical data on the length of the medication period, the dosage, and the length of the interval between the end of medication and the interview. Furthermore, requiring that subjects must have been on medication for at least 6 months should have some basis other than convenience or availability of data and the basis should be described. On the face of it, 6 months seems a very short time, particularly since many children are on stimulant medications for years (Solomons, 1973; Stewart & Olds, 1973). Although national averages on length of drug treatment for hyperactivity are unavailable, local averages could have been determined and an attempt made to match the experimental group mean to the local mean. Altogether, the methodology in this study does not justify generalization of the results to hyperactive adolescents in the general population.

*Interaction Side Effects*

The foregoing short- and long-term effects are *direct* side effects. Recent clinical reports emphasize the possibility of an *interaction side effect* between the stimulants and other medication, including nonprescription medication. Fischer and Wilson (1971) have cautioned that methylphenidate inhibits certain drug-metabolizing enzymes of the liver, thus causing a prolongation of the half-life of such drugs as phenobarbital, dilantin, mysoline, and imipramine, all of which may be used concurrently with the stimulants; as a result therapeutic doses of these drugs can be elevated to toxic level. The possibility of morbidity from such a combination is high, according to Fischer and Wilson (1971), who note that there have been several reports of ataxia in patients who were simultaneously being treated with dilantin and methylphenidate. Huestis and Arnold (1974) have described a case of possible antagonism of amphetamine as a result of the concurrent ingestion of a decongestant-antihistamine compound, in which a hyperactive boy with no known allergy manifested an excellent response to levoamphetamine except when he took cold capsules; during these periods the amphetamine was ineffective. As soon as the cold capsules were discontinued the boy returned to his previous level of improved behavior. Taken together, these findings on short-term, long-term, and interaction side effects suggest that the practice of allowing children to continue on stimulant medication unmonitored for long periods is negligent and potentially dangerous.

## The "Paradoxical" Calming Effect of the Stimulants

The term *paradox* has been defined by Webster (1962) as something inconsistent with common experience or having contradictory qualities, and by Thomas (1973) as an event that seemingly is contradictory but demonstrably true. Examples of psychological effects that are recognized as true paradoxes are *paradoxical warmth,* which refers to a feeling of warmth when the stimulus lies between 29 and 31 degrees Centigrade (typically a cool stimulus), and *paradoxical cold,* which refers to a sensation of coldness when a warm object of 45 degrees Centigrade and above stimulates the receptor for cold (English & English, 1958). An example of a pharmacological paradox is the fact that ganglionic blocking agents can be used to slow the rapid heart beat in tachycardia, and the same agent can be used to effect an increase in the slow heart rate characteristic of bradycardia (Kornetsky, 1970). These effects are truly paradoxical. Note that paradoxical actions can usually be explained, so that a paradox is not synonymous with magic or mystery.

The immediate, dramatic improvement following stimulant medication that Fowlie (1973) described has frequently been called paradoxical (Bradley, 1937; Solomons, 1971; Wender, 1971, 1973), presumably because it is inconsistent with current knowledge that stimulants should exert a calming effect. The validity of the term paradoxical as a descriptor for the positive response to the central nervous system stimulants can be questioned on two counts. First, Kornetsky (1970) has suggested that a true paradoxical effect of stimulant drugs upon the central nervous system would consist of an inhibitory effect on the overaroused child and disinhibitory effects on the child who is either underaroused or in a normal state of arousal. In terms of activity level this suggests that the effects of stimulant drugs should be to reduce activity in the hyperactive and increase activity in the underactive and normally active child. There is little support in the literature for such an effect. One of the few examples occurred in the study (Knopp, Arnold, Andras, & Smeltzer, 1973) referred to previously of the effect of amphetamine on pupillary contraction. Before medication, many of the 22 hyperactive children in the sample manifested pupillary contraction that deviated above or below the normal mean. After medication some of those below the mean showed increased contraction, and some above the mean showed decreased contraction; this is a truly paradoxical reaction to the amphetamine. In the *only* experiment (Shetty, 1971) in which normal children have been given stimulants, both the hyperactive and normals exhibited the same favorable drug response in the form of increased alpha activity. When research on the effects of stimulants on hyperactive children is compared with that on normal adults, there are striking parallels in the physiological and psychological findings. Both groups manifest relatively short-term anorexia and insomnia as a function of medication, and a need for an increased amount of sleep when the medication is withdrawn; both respond with similar patterns of withdrawal and tolerance; both exhibit improvement in motor skills and in performance on routine tasks, particularly those in which sustained attention is of critical importance; and both experience a feeling of increased well-being (Bradley, 1937; Sroufe, 1975; Weiss & Laties, 1962; Wender, 1971). In neither adults nor children are reasoning, problem solving, or learning directly improved, although both groups are capable of increased attention and persistence, which may in turn enhance cognitive performance (Conners, 1972; Sroufe, 1975). Second, the stimulants give the *impression* that a calming effect has occurred in the hyperactive child, but empirical investigations indicate that the actual change in the child's behavior is in more appropriate and better integrated responses in settings characterized by high demands for compliance (Conners, 1972; Werry, 1968; Werry & Sprague, 1970). There is little evidence of a simple reduction in activity level per se, particularly in free-field settings (Ellis, Witt, Reynolds, & Sprague, 1974). Fish (1975) has pointed out that *behavioral change* should not be interpreted as evidence of *pharmacological sedative action*; the action of the stimulant medications could be described accurately as paradoxical only if they were sedative in the pharmacological sense, and there is no evidence that this is the case. She also notes that the stimulant medications' effect helps many children who are not hyperactive even more positively than it does hyperactive children, which is inconsistent with the concept of a paradoxical action. An interesting offshoot of the issue of paradoxical effects has occurred recently with two reports of the paradoxical effects of central nervous stimulants in normal adults. Tecce and Cole (1974) demonstrated paradoxical drowsiness and lowered electrical activity in a group of normal adults given 10 mg of dextroamphetamine. Klein and Salzman (1975) paradoxically lowered average evoked potentials in a group of normal men, but not in women, 2 hours after the ingestion of 300 mg of caffeine.

One problem in establishing evidence for a paradoxical effect is that administering psychoactive drugs to normal children is considered unethical. However, it is interesting that many pediatricians feel no qualms about prescribing a trial of stimulant medication *prior* to seeing the child who has been referred for hyperactivity. If stimulants could be administered to normal children, the photo-Metrazol research by Laufer, Denhoff, and Solomons (1957) would provide the kind of test that is needed to establish the extent to which the stimulants' effect is truly paradoxical. The subjects in this study were two groups of children from a home for the emotionally disturbed; one group was judged hyperactive, the other was not. Metrazol, a drug used to test for the presence of brain dysfunction (Gastaut, 1950), was administered to each subject and a threshold determined (threshold = the amount of Metrazol necessary to evoke an EEG spikewave burst and a myoclonic jerk of the forearms in response to a stroboscope). Analysis of the mean photo-Metrazol thresholds for the two groups prior to medication revealed that the thresholds for the hyperactive children were significantly lower than those of the nonhyperactive. When amphetamine was administered to the hyperactive children and their photo-Metrazol thresholds redetermined, their mean threshold did not differ from that of the nonhyperactive group. A test of the paradoxical effect of amphetamine would be to determine the photo-Metrazol threshold in the nonhyperactive child following the administration of amphetamine. If the nonhyperactive child (who has a higher threshold to the photo-Metrazol test than the hyperactive child) showed a decrease in threshold, it would be evidence that the pharmacologic effect is a true paradoxical effect. However, if the nonhyperactive child showed an increase in threshold following ingestion of amphetamine, as did the hyperactive children in the Laufer, Denhoff, and Solomons study, it would suggest that the amphetamine action was not truly paradoxical. It is unlikely that this specific experiment will ever be used to resolve the paradox issue because there are potential risks in this use of Metrazol with children. Until a definitive experiment is conducted it is a misnomer and is detrimental to progress in the field to use the term *paradoxical* to refer to the more appropriate and better integrated responses that occur in some hyperactive children as a function of stimulant medication, because it suggests a difference in brain functioning of the hyperactive child that has not been established.

## Effects of Guidelines for the Use of Stimulant Medications

One result of the public reaction to the Omaha incident has been a number of publications providing guidelines for the use of medication with hyperactive children (Eisenberg, 1972; Office of Child Development, 1971; Solomons, 1973). The emphasis in these papers is on a conservative approach to the use of medication, careful preliminary evaluation of the child and his environment, the exploration of alternative forms of intervention with the goal of simultaneously using several treatment modalities, careful monitoring and follow-up of drug treatment, and the avoidance of coercion of the parents.

A survey of the literature suggests that these guidelines are being followed by only a minority of practitioners. Although some clinicians are unwilling (Walker, 1974) or reluctant (Stewart & Olds, 1973) to prescribe medication for the hyperactive, most are far less cautious. Browder (1972) reported that pediatricians sometimes make judgments about the use of medication on the basis of only a single brief interview with the mother and child. That such practices are followed is well-documented in the literature; the following excerpt is from a case reported by Divoky (1973, p. 9):

Frank, an attractive but very thin sixth grader, sits quietly in . . . the Learning Disabilities Clinic . . . A clinic doctor checks Frank's cumulative school record. Then he checks the boy's eye movements. Frank has a slight reading problem — a bit below grade level. But the main trouble, according to his mother and teachers, is that he has "trouble concentrating." He's not one to sit still, his mother says . . . At home . . . he can sit and watch TV forever. Frank explains that he doesn't like school, and that's why he won't sit still. The doctor tells Frank: "It's not that you won't sit still. You *can't* sit still." "No," Frank insists, "I won't." "I don't believe you," the doctor says, and continues to question Frank, but the boy stubbornly holds his ground: "I won't because I don't want to." . . . Frank has been on Ritalin in every grade except the fourth, when the teacher said he was fine without it. He doesn't take it in summer, because he doesn't need it when he's not in school. "Do you know what the Ritalin does to him?" the doctor asks. The mother says no, she just knows he doesn't eat much when he's on it . . . and the school says he's a little better on it. The doctor talks rapidly to the mother about hyperactive . . . children . . . Frank's mother nods as the words go over her head. "Keep him on Ritalin," the doctor concludes. "He seems to need it." It is the first time he has seen the boy, and the visit took 15 minutes.

Some physicians are willing to prescribe medication *prior* to seeing a child. There is well-documented evidence that at one private clinic in California children who are referred for "school problems" are *routinely* prescribed a trial dose of stimulant medication *before* they come to the clinic, the rationale for this procedure being that "it saves time for everybody" if the pediatrician has information about how the child responds to medication when he first sees him.

The recommendation of a *careful preliminary evaluation* is often not followed in practice, partly because of an uncritical confidence in the safety and efficacy of stimulant drugs, but also because of the belief that while hyperactivity is difficult to diagnose by examination and psychological tests, drug response is a highly efficient diagnostic tool. There are several problems in relying on the child's response to stimulant medication, as reported by his parents and teachers, to establish the diagnosis of hyperactivity. Although in some cases the immediate and dramatic improvement in quality of response is so distinctive that even experienced observers are satisfied as to the appropriateness of drug treatment, in many cases it is very difficult to distinguish between the responses of the hyperactive and nonhyperactive child (Sroufe, 1975). There is only one direct comparison of the effects of stimulants on hyperactive and normal children (Shetty, 1971). However, the research on the effects of amphetamines in adults (Weiss & Laties, 1962) and heterogeneous groups of problem children (Conners, 1972) suggests that *most* children would show improved attention and classroom behavior and more controlled motor skills. Furthermore, the positive effects of the medication could be enhanced with a placebo effect. Despite these shortcomings, the procedure of using drug response as a diagnostic method is widespread. The following quotation (Snyder, in Ellinwood & Cohen, 1972, p. 919) from a symposium on the use of amphetamines is illustrative of this viewpoint:

Dr. Snyder: This experiment sort of goes on all the time in the child psychiatry department at (Johns) Hopkins. All children with behavior and learning problems are believed to be hyperkinetic until proved otherwise. The hyperkinetic syndrome is not easy to diagnose, and a therapeutic trial is as good a way as any to make the diagnosis. Children whose behavior or learning difficulties are not based on the hyperkinetic syndrome respond, probably, just like a normal adult given an overdose. They don't sleep and don't eat, and occasionally a toxic psychosis develops, with visual hallucinations; this may last for 48 hours after the drug is discontinued. It seems that the children who are going to respond usually show an immediate response — not a sedating effect . . . but a reduction in distractibility . . .

Although many clinicians have strongly advocated a *multimodality treatment* program for the hyperactive child (Fish, 1975; Stewart & Olds, 1973; Werry, 1968), in actual practice for most children on medication, stimulants constitute the *total* treatment program. Furthermore, many clinicians (Oettinger, 1971; Safer, 1971; Wender, 1971) have expressed serious reservations about the potential efficacy of psychological and educational intervention. We are continually astonished at the importance that is attached to the results of a single study by Eisenberg, Gilbert, Cytryn, and Molling (1961) that showed an "indifferent response" in hyperactive children to short-term psychotherapy consisting of an initial interview with a psychiatrist, followed by four 30-minute sessions for both parent and child in the first, third, seventh, and eleventh weeks of a treatment program. Two hours of therapy, spread over an 11-week period, is far too short a period of treatment to provide a fair test of the validity of psychotherapeutic intervention, yet this study is frequently cited as evidence that the hyperactive child is unlikely to benefit from psychotherapy. Many teachers and parents also tend to consider medication alone an adequate form of therapy for the hyperactive child. In a recent description of a group-counseling method for parents of hyperactive children, Schaefer, Palkes, and Stewart (1974) concluded that in principle their counseling procedure could be effectively combined with other methods of treatment; in practice, however, they found that the parents of a child who is being successfully treated with drugs are seldom interested in other forms of intervention.

*Careful monitoring and follow-up* of a child on stimulant drugs is frequently neglected. In a survey of physicians who had at their disposal the facilities and support of an active, concerned university clinic, Solomons (1973) found that almost half of the children being treated by individual practitioners were not being monitored adequately, and that a substantial number of parents were being allowed to juggle the dosage that the child received at their own discretion. This finding is particularly discouraging in view of the fact that the criterion of adequate monitoring was only two patient contacts by the physician in a 6-month period. Similarly, Stewart and Olds (1973) reported children who had been kept on medication for long periods despite the fact that they were not experiencing any beneficial results from the medication and in some cases had suffered negative side effects. These investigators also reported finding adolescents who had been on stimulant medication for 6 years without a trial withdrawal period. Sroufe (1975) has attributed this negligence to heavy patient loads and an uncritical belief in the safety and effectiveness of stimulant drugs. However, there is also the possibility that physicians regard drug intervention as a form of treatment that should routinely require only a minimum of physician time. In a discussion of cost considerations, Wender (1971) points out that with a scarcity of physicians' time, one of the determinants in the choice of treatment modality must be the cost in time per person treated, and he states (1971, p. 131):

Adequate evaluation and treatment of the average minimal brain dysfunction child requires approximately four to six hours for the first year and less thereafter.

Another facet of the medication problem concerns the use of *coercion in initiating drug intervention*. The Office of Child Development report (1971, p. 27) stated that:

Under no circumstances should any attempt be made to coerce parents to accept any particular treatment . . . It is proper for school personnel to inform parents of a child's behavior problems, but members of the school staff should not directly diagnose the hyperkinetic disturbance or prescribe treatment.

Many parents are directly or indirectly coerced into accepting a period of trial medication for their children and much of this coercion originates with the school personnel (Grinspoon & Singer, 1973; Stewart & Olds, 1973). Parents have often reported receiving ultimatums from the school authorities that disregarded the recommendations of the child's pediatrician. One California mother stated that she had been pressured for 4 years to put her son on medication despite the fact that two pediatricians supported her antimedication stand (Hunsinger, 1970). Another mother reported that every parent with a child believed to be hyperactive was referred to the same pediatrician "because that doctor knows what the school wants" (Grinspoon & Singer, 1973, p. 518). An elementary school teacher pointed out three active 8-year-old boys in her class in September to one of the authors and said, "I'll have those three on medication by Thanksgiving or they won't be in this class," and in November all three boys were on medication. When asked how she had accomplished it she replied smugly that "it took a bit of pressure." Sometimes the pressure is less direct: it is suggested to the parent that drugs will help the child perform better in school, or the parents are bombarded with information about the prevalence of hyperactive children and the simplicity of the drug solution

(Sroufe, 1975). The source of the pressure may also be the physician. For parents who regard psychotherapy as the treatment of choice, express a desire to get to the bottom of the problem, and are unwilling to embark on a course of drug treatment for their child, Wender (1971, p. 114) says:

Parents must sometimes be seduced into accepting drug treatment. It is sometimes necessary to obtain full diagnostic batteries and offer brief "psychotherapy" to meet the family's needs. Otherwise, they are apt to withdraw and search for "real therapy" elsewhere.

Although the majority of parents are probably the blameless victims of pressure, propaganda, and professional advice in the matter of approving stimulant medication for their children, we have been dismayed at the number of parents, particularly mothers, who would like to have their children on drugs. As supportive evidence for this statement, consider the following finding. In 1972 Levin published *The Stepford Wives*, a widely-read novel about a group of young suburban business and professional men who developed a chemical formula that almost instantly enabled them to turn their wives into forever young, docile robots who worked industriously and tirelessly to please their husbands. We asked a group of young mothers ($n = 109$) who had read the book a number of questions related to school problems, literary preferences, and other topics. Embedded in the interviews were two questions, one to determine whether the respondent agreed or disagreed with the use of drugs for classroom behavior problems, the other to determine how the respondent felt about the use of chemical intervention to turn women into docile, industrious wives. The majority of these young mothers saw nothing wrong with using drugs to turn children into docile students: 98 respondents approved and 11 disapproved of the use of classroom drugs. However, 90 of the respondents objected to the use of drugs to effect such a change in wives, and only 19 approved this. It is a measure of our drug-oriented society that a number of these young women ($n = 14$) not only approved of the drug transformation in *The Stepford Wives*, but also added wistfully that if there were a pill that would turn them into good wives and mothers they would be all for taking it, despite its robot-like aspects.

## Research on Stimulant Drug Treatment with Hyperactive Children

A question that occurred frequently in the spate of editorials, informal debates, and official investigations that followed the Omaha incident concerned the validity of the evidence for the efficacy of stimulant drug treatment. Although proponents of this treatment cited the extensive clinical and experimental evidence of the positive effects of stimulants on hyperactivity, in fact, the majority of experimental studies in the stimulant drug literature do not stand up well under critical scrutiny (Sroufe, 1975). Most studies are characterized by such methodological faults as failure to assign subjects randomly to drug and placebo conditions, use counterbalancing of treatment conditions, control relevant stimulus and response variables, ensure fulfillment of experimental condition requirements, and obtain objective, valid, and reliable measurements. Evidence of the relative lack of definitive research data is contained in a 1971 review of the drug research literature by Sulzbacher (Wiens, Anderson & Matarazzo, 1972): of 1100 drug studies reviewed, only 210 were considered to have adequate controls. When this latter group of studies was categorized in terms of objectivity of the measures of behavior change used, it was found that 133 studies had used *subjective measures,* such as clinical opinion or inadequate rating scales, whereas only 77 had employed *objective* criteria of behavior change, such as psychological tests and direct behavior measures of hyperactive behavior. Of the 133 subjective studies, 86 reported significant improvement on the measures obtained, and 47 studies found no differences between drug and placebo groups. Of the 77 objective studies, only 20 studies showed evidence of positive effects of drug administration, whereas 57 studies reported no difference. It can be seen from Table 4 that the use of subjective measures results in a preponderance of positive drug

**Table 4. Categorization of Behavior-Modifying Drug Studies According to their Objectivity and to the Significance of Change**

| Dependent Variable | Significant Difference | Nonsignificant Difference |
|---|---|---|
| Clinical opinion | 30 | 4 |
| Rating Scales | 56 | 43 |
| Psychological tests | 8 | 38 |
| Direct behavioral measure of hyperactivity | 12 | 19 |
| Total | 106 | 104 |

From Wiens, A. N., Anderson, K. A., & Matarazzo, R. G. Use of medication as an adjunct in the modification of behavior in the pediatric psychology setting. Professional Psychology, 1972, Spring, 157-162. Copyright 1972 by the American Psychological Association. Reprinted by permission.

effects; however, when objective measures are used the number of studies showing positive effects drops sharply.

Although the Sulzbacher review is representative of the current status of drug research, the substantial drug research literature does include a number of well-designed studies that have used objective and reliable measures of behavior, and have provided evidence of the potential of stimulant drug treatment in the control of hyperactivity. The research to be discussed here concerns only the *short-term* effect of the stimulants on such dependent measures as activity level, motor performance, and cognitive tasks because there is a paucity of objective and rigorous data on the *long-term* effects of these drugs. Most of the information that is available consists of clinicians' reports, school achievement data, and global impressions of parents and teachers. A notable exception is a long-term follow-up study (Weiss, Kruger, Danielson, & Elman, 1974) that showed that children who were given methylphenidate over a three to five-year period were more manageable at school and at home while on drugs but did no better five years later than a carefully matched hyperactive control group (who had not been given medication) on objective measures of intelligence, academic performance, emotional adjustment, and delinquency. Before reporting the findings on the effect of drug treatment on such measures as activity level, motor performance, and cognitive tasks, we will discuss some of the general methodological procedures, factors in drug effects, and the problems inherent in drug research with children.

### Double-Blind Cross-Over Design

One of the best experimental procedures for assessing the efficacy of drug intervention is the *double-blind cross-over design*. The term *double-blind* implies that neither the subject, the observers, nor any others involved in assessment know whether the child is in the active drug group or the placebo group. In the cross-over procedure each subject serves in every experimental condition including the placebo condition. In an experiment in which dosage level is parametrically manipulated each subject would be administered two or more dosages of medication and would also be given a placebo, all for specified blocks of time. Counterbalancing of order of participation in the various drug and placebo conditions would be used. The *advantages* of this design are that it reduces subject variance and thus permits the use of smaller samples than does a simple randomized group design. Also, the cross-over design provides information about each subject's response to the drug being investigated, and this information is of considerable value for the child, his parents, and his pediatrician. The *disadvantages* are that the time required to complete such a study is extended because of the cross-over feature and thus the probability of subject attrition is increased. Multiple testing is required and so there may also be practice effects. The "blindness" of observers is sometimes difficult to maintain due to the dramatic and immediate change in behavior that often occurs in hyperactive children who respond well to stimulant medication, and also to the occurrence of the more common and observable side effects (Weiss, Minde, Douglas, Werry, & Sykes, 1971). Main effects for condition may be confounded with sequence effects. For example, there could be a carry-over effect from drug to placebo in which a subject's placebo scores following his participation in a drug condition are higher than those of a subject who is assigned to a placebo-drug condition. In addition, in the placebo-drug sequence there may be a suppression of drug condition performance, and in the drug-placebo condition the subject may experience rebound effects as a function of drug termination. All of these sequence effects make the interpretation of main effects for drug condition difficult (Sprague & Werry, 1971; Sroufe, 1975).

An example of a methodologically sound double-blind cross-over design is the study of Steinberg, Troshinsky, and Steinberg (1971) in which elementary school children with behavior or learning problems were randomly assigned to either a drug (dextroamphetamine) or placebo condition for a period of 4 weeks, followed by a 10-day drug vacation period to minimize sequence effects, after which subjects were crossed over to the other condition for a second 4-week period. The administration of the dextroamphetamine and placebo was carried out every school day morning by the public health nurse and both the drug and placebo were given in liquid form because young children sometimes experience difficulty in swallowing tablets and they sometimes conceal tablets and discard them later. Baseline behavior ratings by each of the subjects' teachers (each child had two or three teachers, all of whom independently rated his behavior) on a scale similar to that of Conners (1969) were obtained for each subject 1 week prior to starting the medication and at weekly intervals during each of the two 4-week blocks. No subjects were dropped or lost from the study. Although Steinberg, Troshinsky, and Steinberg (1971) refer to this study as a double-blind, technically it is a triple-blind, because neither the raters nor the public health nurse were aware of the design of the study or the drug status of the children, and the psychiatrist who interviewed the parents concerning their children's participation was aware of the design but not of the drug status of any given patient. Notice in Figure 4 that in the second 4-week period there was a positive sequence effect for the subjects in the drug-placebo condition, with the placebo scores following the drug condition indicating less hyperactive behavior than those of the group who were given placebo prior to drugs.

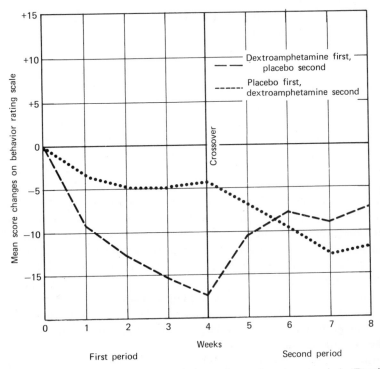

**Figure 4.** Comparison of behavior ratings in first and second treatment periods. (Reprinted, by permission, from Steinberg, G. G., Troshinsky, C., & Steinberg, H. R. Dextro-amphetamine-responsive behavior disorder in school children. *American Journal of Psychiatry*, 1971, Vol. 128, 174–179. Copyright 1971, the American Psychiatric Association.)

### Randomized Group Design

A less commonly used design is the simple *randomized group design* in which the subjects are randomly assigned to the treatment conditions so that there are independent groups of subjects for each treatment. An example of this design is the comparative test by Conners, Taylor, Meo, Kurtz, and Fournier (1972) of the efficacy, side effects, and safety of pemoline and dextroamphetamine. The *advantages* of this design are that there are no sequence effects, multiple testing is not required, and specific drug conditions may be subjected to longer periods of experimental scrutiny than is usually possible in the cross-over design. The *disadvantages* are that random assignment to groups may lead to pre-treatment differences whose relationship to the problem being investigated creates difficulties that may not be eliminated with covariance techniques; larger sample sizes are needed than in the cross-over design; and subjects in the placebo condition generally reap few benefits for their participation.

## Placebo Effect

Regardless of the type of research design selected, the drug effect that is achieved cannot be attributed solely to the chemical action of the drug. The placebo effect is an important nonchemical factor that often serves as a determinant of drug effects and, as such, may confound the results. A placebo is a dummy pill made of some inert material such as milk sugar, but identical in appearance to the active medication. Its purpose is to make the patient and the observers feel that he is being given medication. Under placebo conditions any improvement that occurs or is seen by others to occur in a patient can be attributed to the expectation of the patient and others that improvement would occur as a function of medication. An astonishing range of placebo effects has been reported (Beecher, 1955). Placebos have been found to modify successfully problems such as asthma, toothache, headache, and nausea; and Sroufe (1975) has reported the case of a subject whose tic was exacerbated by placebo but then responded to a modification of the dosage. The specific placebo effect that occurs is largely a function of the expectation of the parent or child concerning the outcome of the use of the drug. McDermott (1965) reported a case in which a hyperactive child's parents discontinued the use of dextroamphetamine because they misinterpreted their pediatrician's instructions and thought that only a short period of drug treatment was required. Although all medication had been discontinued, the dramatic improvement in the child's activity level, general behavior, and school performance that the parents expected persisted for a 6-month period.

## Problems in Drug Research with Children

Although there are many genuine inadequacies in the literature on drug research with children that are valid targets of criticism (see, for example, the reviews of Baker, 1968; Conners, 1972; Freeman, 1966; Sprague & Werry, 1971), it is important to keep in mind that drug research with children, particularly long-term research, is beset with more than the usual problems that occur in research with children in naturalistic settings. Minde and Weiss (1970) cite as one problem the fact that changes attributed to drug effect must be carefully evaluated within the context of the child's sphere of activity because children typically are more responsive than adults to minor environmental fluctuations. Because of a seasonal variation (Eisenberg, 1959) in the frequency and reason for referral, comparisons between children referred in the winter and those referred in the summer should be avoided. It is a well-established fact (Sprague & Sleator, 1973; Sroufe, 1975) that subjects often fail to take their medication so it is essential that the procedures allow for careful monitoring by the experimenter of drug intake. Hyperactivity varies in its response to a specific type of medication depending on the intellectual status of the subject, severity of the problem, and certain etiological factors (Fish, 1969). It is therefore important to obtain as precise a description as possible of the subjects. In the experience of Minde and Weiss (1970) children respond with more variation to an identical mg per kg dose and require a larger dose per kg than do adults, and for this reason the use of individually titrated dosage is favored by these investigators. Sprague and Werry (1971) do not agree with the use of this procedure in research and, instead, recommend a standardized dose. Finally, the natural growth and development of the child may confound the assessment of change, particularly in a long-term study.

## Stimulant Drug Effects on Specific Aspects of Behavior and Performance

### Activity Level

One concern that is frequently expressed by parents is that the calming effect of the stimulant medications will turn their children into zombies. This concern appears to be unwarranted, the general finding being that the drug action is *situation-specific* and thus has little effect on the energy expenditure of the child in free-field settings, while consistently decreasing activity level and task-irrelevant behavior in settings, such as the classroom and laboratory, where the tasks are structured and the demands for compliance are high. Ellis, Witt, Reynolds, and Sprague (1974) used a double-blind cross-over design to study the effect of a range of dosages (0.10, 0.30, and 1.00 mg per kg of methylphenidate and placebo) on the activity of hyperactive elementary school boys in a playroom setting. The finding that methylphenidate did not influence activity level as measured by observational ratings and analysis of the position and movement of the subjects on photographs taken every 4 seconds was consistent with previous results (Witt, Ellis, & Sprague, 1970) from the same laboratories. Further evidence that methylphenidate effects little change in free-field behavior is contained in studies of preschool (Conners, 1973; Schleifer, Weiss, Cohen, Elman, Cvejic, & Kruger, 1975) and school-age children (Knights & Hinton, 1969; Millichap & Boldrey, 1967; Sprague, Barnes, & Werry, 1970). However, there is substantial support for a decrease in extraneous activity and task-irrelevant behavior in playroom (Rapoport, Lott, Alexander, & Abramson, 1970), classroom (Hoffman, Engelhardt,

Margolis, Polizos, Waizer, & Rosenfeld, 1974; Knights & Hinton, 1969; Sprague, Barnes, & Werry, 1970), and laboratory settings (Cohen, Douglas, & Morgenstern, 1971; Sroufe, Sonies, West, & Wright, 1973) characterized by high demands for compliance. Evidence of a drug-with-situation interaction receives strong support from the Sprague, Barnes, and Werry (1970) finding that teachers' global impressions of the effects of methylphenidate in a formal setting were reliably sensitive to dosage, whereas parents' reports obtained during the less formal weekend activities were not sensitive to drug, placebos, or dosages. In the study by Hoffman et al. (1974) there was evidence that an interaction between drug response and aspects of the child's symptomatology produced an unstable treatment response. When children with an uneven, erratic response to medication were compared with those with a more consistent response, the variable responders were characterized by a cluster of difficulties including problems with peers, negative attitudes to school and authority figures, and reluctance to admit errors. The empirical demonstration of interaction effects coupled with clinical reports of these effects underlines the importance of isolating these factors and determining their relative strengths. Knowledge of the extent to which such factors might influence the clinical usefulness of the stimulant medications would have predictive value in making decisions about prescribing stimulant drugs for specific individuals (Ellis, Witt, Reynolds, & Sprague, 1974).

## Motor Performance

A variety of measures has been used to assess the effects of the stimulant drugs on fine motor skills performance. The results suggest that the stimulants generally improve performance on these tasks and that this improvement occurs partly as a result of the acquisition of more selective control of motor behavior. Increased visual-motor coordination and motor steadiness following stimulant drug treatment has been reported by Lasagna and Epstein (1970), and Millichap, Aymat, Sturgis, Larsen, and Egan (1968). Knights and Hinton (1969) also reported significant improvement in motor steadiness on two tasks. One was a maze test, a measure of steadiness in motion, in which the child was required to move a stylus through a maze, twice with each hand. The second task was a holes test, a measure of steadiness while resting, the task being to hold a stylus for 10 seconds in each of a series of progressively smaller holes, without touching the edge. On both tasks the children showed improvement in terms of duration of contacts with the sides of the maze. Zimmerman and Burgemeister (1958) demonstrated increased speed of performance on the Seguin Form Board and block-tower tasks, and a series of studies from the McGill University laboratories showed improvement in performance on the Lincoln-Oseretsky Motor Test (Douglas, 1972), a reduction in motor impulsivity (Sykes, Douglas, & Morgenstern, 1972), and a decrease in the frequency of redundant motor responses (Cohen, Douglas, & Morgenstern, 1971). However, in other investigations no effects of stimulant medication over placebo have been found on a diverse group of motor tasks including a Luria-type tremorgraph (Conners, 1966), key tapping (Millichap, Aymat, Sturgis, Larsen, & Egan, 1968), pegboard performance (Knights & Hinton, 1969), and motor control (qualitative scores) on the Porteus Maze Test (Conners & Eisenberg, 1963; Conners & Rothschild, 1968). Some of these divergent findings almost certainly reflect variability in the subjects' degree of motor control prior to drug intervention, other kinds of subject heterogeneity relevant to fine motor performance, and the variety of measures used. Research is needed to determine whether the stimulant drugs effect a change in specific motor components affecting performance (for example, speed of response and selectivity of control) or in general performance by improving such factors as motivation (Epstein, Lasagna, Conners, & Rodriguez, 1968), improved attention (Conners & Rothschild, 1968), or persistence (Sprague & Werry, 1971).

*Classroom Behavior*

There have been relatively few studies on the effect of drug treatment on classroom performance and many of those that have been conducted have failed to use objective measuring techniques. One of the best classroom studies was a triple-blind, cross-over, placebo control study (Sprague, Barnes, & Werry, 1970) in which 12 elementary school boys described as "antisocial, distractable, and hyperactive" served as their own controls in a three-factor study: drug (methylphenidate, thioridazine, and placebo), dosage (low and high), and task complexity as determined by number of stimuli to be processed. Time sampling methods and teacher ratings were used and measures were obtained in both the laboratory and classroom. The results showed that certain deviant classroom behaviors, attention to task, and points earned for good behavior were significantly improved with methylphenidate as compared with placebo. Other studies have used ratings to confirm the superiority of the stimulant medications over placebo on symptoms of hyperactivity, distractability, and impulsivity (Conners & Eisenberg, 1963; Conners & Rothschild, 1968; Knights & Hinton, 1968; Weiss, Minde, Douglas, Werry, & Sykes, 1971). Sroufe (1975) has emphasized that with rating scales there are several potential problems: the raters may exert a halo effect by rating a child who shows specific improvement in one area as also improved in other areas, the double-blind may be broken by teacher and parental recognition of side effects of the drug, and there is a lack of any reliable information about what factors parents and teachers are actually responding to when they assign ratings. A good example of the strong effect of rater expectations was reported in a study by Knights and Hinton (1968) in which both teachers and parents were aware that the children were participating in the investigation of a drug (methylphenidate) considered helpful with behavior problems. Their positive attitudes concerning drug treatment were probably a major determinant of the strong placebo effect: 88 percent of the children on drug and *67 percent of those on placebo* were rated as improved by their teachers, and 73 percent of the drug group and *54 percent of the placebo group* were perceived as improved by their parents.

In considering the efficacy of stimulant medication for classroom behavior, it is important to emphasize that very little attention has been given to the effects of drugs on the kinds of learning and cognitive skills, such as achievement in the basic academic subjects and problem solving, that normally occur in the classroom. As Sroufe (1975) has pointed out, the types of tasks that are most often studied and have yielded positive results of drugs are ones that are "repetitious, mechanical, and/or of long duration, and seem to require concentration, care, and sustained performance." It is time for researchers to turn their attention to the efficacy of stimulant medication for the acquisition of learning that is required in the classroom. In addition to the foregoing, what is urgently needed in classroom research are two kinds of study, one in which drug effects are compared with special educational procedures, and the other of the effect on classroom performance of the interaction between drug effects and special educational procedures. Unfortunately these important topics have attracted little research interest although Ayllon, Layman, and Kandel (1975) have recently demonstrated a behavioral-educational procedure that resulted in control of hyperactivity equal to the effect of drug intervention, and academic gains superior to those achieved while the subjects were on medication. This study is described in detail in Chapter 6. Also, Stewart and his associates at the University of Iowa are currently comparing the relative efficacy of stimulant drug treatment with management by behavioral counseling of teachers and parents of the hyperactive child (Smithsonian Science Information Exchange, 1975). Apart from these two studies the only research in the area was a study in which Conrad, Dworkin, Shai, and Tobiessen (1971) assigned groups of lower socioeconomic class children to four conditions: dextroamphetamine alone, placebo alone, drug plus 40 sessions of prescriptive tutoring, and placebo plus prescriptive tutoring. The tutors were adult volunteers who were trained for the task and carefully supervised. Measures obtained prior to and following the 4- to 6-month treatment period provided little support for the efficacy of drug treatment alone over tutoring. However, both parents and teachers rated children in the drug-plus-tutoring group as more improved than those in the placebo-plus-tutoring, which suggests that drug treatment may interact with classroom intervention strategies such as tutoring on behavioral measures. There was no firm evidence of the efficacy of either of the two drug conditions over either of the two nondrug conditions on a variety of cognitive, perceptual, and achievement measures. Unfortunately the results were somewhat confounded by two features of the study: one was the use of the Wide Range Achievement Test (WRAT) as the measure of academic achievement (for a discussion of this point see page 269 in Chapter 8); the other was the fact that half of the children in the drug-plus-tutoring group received their medication irregularly, which serves to emphasize the importance of control of experimental procedures.

*Standardized Tests*

Although hyperactive children are not generally referred primarily for the assessment of intelligence or academic achievement, standardized tests in these areas frequently have been used as dependent measures in research on drug effects, probably because they provide an objective and reliable assessment of performance that permits between-study and long-term within-subject comparisons. Studies that have used these measures as dependent variables have varied markedly in research design, dosage level, duration of drug treatment, and subject variables. Despite this variability, the results have been remarkably consistent in demonstrating short-term improvement in intelligence test performance as a function of stimulant medication and, where improvement has not occurred, the duration of drug treatment has been so short as to preclude any reliable change in performance (Sroufe, 1975).

Improvement in intelligence test performance has been consistently demonstrated on the Performance Scale of the Wechsler Intelligence Scale for Children (WISC), Porteus Maze IQ score, and the Goodenough Draw-A-Man Test (see, for example, Conners, 1971; Conners & Rothschild, 1968; Knights & Hinton, 1969; Millichap, Aymat, Sturgis, Larsen, & Egan, 1968; Zimmerman & Burgemeister, 1958). Using methylphenidate with 6- to 12-year-old children, Butter and Lapierre (1974) reported improvement on sensory perception and integration as measured by the Illinois Test of Psycholinguistic Abilities. Standardized achievement tests have rarely been used but the data available are consistent with those on intelligence test performance, with short-term improvement occurring in the basic academic subjects (Conners, Rothschild, Eisenberg, Stone, &

Robinson, 1969; Sroufe, 1975). However, these findings should not be interpreted as evidence that intelligence or learning ability can be increased with drug intervention, particularly with the short-term intervention that is used in most drug studies. It is generally agreed (Conners, 1972) that improvement in performance could be a function of increased motivation and attention, which are of critical importance in test situations. Support for this interpretation is contained in the finding that the stimulant drugs facilitate sustained attention to visual and auditory stimuli (see, for example, Douglas, 1972; Knights & Hinton, 1969; Sykes, Douglas, & Morgenstern, 1972) and improve performance on simple and choice reaction time tasks (Cohen & Douglas, 1972; Sroufe, Sonies, West, & Wright, 1973; Sykes, Douglas, & Morgenstern, 1973). Furthermore, Creager and Van Riper (1967) have documented another response to methylphenidate that could be expected to enhance performance on complex cognitive tasks. They found that the verbal output and qualitative verbal response of children were significantly improved with drug intervention. It follows that an improvement in these components of intellectual performance could account for the reported improvement on many standardized tests. Also, in many studies the interval between pre- and posttesting is so short that improvement as a function of memory effects rather than of drug effects should not be discounted, particularly for the intelligence tests.

## Performance on Laboratory Tasks

The positive effect of stimulant medication on paired-associate learning has been demonstrated by Conners and his colleagues (Conners & Eisenberg, 1963; Conners, Eisenberg, & Sharpe, 1964; Conners & Rothschild, 1968). In the latter study, associative strength of lists was varied and there was no interaction between drug condition and associative strength of list. This finding, coupled with a significant effect of drug in the form of error reduction on the paired-associate learning tests only in the last block of trials in the Conners and Eisenberg (1963) study, points to an attention factor rather than a change in associative learning ability. In laboratory studies of short-term memory, in which the task was to look at a matrix of pictorial stimuli and then look at a single test picture and indicate whether that picture had appeared in the matrix presented a few seconds before, one study showed a significant increase in the stimulant drug condition in number of correct responses and speed of responding (Sprague, Barnes, & Werry, 1970). A second study (Sprague & Werry, 1971) demonstrated an inverted "U" dose-response curve with placebo increasing correct responses over no-drug, and 0.20 and 0.30 mg per kg of methylphenidate increasing number correct over placebo, but further increases in drug to 0.40 mg per kg resulted in a *decrease* in number correct.

Stimulant drugs improve performance when *sustained attention* is required. The measure that is frequently used here is the Continuous Performance Test, a measure of vigilance to monotonous visual or auditory stimulation. On the visual presentation the child's task is to monitor a visual display of letters, each presented for only a fraction of a second, and to signal whenever he sees a specific letter. In a summary of a series of experiments, Douglas (1972) presented evidence of the facilitative effect of the stimulants on sustained attention. Conners and Rothschild (1968) also reported a drug-induced reduction in impulsivity and fewer errors of omission on this task. A general finding in reaction time tasks is that the stimulants reduce response latency (Cohen, Douglas, & Morgenstern, 1971), and where reflectivity is important for success, the stimulants increase response latency (Campbell, Douglas, & Morgenstern, 1971), which is consistent with the conclusion that stimulants generally result in a more controlled, integrated performance (Conners, 1972).

## Retention of Learned Material

One extremely important area of investigation concerns the possibility of a reduction in ability or a failure to transfer learning that occurred under a drug state to a nondrug state, or vice versa. The fact that a response learned under the influence of a particular drug may recur with maximum strength only when that drug condition is reinstated is referred to as *state-dependent learning* or *learning dissociation* (Overton, 1968). The assumption underlying this phenomenon is that if a specific drug was present during the initial acquisition of a response, later absence of the drug would constitute a novel stimulus environment and the previously learned response would not occur. This phenomenon has been the subject of extensive infrahuman investigations (see, for example, Barrett, Leith, & Ray, 1972) but has attracted surprisingly little research attention at the human level in view of the fact that hyperactive children on medication usually spend a substantial amount of time in learning academic material. If state-dependency could be demonstrated to occur in children learning cognitive tasks, this finding would have potentially serious implications for pediatric psychopharmacology because it would mean that children might lose an indeterminate amount of what they had learned while they were on the medication that was intended to facilitate their learning. Only limited research on the possible state-dependent effects of stimulant drugs in humans has been reported. Bustamente and his colleagues (Bustamente, Jordan, Vila, Gonzalez, & Insua, 1969; Bustamente, Rossello, Jordan, Pradera, & Insua, 1967) demonstrated a significant state-dependent effect in subjects who were required to learn items in one experimental session for recall during that session and subsequent sessions under constant or changed drug state; but their findings were weakened by methodological faults, such as biased sampling procedures, and the allowance of insufficient time for drug absorption. Hurst, Radlow, Chubb, and Bagley (1969) conducted a study similar to those of Bustamente and his colleagues (1967, 1969) but found no evidence of state-dependent effects. An unpublished study by Hallsten and Sprague (1971) of short-term memory in young mentally retarded boys showed no evidence of state-dependent effects and some of the retention means were higher for groups tested on a drug different from that employed in the original training period. In an extensive study of state-dependent learning effects, Aman and Sprague (1974) tested a group of hyperactive children using methylphenidate and dextroamphetamine on three different learning tasks: short-term memory, paired-associate learning, and fine motor performance on a maze task. Each subject learned the tasks under one condition and was then tested for retention under each of the drug conditions, that is, methylphenidate, dextroamphetamine, and placebo. The results showed no evidence of state-dependent learning, with reasonable clinical dosages of stimulant medication. Some transfer data were in the direction *contrary* to what state-dependent effects would predict. This study represented a stringent test of state-dependency because the dosages used were larger than the regular therapeutic dosage. The fact that no evidence of state-dependent learning was observed with this moderately heavy dosage reduces the probability that state-dependent learning might occur with the clinical use of stimulant medication. The findings were consistent with those of Sprague, Werry, Greenwold, and Jones (1970) with emotionally disturbed children. Evidence of transfer of a benefit of drug therapy to the nondrug state is contained in a study of the effects of methylphenidate on reaction time by Cohen, Douglas, & Morgenstern (1971) who reported that subjects who were tested first on methylphenidate became less variable while on medication and continued to exhibit more stable performances when they were subsequently tested on placebo.

Although the research presented here provides little support for the occurrence of state-dependent learning in hyperactive children, until this possibility has been subjected to more intensive experimental investigation, clinicians might be wise to consider a precautionary procedure advocated by McCabe and McCabe (1972). The basis for their suggestion was a study by Barrett, Leith, and Ray (1972) in which dextroamphetamine produced a dose-dependent facilitation of avoidance behavior in rats in a Y-maze situation. Abrupt termination of the stimulant was followed by a decrement in the avoidance response, and a gradual reduction of the dosage on consecutive training days produced a permanent avoidance facilitation that continued into the no-drug condition of the experiment. This result suggests that withdrawal of the drug in a way that allowed the transfer of stimulus control of the avoidance response from drug to nondrug related cues was important for retention of the learning. McCabe and McCabe (1972) have recommended a gradual, step-wise withdrawal of stimulant medication in children to facilitate the transfer to the nondrug state of response patterns acquired while on medication. Such a therapeutic strategy would serve two purposes: it would decrease the probability of state-dependent learning and minimize the possibility of undesirable effects occurring as a function of abrupt termination of long-term stimulant therapy.

## Other Drugs Used in the Treatment of Hyperactive Children

Although the amphetamines and methylphenidate are by far the most widely used drugs with hyperactive children, two other *central nervous system* stimulants, caffeine and magnesium pemoline (Cylert) have recently gained clinical and research attention in the treatment of this problem. One *antidepressant,* imipramine, and one *major tranquilizer,* phenothiazine, have also been used with some success. Each of these psychoactive drugs will be briefly described.

### Caffeine

Caffeine is one of the xanthines, which are among the oldest central nervous system stimulants known to man. Caffeine is the only psychoactive drug that is legally available without prescription and is found in coffee, tea, colas, chocolate, and cocoa (see Table 5). It is not considered addictive in the sense that narcotics are (Goodman & Gilman, 1970). A therapeutic dose of caffeine for a child is from 100 to 150 mg. The absorption of caffeine administered orally occurs rapidly and peak blood levels are usually reached within an hour after ingestion. In terms of central nervous system

**Table 5. Amount of Caffeine in Selected Beverages**

| Beverage (8 oz) | Caffeine (mg) |
| --- | --- |
| Regular coffee | 150 - 200 |
| Instant coffee | 100 - 130 |
| Tea | 50 - 110 |
| Coca-Cola | 30 |
| Pepsi-Cola | 20 |
| Cocoa | under 10 |

potency 150 mg of caffeine is equal to 6 mg of dextroamphetamine. The most common behavioral effects of a therapeutic dose of caffeine are an increase in attention and well-being, a slowing of the development of boredom, and a general increase in mental and motor efficiency. When tolerance occurs it is low grade and does not seem to be a problem. In a review of the research on the amphetamines and caffeine in adults, Weiss and Laties (1962) noted that the amphetamines produced more subjective positive behavioral effects, such as alertness, talkativeness, excitement, and feelings of exhilaration, and fewer subjective negative effects, such as difficulty in concentrating, exhaustion, dizziness, sleepiness, and tremor, than did caffeine. They concluded that "the superiority of the amphetamines over caffeine is unquestionable."

Despite the apparent superiority of the amphetamines over caffeine in adults, there is some evidence that caffeine may be an effective alternative to dextroamphetamine and methylphenidate in the treatment of hyperactive children. In a pilot study by Schnackenberg (1973), 11 hyperactive children who had developed annoying side effects from methylphenidate were given a 3-week medication holiday and then put on 200–300 mg per day of caffeine in the form of one cup of coffee at breakfast and a second cup at lunch. Their teachers, who had not been informed of either the drug holiday or the change in medication, were interviewed and were also asked to rate the children's classroom behavior during the child's last month on methylphenidate, last week off all medication during the 3-week drug holiday, and third week on caffeine. The scale used was the Rating Scale for Hyperkinesis (Davids, 1971); a score of 24 or more on this scale suggests the presence of hyperactivity, scores ranging from 19 to 23 are regarded as suspicious, and scores of 18 or less are viewed as indicative of an absence of significant hyperactivity. It can be seen from Table 6 that the mean scores for the methylphenidate and caffeine periods were almost identical and generally signified an absence of hyperactivity, whereas those obtained during the drug holiday were clearly in the hyperactivity range. Schnackenberg (1973) could see no difference between the response to treatment of the 11 children on caffeine and that of approximately 300 children whom he had treated with dextroamphetamine and methylphenidate. There was no appreciable change in the 11 children on caffeine when the daily dosage was doubled (400–600 mg of caffeine) or halved (100–150 mg). One other brief pharmacological study and one case study report provide further evidence of the efficacy of caffeine. Firestone (1974) found that caffeine improved the performance of hyperactive children on reaction time tasks. There was a marked decrease in the tendency to respond impulsively. However, the amount of improvement was not as striking as that which had occurred with methylphenidate in previous studies in the McGill labora-

**Table 6. Patients' Side Effects on Methylphenidate and Scores on Rating Scales for Hyperkinesis**

| Patient | Age (Years Months) at which Methylphenidate Started | Discontinued | Side Effects Attributed to Methylphenidate* | Scores on Rating Scales for Hyperkinesis Methyl-phenidate | No Drugs | Caffeine |
|---|---|---|---|---|---|---|
| 1 | 8-4 | 8-5 | Insomnia | 18 | 26 | 19 |
| 2 | 7-6 | 8-6 | Anorexia, no weight gain | 16 | 27 | 16 |
| 3 | 8-0 | 8-9 | Anorexia, weight loss | 19 | 26 | 18 |
| 4 | 7-3 | 7-5 | Insomnia | 19 | 26 | 17 |
| 5 | 7-10 | 8-4 | Anorexia | 16 | 25 | 16 |
| 6 | 7-6 | 8-1 | Anorexia | 14 | 24 | 15 |
| 7 | 6-7 | 7-0 | Anorexia, weight loss | 19 | 26 | 17 |
| 8 | 8-5 | 8-8 | Anorexia, weight loss | 18 | 26 | 17 |
| 9 | 8-3 | 8-9 | Insomnia | 13 | 24 | 15 |
| 10 | 7-9 | 8-4 | Anorexia, no weight gain | 19 | 29 | 18 |
| 11 | 7-4 | 8-3 | Anorexia | 18 | 26 | 17 |

* All side effects listed disappeared during treatment with coffee.
Reprinted, by permission, from Schnackenberg, R.C. Caffeine as a substitute for Schedule II stimulants in hyperkinetic children. *American Journal of Psychiatry*, 1973, Vol. 130, pp. 796-798, Copyright 1973, the American Psychiatric Association.

tory. Fras (1974) reported that caffeine in the form of whole coffee alternated with stimulant medications was an effective procedure for the control of hyperactivity.

Three other studies have failed to find evidence of the efficacy of caffeine in the control of hyperactivity. In a 9-week double-blind cross-over design with eight hyperactive boys who were full-time day-treatment hospital patients, Garfinkel, Webster, and Sloman (1975) reported that 20 mg of methylphenidate daily was significantly more effective in controlling hyperactivity than was 160 mg of caffeine. The measure of improvement used was daily ratings on the Conners Teacher Rating Scale of each child by child care workers. A comparison of methylphenidate with decaffeinated coffee showed that methylphenidate was superior in attenuating hyperactivity. Decaffeinated coffee did not differ from placebo. It is important to note that the dosage of pure caffeine used was approximately two-thirds of the caffeine content of the whole coffee used in the Schnackenberg (1973) study. Huestis, Arnold, and Smeltzer (1975) used a double-blind cross-over design to compare the effects of caffeine with methylphenidate and dextroamphetamine. The subjects were 18 hyperactive elementary school children (M = 12, F = 6). Each of the three drug conditions lasted for 3 weeks. The subject selection criteria and evaluation procedures used were excellent. The results showed significant improvement with methylphenidate and dextroamphetamine, both of which were significantly superior to caffeine. The slight improvement that occurred with caffeine was not significantly better than placebo. Huestis et al. concluded that caffeine did not offer the same therapeutic benefits as the other two stimulant medications. However, they note that the discrepancy between their findings and those of Schnackenberg (1973) could reflect some important difference between the *pure caffeine* used in this study and the whole coffee used by Schnackenberg. Conners (1975) also reported negative results in all but one case with pure caffeine in a double-blind cross-over study of caffeine treatment of hyperactive children (n = 8). His dosage levels were fixed and did not approach the levels used by Schnackenberg (1973) until the last week of the 3-week dosage period.

Huestis, Arnold, and Smeltzer (1975) state that caffeine does not offer the same therapeutic benefits as the other stimulant medications. This conclusion seems, at best, premature in view of the fact that in the group of five studies and one case report discussed here not one of the studies has been replicated, and marked variation in the independent variables occurs across studies. Whole coffee was used in some studies and pure caffeine in others; marked variation in dosages occurred as well as differences in length and locus of study, method of assessment, and type of subject. Some subjects were children in a private practice and others were day-treatment patients in a hospital clinic. Also, in some studies the children were on caffeine because they could not tolerate the stimulant medications, whereas in others the children had previously responded favorably to these drugs. Each investigator has, in effect, conducted *noncomparable variations* on the initial research by Schnackenberg (1973). To advance the current status of our knowledge of the efficacy of caffeine, Schnackenberg's study (1973) should first be replicated by others in the field, with strict adherence to *all* of the requirements defining a replication. Then, keeping any one of Schnackenberg's main independent variables constant, the effects of systematic variations in each of the other independent variables should be studied. With this approach a body of research findings could be built up that would permit new studies to build on existing data and allow between-study comparisons to be made. The possibility that there are distinct subgroups in the response to medication should not continue to be ignored in the design of experiments. Schnackenberg's positive findings may be directly related to the fact that the children in his group had all developed troubling side effects as a result of medication. Research is needed to determine the long-term effects of administering significant amounts of caffeine in the form of coffee to children.

The advantages of caffeine over the other stimulant medications are that there is no known risk of drug abuse; caffeine apparently produces fewer annoying short-term side effects in children (contrary to Weiss and Laties' [1962] report of more subjective negative effects in adults); no stigma is attached to drinking coffee; and the necessity for it can be minimized by such strategies as including a chocolate-mocha milkshake in the child's lunch. Furthermore, the cost of coffee per year is approximately one-tenth that of the stimulants, and this can be an important consideration for a family that must maintain a child on medication for several years.

## Magnesium Pemoline (Cylert)

Pemoline is a mild central nervous system stimulant that has been reported to have significant anti-fatigue and performance-enhancing properties in studies with adults, children, and animals (Plotnikoff, 1971). The major difference between pemoline and the more commonly used central nervous system stimulants is its long duration of psychostimulant activity without sympathomimetic cardiovascular effects; a single daily dose of 25–100 mg of pemoline given in the morning is sufficient to maintain satisfactory behavior. This relatively long duration of action offers an important advantage over dextroamphetamine and methylphenidate. In addition, unlike the amphetamines, pemoline has not proven addictive in monkeys (Plotnikoff, 1971).

Preliminary clinical studies have suggested that pemoline may effect improvement in school performance in hyperactive children, particularly on tasks involving short-term memory, and may facilitate attentiveness to school tasks. In a comparative test of the efficacy, side effects, and safety of pemoline and dextroamphetamine, Conners and his colleagues (Conners, Taylor, Meo, Kurtz, & Fournier, 1972) randomly assigned 84 6- to 12-year-old children (M = 74, F = 10) of normal intelligence to groups receiving pemoline, dextroamphetamine, or placebo for 8 weeks. The children, whose major complaints were severe overactivity, poor attention, distractibility, low frustration tolerance, disruptive behavior, and failure to progress in school at a rate consistent with intellectual potential, were given a battery of psychological tests before treatment and at the end of 8 weeks, and clinician, parent, and teacher ratings of behavior were also obtained throughout the study using both global and factored ratings. The ratings consistently showed that both pemoline and dextroamphetamine resulted in a significant reduction in symptoms as compared to placebo, with dextroamphetamine producing a more immediate and dramatic improvement and pemoline resulting in fewer anorexic side effects. There were few differences between the drugs on psychological test performance or in side effects other than anorexia, and a laboratory battery showed no short-term toxic effects. Conners et al. (1972) concluded that pemoline is an alternative that can be safely used in the treatment of the minimal brain dysfunction syndrome.* Millichap (1973) reported that pemoline alleviated hyperactivity and was associated with increased scores on the Performance Scale of the WISC. Knights and Viets (1973) also reported that the onset of effectiveness of pemoline was slower than that of some of the other central nervous system stimulants, with maximum therapeutic effect not being apparent for 3 to 4 weeks. These investigators also noted that pemoline was effective when given in a single daily dose, there were very few side effects, and almost all of the children showed improvement in mood and communication skills, in addition to marked improvement in behavior and school performance. Although the research to date on this stimulant has been limited, the consistency of improvement over placebo, coupled with the absence of troubling side effects, is very encouraging.

*Tricyclic Antidepressants*

Imipramine (Tofranil) is one of a series of antidepressant compounds called tricyclic because of its chemical structure. It has been extensively and successfully used in a variety of clinical conditions, such as enuresis (see, for example, Alderton, 1970, and Tec, 1963). Several investigators have found imipramine to be effective in treating hyperactive children. Waizer, Hoffman, Polizos, and Engelhardt (1974) treated hyperactive elementary school boys in an outpatient clinic with imipramine for 8 weeks followed by 4 weeks of placebo. Ratings by a psychiatrist, parents, and teachers indicated significant improvement in hyperactivity, attention span, and sociability in the drug group, whereas a noticeable deterioration of behavior occurred in the placebo group. The conclusion that imipramine was highly

---

* According to Schrag and Divoky (1975, pp. 95–105) serious criticisms concerning the subject characteristics, evaluation procedures, and completeness of data in the Conners studies (1970, 1972) were raised by FDA medical officer Carol S. Kennedy after she had examined the *raw data* and *procedural records* from the two studies. Schrag and Divoky state that the Kennedy criticisms were upheld by an outside committee appointed by the FDA to conduct a second review of the pemoline data, the committee members being Gerald Solomons, Eric Denhoff, and Roger D. Freeman, all of whom are highly respected for their knowledge of pediatric psychopharmacology. The account of the controversy about Conners' pemoline data appears to be well documented with memos, letters, and documents from the FDA files that Schrag and Divoky state they obtained from an unidentified source. We assume that their account is accurate, and, as such, it gives a chilling picture of the procedures used in validating a drug for use with children and the pressures on the FDA for their approval.

effective in the treatment of hyperactive children corroborated the findings of Huessy and Wright (1970), whose success in treating hyperactive children with this drug was so marked that they recommended it be used instead of the amphetamines. Winsberg, Bialer, Kupietz, and Tobias (1972) also found imipramine to be as effective or more so than dextroamphetamine with hyperactive children, but cautioned that imipramine required close surveillance for possible systemic toxicity. In the Gross and Wilson study (1974), 86 percent of the children on imipramine showed a significant amount of improvement, and there were significantly fewer side effects than with the stimulant medications. Some children did best with a combination of imipramine and one of the stimulants, possibly due to one drug enhancing the blood level of the other (Perel, Black, Wharton, & Malitz, 1969). One major deterrent to the use of this drug is that there has been relatively little documentation of the range of safety and side effects of imipramine in children, and in 1970 the Food and Drug Administration specifically warned against the use of this antidepressant and similar drugs in children. Furthermore, several recent studies suggest that the prolonged use of imipramine requires very careful monitoring. Saraf, Klein, Gittelman-Klein, and Groff (1974) reported the sudden death of a 6-year-old girl during imipramine treatment. Brown, Winsberg, Bialer, and Press (1973) reported three cases of children who developed seizures while receiving imipramine treatment for hyperactive-aggressive behavior disorders. All three children had organic brain disease but no previous history of seizures. Only two of the children remained seizure-free after anticonvulsant medication was added to the treatment regimen. These investigators suggest that clinicians prescribing imipramine be alert to the possible complication of seizures. Fromm, Amores, and Thies (1972) found that the drug was helpful in some patients with seizures but exacerbated major seizures in other patients. Evidence of electrocardiographic abnormalities has been described by Winsberg, Goldstein, Yepes, and Perel (1975), leading to the recommendation (Hayes, Panitch, & Barker, 1975) that the Food and Drug Administration issue another warning about the risks in using imipramine for children. The severity of some of these side effects suggests that extensive laboratory investigations must be carried out before imipramine can be considered superior to the stimulant medications in the treatment of hyperactivity.

*Phenothiazines*

The two phenothiazines that have been most extensively investigated are chlorpromazine (Thoradazine) and thioridazine (Mellaril). As with the stimulant medications, there is a lack of adequately controlled studies of the efficacy of these drugs, although Grant (1962) considered that there was sufficient empirical support for chlorpromazine to describe it as "an effective and useful inhibitor of hyperactivity." Werry (1970) formulated the most comprehensive statement on the efficacy of the phenothiazines for hyperactive children. He concluded that in naturalistic settings, such as the home and classroom, these drugs have no consistent effect on attention and cause children to be perceived by their mothers as improved particularly in respect to their hyperactivity. The reactions of teachers were inconsistent, with some reporting reduction in motor activity and others reporting *decreased* positive teacher-pupil interactions. In laboratory situations these drugs increased response latency, had no consistent effect on motor activity, and effected a deterioration in several kinds of task performance, such as repetitive tasks. Only one study has systematically investigated retention of learned material and the results suggest a reduction in retention when learning occurs under the thioridazines (McArdle, 1968). Werry (1970) concluded that the phenothiazines were generally inferior to the stimulant medications in effects on behavior and cognitive functioning.

Side effects are reported more frequently with the phenothiazines than with other tranquilizing agents (Millichap & Fowler, 1967); some of the most common effects are increased daytime drowsiness and weight gain as a function of increased appetite. Less frequently reported effects include bedwetting, lowered blood count, and with high dosages, tremors or uncoordinated movements.

### Research Needed on Stimulant Drug Effects

It is clear that the stimulant drugs have gained considerable interdisciplinary acceptance despite a paucity of objective experimental support in some areas, conflicting research in others, and considerable dissent among the experts concerning the efficacy of drug intervention for the hyperactive child. Given the uncritical acceptance that presently exists, it is essential that future research be directed towards the intensive examination of some of the major issues in child psychopharmacology rather than continuing to demonstrate simple drug effects. Some of these issues have already been identified, for example, there is widespread concern about the lack of information that we have about the *long-term psychological and physiological consequences* of stimulant drug intervention. We have only limited knowledge about the extent of *misuse* of the stimulants during the therapeutic period. The authors know of instances of children taking extra pills before an examination under the erroneous assumption that if one helps with schoolwork, two will be even better, and of children selling pills to other children for the same purpose. The potential of the stimulants for *drug abuse* has not been empirically established, although one of the few relevant studies (Laufer, 1971) is often treated as the definitive study despite serious methodological flaws. Several clinicians have made totally unsupportable statements, presumably on the basis of their clinical experience; for example, Gross and Wilson (1974, p. 108) say that "we can categorically state that the risk of addiction is zero." In contrast to these optimistic statements, Williams (1970) testified before a House subcommittee that a number of students in her high schools who were no longer formally on stimulant medication still came back regularly on their own initiative to get the drugs. Another important area of research concerns the lack of *an adequate physiological explanation for the efficacy of the stimulants* in modifying hyperactivity. There is some empirical support for the Wender model (1971) and there is in progress a major study of a neurochemical-neurophysiological model (Stern, 1975). If the therapeutic value of the central nervous stimulants could be adequately explained, such information might provide leads toward the prediction of drug response and the identification of etiological subgroups, both of which would represent major contributions to the management of hyperactive children.

Although the foregoing issues are clearly of major importance, we would assign priority to the comprehensive study of the effects of stimulant drug intervention on attention, with the two main research areas being a *comparison* of the effects of the stimulants with those of other treatment modalities and study of the *interaction* between the stimulants and other forms of treatment. Educators commonly assume that the stimulants make the child more amenable to remedial procedures, an assumption that is possibly the result of the Office of Child Development (1971) statement that the stimulants do not *cure* the hyperactive child, but they may make him more accessible to educational and counseling efforts. There is no evidence for this interaction, but it is an area that demands intensive investigation. The importance of the role of attention in hyperactivity has gained increasing support from two sets of empirical findings. One concerns the positive effects of drug intervention on indices of attention such as reaction time and cardiac deceleration (Douglas, 1972; Porges, Walter, Korb, & Sprague, 1975; Sroufe, Sonies, West, & Wright, 1973); the other is the fact that the short period of drug intervention required to effect improvement on a diverse group of academic and performance tasks, coupled with the inconsistent nature of the findings, suggests an attentional factor rather than an improvement in specific abilities per se (Alabiso, 1972; Conners, 1972; Douglas, 1972). If stimulant drug intervention did prove to make the child more amenable to attentional training, this finding would have major implications for special education.

A two-phase research strategy would be required to investigate the efficacy of drug intervention on attention. In the first phase, baseline data would be collected on the effects of drugs and other treatment modalities on (1) tasks that measure *components of attention,* such as temporal and selective attending, and (2) *indices of attention,* such as reaction time and cardiac deceleration. The *temporal* component of attention is the ability to respond consistently and it is an attention-span or duration of attention skill that can be measured on vigilance tasks such as continuous performance tasks. The *selective* component is an information-processing skill that involves the ability to focus on the relevant or central aspect of a task and to exclude the irrelevant or peripheral aspects. It is best assessed within the context of the Type II incidental learning paradigm, in which certain aspects of an activity are designated as relevant or central task performance and others are classed as irrelevant or peripheral. Measures are obtained of the amount of relevant and irrelevant learning and retention, and these two scores provide a basis for inferring selective attention. Baseline data for these attentional variables would be obtained for drug intervention, direct training using operant reinforcement and modeling procedures, and training in self-instructional techniques for inducing and maintaining attention. Previous research has demonstrated the effect on attention of the reinforcement-modeling procedure with young mentally retarded children (Ross, 1970; Ross & Ross, 1972), and the efficacy of self-instructional procedures for hyperactive children (Palkes, Stewart, & Kahana, 1968). Between-group comparisons would establish the relative efficacy of the three modes of intervention. It would be particularly interesting to determine if self-instructional procedures could be used to induce cardiac deceleration; our experience has shown that young mentally retarded children frequently use spontaneous overt verbal commands to induce attentional readiness prior to the onset of a competitive task (Ross & Ross, 1972), and there is abundant anecdotal evidence to suggest that in competitive situations many adults use covert self-commands for the same purpose. Certainly this possibility is consistent with biofeedback research (Schwartz, 1973).

In the second phase of this proposal research on a variety of tasks would be used to study the interaction between drug intervention and the other treatment modalities to determine if the stimulant drugs do, in fact, make hyperactive children more accessible to other forms of intervention. The interaction between these interventions is an area of major importance that has been almost completely bypassed by researchers, despite the fact that there is a great potential for a positive interaction between techniques such as drug intervention and behavior modification (Bandura, 1969; Sprague & Werry, 1971). One possibility is that the stimulant drugs would facilitate operant conditioning by reducing task-irrelevant behavior. The possibility that learning which occurs as a function of a combination of interventions might then prove to be state-dependent would also have to be investigated.

In his critical review of drug treatment with hyperactive children, Sroufe (1975) has noted the almost complete lack of theory and models of attention in most of the drug experiments. The two-phase research strategy proposed here is more than adequate in this respect, since the proposed research stems from reinforcement theory (Bijou, 1965; Skinner, 1953), observational learning theory (Bandura, 1969), and the filter model of selective attention proposed by Broadbent (1958); as such, it could result in the progress in understanding drug effects that Sprague and Werry (1971) say will occur when research is based on theoretical formulations rather than "a shotgun empirical approach."

# CHAPTER 5

# *Psychotherapy*

Psychotherapy is a nonspecific term used to describe techniques for helping the individual achieve acceptance of his own behavior, as well as for modifying or eliminating behavior that is creating interpersonal difficulties, is potentially harmful to the individual or others, or deviates markedly from accepted social and ethical norms. The term *psychotherapy* is generally limited to treatment that has been designed and implemented by a professionally trained person such as a psychiatrist or psychologist; it conveys no information about the severity of the maladaptive behavior, the duration or intensity of the treatment process, or the theoretical background and affiliation of the therapist (Ullman & Krasner, 1969). It includes a diverse group of techniques; for example, psychoanalysis, hypnosis, operant conditioning, modeling, and psychodrama are all subsumed under its general rubric.

Two fundamentally different approaches, traditional psychotherapy and behavior therapy, have dominated the field of psychotherapy (O'Leary & O'Leary, 1972). The differences between the two approaches center around beliefs and assumptions concerning the nature, causes, and treatment of maladaptive behavior. *Traditional psychotherapy* is based on a psychoanalytic or medical model that embraces the disease concept of behavior abnormalities (Bandura, 1969). According to this concept, abnormalities of behavior are symptoms of an underlying psychic disturbance or neurosis. The therapist's task is to identify the underlying cause of the behavior and modify or eliminate the behavior by effecting changes in the intrapsychic organization of the individual through the restructuring of some of his internal mediating processes. Central to the disease concept is the assumption that long-term benefits from treatment can only be achieved if the individual gains some understanding of the psychic forces that underlie his maladaptive behavior, so that the development of such insight becomes one of the primary targets of treatment. The assumption is that insight will increase the individual's ability to deal effectively with his own behavior and control his life situation. *Behavior therapy* is based on a sociopsychological model that assumes that maladaptive behavior is a learned response acquired as a method of coping with the demands of the

146

environment (Ullman & Krasner, 1969). Because the maladaptive behavior is learned, it is potentially modifiable. The therapist's task is to effect a change in the behavior through the application of general learning princi-ples, the emphasis in treatment being on a direct attack on the problem behavior. The treatment process has an empirical basis and consists of the teaching of specific responses. The use of behavior therapy does not preclude the spontaneous acquisition of insight; in the process of using newly learned responses, clients sometimes achieve an understanding of the reasons for their previously maladaptive behavior (Bandura, 1969; O'Leary & O'Leary, 1972).

In the first half of this century the proponents of these two conceptually different approaches to the modification of behavior were polarized, with each faction strongly rejecting the viewpoint of the other. Traditional psychotherapy was firmly entrenched and its proponents were highly criti-cal of the sporadic and unsuccessful attempts of behavior therapists to put the treatment of behavior problems on a more objective base. However, the next two decades were characterized by a sustained attack in the form of criticisms of traditional psychotherapy (see, for example, Skinner's 1953 text, *Science and human behavior*) and empirical demonstrations that forced a reconsideration of some of the basic tenets of these therapeutic procedures (Bandura & Walters, 1963). Concomitant with these events was a series of publications such as Eyesenck's (1960) text, *Behavior therapy and the neuroses*, and empirical demonstrations of reinforcement and other procedures for effecting behavior change (Bijou, 1965), that strengthened the position of behavior therapy. One effect of all these events has been a convergence of traditional psychotherapy and behavior therapy so that now there is some overlap, with some clinicians using methods based on learning theory and some behavior theorists incorporating concepts and variables central to traditional psychotherapy in their approaches to be-havior change (Urban & Ford, 1971).

The modification of behavior has become a major area of experimental investigation, one result being the development of a set of therapeutic procedures with demonstrated efficacy for behavior problems that previ-ously had defied treatment. These treatment procedures have certain characteristics in common: they emphasize current behavior problems within a learning context, attach little importance to the patient's history and family background, consider concepts such as insight unnecessary, avoid the use of diagnostic categories, regard labels as potentially harmful to progress, and generally aim for a short duration of treatment. At the same time they differ on several major dimensions, including the extent to which they reflect a psychoanalytic or learning theory approach, the amount of training required for their effective use, the degree of involvement of agents of socialization such as parents, and the duration of treatment.

The purpose of this chapter is to describe some of the therapeutic methods relevant to the treatment of hyperactivity rather than to provide a comprehensive review of the field. The methods to be discussed have proven effective in treating hyperactivity, or clearly have potential for the modification of this problem, or have been advocated for use with hyperactive children. They reflect the convergence of psychoanalytic and learning theory, and in most cases have the latter's advantage of describable steps in its application to specific problems. The first section describes reinforcement procedures that have been used successfully in the problem of hyperactivity. In a traditional psychotherapy-behavior therapy dichotomy, these procedures and those in the second section, modeling, would be more appropriately categorized as behavior therapies rather than as traditional therapies although some overlapping exists, particularly in some of the modeling procedures.

## BEHAVIOR THERAPY APPROACHES

### Reinforcement Procedures—Operant Conditioning

One of the major behavior therapy techniques, operant conditioning, uses reinforcement procedures to modify behavior. The specific reinforcement procedures used were developed by Skinner and his colleagues (1953, 1968) and have since had extensive use in remedying behavior deficits, eliminating maladaptive behaviors which are maintained by their rewarding consequences, and strengthening existing patterns of behavior. Operant conditioning has also had widespread and successful use, both alone (O'Leary & O'Leary, 1972) and in combination with other behavior therapy techniques (Daniels, 1973), in effecting changes in the behaviors characteristic of the hyperactive child. The *ABAB* procedure is the design that is used in most operant conditioning studies and in some therapeutic settings (in others, only the first two steps, *AB*, are used). In the four-step procedure the occurrence of the problem behavior in naturalistic settings is measured in the *baseline period, A*; then in the *reinforcement period, B*, the behavior is eliminated with the systematic use of reinforcement procedures; in the *nonreinforcement period, A*, there is a return to baseline conditions, that is, the reinforcement procedures are omitted and the behavior is reinstated; and finally in the *return to reinforcement period, B*, the behavior is eliminated again with reinforcement procedures.

The following example (Allen, Henke, Harris, Baer, & Reynolds, 1967) shows how the *ABAB* procedure was used to increase the attention span of a hyperactive preschool boy. The boy moved constantly from one activity to another exhibiting a level of activity far in excess of that expected in a 4-1/2 year old child; the average duration of time spent at any one activity was less than 1 minute. Concomitant with the frequent changes in activity were short periods of attending. The goal was to increase the attending behavior.

In the *first stage* the child was observed for 21 successive 50-minute periods of free play (usually two a day) to determine the actual frequency of activity changes, the contexts in which they occurred, and the reactions of the teachers and other adults present. With these observations a baseline was established of the level of activity changes prior to any intervention. The goal of the *second stage* was to increase the duration of time spent on any activity. The procedure used involved making social reinforcement, in the form of teacher attention, contingent on continuous attention of one minute to an activity. Teacher attention included talking to the child, using his name, touching him, and giving him materials relevant to the ongoing activity; withdrawal of attention consisted of turning away from the child, neither looking at nor speaking to him, and clearly attending to some other child. In this reinforcement stage teacher attention was given immediately when the child spent 1 minute at an activity and was continued for as long as the child remained at the activity. As soon as the child left the activity teacher attention was terminated until he again remained at an activity for 1 minute. This procedure was continued for seven 50-minute periods, at which time attending behaviors had markedly increased. The *third stage* was a reversal stage designed to determine if the crucial factor in modifying the attending behavior was indeed adult social reinforcement in the form of teacher attention. In this stage teacher attention was delivered on the same random noncontingent basis as it had been during the baseline period. This reversal of contingencies was conducted for a sufficiently long period (four 50-minute periods) to provide a clear assessment of the effects of the changed conditions. In the *fourth stage* the reinforcement procedures used in the second stage were reinstated, but with one change: the criterion for teacher attention was raised to 2 minutes of continuous attending. Duration of attending behaviors again increased. Thus, by varying the social consequences, the child's attending behavior was successively extended, shortened, and then further extended. The supporting observational data shown in Figure 5 were collected under objective conditions.

In reinstating the *A* stage to demonstrate that the maladaptive behavior has been controlled by environmental contingencies, the *ABAB* design

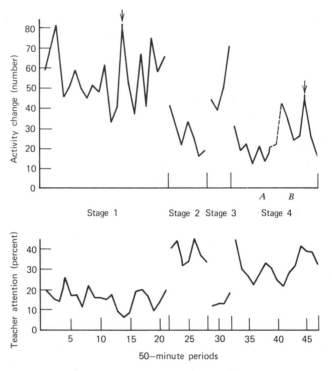

**Figure 5.** Activity changes of subject over the four stages. (From Allen, K. E., Henke, L. B., Harris, F. R., Baer, D. M. & Reynolds, N. J. Control of hyperactivity by social reinforcement of attending behavior. *Journal of Educational Psychology*, 1967, **58**, 231–237. Copyright 1967 by the American Psychological Association. Reprinted by permission.)

frequently is criticized for giving priority to scientific goals at the expense of therapeutic goals. Critics question the effect on the child of returning his behavior to its original undesirable form and also question the effectiveness of the method if the behavior returns so readily to its undesirable baseline frequency. In rebuttal, it is unlikely that the child is harmed by this experience. After several days of experiencing the reinforcement that is being used, he is reminded of how much less enjoyable his experiences are when he exhibits the undesirable responses or misbehavior. In this respect the treatment contrast could even be beneficial. In operant studies using the *ABAB* design the rate of responding with the maladaptive behavior during the second *A* period rarely returns to the level of the first *A* period. In fact, when the *ABAB* design is extended through additional series of reversals (e.g., *ABABABAB*) the desirable behaviors occurring in the *B* periods show less and less decrement as the contingencies are reversed, because these behaviors are increasingly strengthened by the reinforcement that occurs in the natural environment. In addition, the *ABAB* design constitutes a dramatic demonstration to the parent, teacher, or peer that his behavior is influencing the subject's behavior. This kind of feedback is in itself a reinforcer of change in the key environmental figures (Bandura, 1969; Bijou & Baer, 1966).

Several single-subject studies have proven the efficacy of operant conditioning for the modification of hyperactive behavior in young children (Anderson, 1964; James, 1963; Patterson, 1964; Patterson, Jones, Whittier, & Wright, 1965). In the studies by Patterson and his colleagues (1964, 1965) a *differential reinforcement of other behavior* (DRO) method was used in which candy was delivered to the child contingent on the absence of such nonattending behaviors as arm and leg movement, fiddling, and shuffling of feet. This study was criticized by Doubros and Daniels (1966) because the reinforcement contingency was announced to the hyperactive child and his classmates, thus contaminating the independent variable with social reinforcement and conditioning awareness. These awareness factors were carefully controlled in a subsequent study by Doubros and Daniels (1966) in which the DRO procedure was used in a playroom setting to modify the overactivity of six mentally retarded boys whose ages ranged from 8 to 13 years. The DRO treatment method focused on the absence of overactivity and provided reinforcement, in the form of tokens that could later be exchanged for candy, contingent on the *nonoccurrence* of overactive behavior and the occurrence of any constructive activity during the absence of overactive behavior. It was predicted that the level of undesirable verbal and motor activity would be reduced and constructive play activity increased as a function of the conditioning process. In order to construct a checklist of overactive behavior, the subjects were observed in the playroom prior to the study. Their responses fell into four general classes of behavior: stationary body movements, locomotive behavior, destructive behavior, and inappropriate types of communication, such as shouting. The study itself consisted of fifty-six 10-minute sessions divided into 5 groups: pre-conditioning (baseline) for 8 days, conditioning for 30 days, phase-out for 4 days to maintain resistance to extinction at a higher level, extinction for 8 days, and a follow-up of 6 days, during which time post-conditioning observations were made. It can be seen from Figure 6 that DRO is an effective method for reducing hyperactive behavior and increasing constructive play in young children. The frequency of hyperactive responses during the extinction and follow-up periods was less than one-third of that during the baseline period and this effect occurred in both verbal and motor overactivity. In addition, there was a substantial reduc-

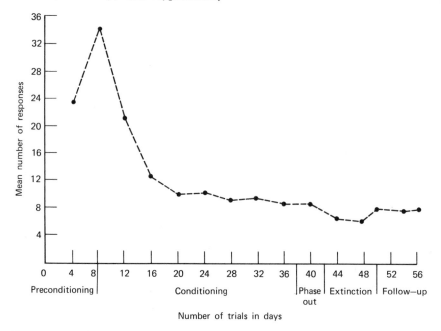

**Figure 6.** The effective control of motor and verbal overactivity as a function of conditioning. (Reprinted with permission from Doubros, S. G., & Daniels, G. J. An experimental approach to the reduction of overactive behavior, 1966, Pergamon Press.)

tion, particularly in the latter part of the conditioning period, in the random, purposeless play that Doubros and Daniels (1966) fittingly called "grasshopper" play.

The use of operant conditioning in single-subject studies or studies with a small number of subjects has two important advantages: the reinforcement procedure used can be designed precisely for the problems and environment of individual children and typically there is close and detailed surveillance, which results in the identification of side effects that might pass unnoticed in a larger group. One such side effect has been described by Miklich (1973) in a report on the use of operant conditioning procedures in modifying asthma panic in a hospitalized 6-year-old hyperactive asthmatic boy. Operant conditioning procedures were successfully combined with modified systematic desensitization (Wolpe, 1958) to treat the asthma panic reaction. In the first few months after the relaxation training there was also a marked reduction in the hyperactivity. The factor responsible was not clearly identifiable but Miklich has speculated that the improvement was a generalization from the relaxation training. The occurrence of side effects, both positive and negative, has been reported by other investigators (see, for example, Sajwaj, Twardosz, & Burke, 1972) and the single-subject study provides an excellent context for the investigation of such phenomena.

Of relevance here is a phenomenon described by Patterson, McNeal, Hawkins, and Phelps (1967) that they have labeled as a *chain reaction* or *avalanche effect*. These terms refer to the consistent finding in their research that the successful use of behavior modification procedures in changing a specific response is often followed by changes in a wide spectrum of behavior not only in the child but also in the behavior of others in his environment. The following is an example of the chain reaction in the family of a hyperactive boy treated by these investigators (Patterson, McNeal, Hawkins, & Phelps, 1967, p. 193):

. . . the contribution of the behavior modifier was simply that of providing a "time out" procedure for a very anxious angry mother to use in controlling the behavior of a hyperactive boy. When the behavior of the child was out of control she placed him in the bathroom, and thus effectively removed him from reinforcement for such behavior. In his case, his younger brother offered a plentiful supply of social reinforcers for his obstreperous behavior. The technique was immediately effective in this respect. This was followed by a reduction in the output of the mother's shrill, scolding, punitive behavior directed toward all her children . . . this, in turn, probably produced a somewhat more pleasant household so that the father was inclined to spend more time there . . . [and] he could now be more positively reinforcing to her. From her reports, she eventually felt less deprivation of social support and experienced a marked reduction in anxiety. We observed an increase in her use of positive social reinforcers to control the [children's] behavior . . . For the first time in months she felt safe in leaving the house to go shopping; . . . terminated her use of tranquilizing medication and enrolled in a ladies' club. Obviously many variables could have contributed to these changes . . . [and] teaching the mother to use a "time out" procedure could not directly produce all of these dramatic changes. The procedure merely *initiated the first step in a chain reaction*. The (unpredictable) end result of this program was the dramatic remission of symptoms of both mother and child.

The foregoing account suggests that although changes must be made in the sources of reinforcement controlled by the therapist, the process of change itself generates environmental reinforcers that serve to maintain and extend the positive behavioral changes that have occurred as a result of direct intervention.

### Selection of Reinforcer

Several conditions are essential for the successful use of operant conditioning, the first being the selection of an effective reinforcer. A reinforcer can be anything that increases or decreases output of behavior, but the reinforcement procedure or incentive system used must be capable of maintaining the child's responsiveness over a relatively long period of time (Bandura, 1969). This requirement is complicated by the possibility that a reinforcer may lose its effectiveness over time. Selection of a reinforcer for a specific individual or group should be determined in a systematic fashion. Some investigators have had their subjects choose their own reinforcers. Staats, Minke, Finley, Wolf, and Brooks (1964) had subjects with reading problems preselect toys which were then used as reinforcers; in advance of treatment, Barrett (1962) asked her patient with multiple tics what music he liked; Hutchinson and Azrin (1961) ascertained that their subjects were heavy smokers before using cigarettes as reinforcers; and Cautela and Kastenbaum (1967) developed a checklist of reinforcers for subjects to fill out before starting to work.

Although the assumption underlying these procedures is that the *subject* knows what he will work for, the subject will not necessarily choose the most effective reinforcer because he generally does not analyze his own behavior and its context objectively. It is important that the investigator try to identify the reinforcers that will most effectively maintain the child's behavior. In a clinical situation it is often difficult to identify the optimum reinforcers solely by observation. For example, in one group of primary grade boys described as impulsive, extensive discussion combined with observation revealed that one boy had acquired the habit of answering almost without a second of contemplation because being first was enormously important to him. The desire to be first pervaded his school activities whether it was being first to answer, complete a written assignment, or line up for the school bus and cafeteria meals; whereas a second boy answered quickly because he was rewarded with positive teacher attention in the form of comments such as "Here's a boy whose hand always goes up the minute I ask a question" or "X always tries hard." Although both boys had chosen toys as reinforcers for an experimental program whose goal was the modification of impulsivity, the most effective reinforcer for the first boy would likely have been being first in specific classroom activities, and for the second boy, teacher attention. The need for an adequate incentive was demonstrated by Levin and Simmons (1962) in a study of hyperaggressive disruptive boys. When the boys were praised for appropriate behavior, not only did they terminate that behavior, they immediately behaved in a highly disruptive way, tossing the task materials out the windows, climbing on filing cabinets, and exhibiting other undesirable behaviors. As soon as food was introduced as a reinforcer, the boys worked steadily at their assignments and maintained this good behavior pattern even though the food reinforcement was progressively reduced and eventually discontinued.

*Immediacy of reinforcement*

The second condition of critical importance for the effective use of operant conditioning is that the reinforcement be made contingent on the occurrence of the desired behavior and occur immediately following the emission of the response (Bandura, 1969). The need for immediacy is particularly relevant for hyperactive children because their verbal capacity is often limited and, consequently, they cannot effectively mediate a delay or inconsistency in reinforcement.

*Eliciting the desired behavior*

The third condition concerns the need to find a reliable way of eliciting the desired behavior, because the behavior, if it seldom occurs, is unlikely to be strengthened through association with a new reinforcer (Bandura, 1969). In most cases the hyperactive child is a socialized child who already has the desirable responses in his behavioral repertoire. He does not have the *major* behavioral deficits that characterize some other groups of children with learning difficulties. However he may exhibit a response so infrequently that it is sometimes necessary to use environmental stimulation to elicit it so that it can be strengthened by reinforcement. Bensberg (1965) increased the attending behavior of severely retarded children, who were totally unresponsive to verbal prompts, by flashing lights on a wall while simultaneously instructing the child to look and immediately rewarding him for directing his attention to the light spot. In this way the children's attending responses were brought under verbal control and the light flashes were then withdrawn. Another method of ensuring that the responses to be rewarded will be emitted with sufficient frequency to facilitate acquisition is to break down tasks into subskills simple enough to elicit rewardable behavior at each successive step (Ross & Ross, 1972).

*Maintaining the behavior*

The fourth condition concerns the problem of maintaining the behavior after the reinforcement procedures are terminated, a problem of great concern to teachers, parents, and others closely connected with the child. To maintain the behavior after ending the reinforcement, the reinforcement system must be altered *during* the course of treatment. To accomplish the transition from reinforcement to no reinforcement the following procedures should be incorporated (Bandura, 1969). *The frequency and magnitude of reinforcement should be reduced.* As soon as response patterns are established with continuous reinforcement the schedule should change to intermittent reinforcement (a schedule that is extremely resistant to extinction) and the amount of work required for reinforcement to occur should be increased (e.g., score cards with more squares should be introduced). *The locus of reinforcement should change.* As adult reinforcement is reduced the child should be enjoying increased reward from peers. The point here is that when treatment is successful the behavior will be maintained by rewards from the child's own social environment and from the self-reinforcement that follows from the internalization of standards which permits the child to evaluate his own behavior. For example, one child on finishing a page of seatwork looked critically at it, shook her finger and said, "This simply won't do," proceeded to correct the paper, and then handed it in with great satisfaction. She had internalized the teacher's standards for correct work and also, through imitation, had acquired the teacher's verbal habits. *The form of reinforcement should change.* To start with, a combination of tangible rewards and social approval are likely to be most effective. As the behavior is established, tangible rewards gradually can be dropped as social rewards increase. Intrinsic satisfaction will also become reinforcing. One child who had learned to read with the help of tangible rewards in the form of small prizes gained such immense satisfaction from her new accomplishment that she brushed aside the tangible rewards, which could be kept, and chose instead to borrow additional books. Research by Parry and Douglas (1975) suggests that it is important to proceed cautiously in making any change in the pattern of reinforcement. In this study the hyperactive elementary school children who served as subjects showed a number of unique reactions to reward: their performance was disrupted under partial and noncontingent reward conditions, and there was evidence that they were overresponsive to rewards and unusually sensitive to the withdrawal of reward. Further research by Douglas and her associates (Douglas, 1975) has confirmed the existence of differences between hyperactive children and normal controls in their response to reinforcement contingencies. These findings, which are discussed in Chapter 6, have led Douglas to advocate special care in the use of behavior modification techniques with hyperactive children.

## Reinforcement Procedures—Differential Reinforcement of Related Operants

This conditioning procedure is a more complex variation of the standard operant conditioning procedure described in the preceding section. Its goal is to eliminate an undesirable behavior and *simultaneously* work toward replacing it with a more desirable related response. Note that the elimination or weakening of an undesirable response does not automatically guarantee the occurrence of the desirable related response; the new response must be elicited and strengthened through reinforcement. The crucial difference between the differential reinforcement of related operants and the standard operant conditioning procedure is that in the former paradigm the therapist is actively working on two related but not necessarily reciprocal target behaviors, one that is to be eliminated and one that is to be strengthened or introduced. In the standard operant conditioning procedure, he is usually working on strengthening *or* weakening one behavior or a set of behaviors, but he is not actively and simultaneously trying to strengthen a related behavior. In operant conditioning change may occur in a related behavior, but it is basically a side effect and, because it has not been directly reinforced, the behavior is not as strongly established as it would be with the differential reinforcement procedure. The two conditioning procedures *appear* to achieve the same result when the elimination of one behavior automatically ensures the emission of another. For example, if all inappropriate out-of-seat behaviors in a classroom situation are eliminated, the desirable behavior of remaining in one's seat will occur automatically; however, the strength of the new response would be greater with differential reinforcement as a function of the direct reinforcement used. But the desired behavior does not always automatically occur as a function of the nonoccurrence of the problem behavior, for example, the elimination of impulsive behavior increases the latency of response but does not guarantee that the child will then reflect on the task in the latency period. Usually, he must be taught a reflective strategy, and it is in this type of situation that the difference between the two procedures and the superiority of differential reinforcement are clearly demonstrated.

The prerequisites to the use of differential reinforcement are similar to those described earlier for operant conditioning. The behavior that is bringing the child into conflict with his social environment must be clearly defined and its frequency determined; the situations in which this behavior occurs must be identified; the social and nonsocial factors in the environment that elicit and maintain this behavior must be noted; and procedures to elicit and strengthen the desired related behavior must be planned. One phase of the therapeutic strategy concerns the elimination of the problem behavior by removing eliciting cues, such as attention from the peer group, and ensuring that the behavior is not reinforced when it does occur. As in operant conditioning, punishment may be used to diminish the frequency of the problem behavior if the therapist makes sure that the attention aspect of the punishment is not rewarding to the child. Time-out from a reinforcing situation, response cost, and loss of privileges are all likely to be more effective than physical punishment. A good example of the effective use of such procedures is contained in a study by Lovaas and Willis (1975) of the modification of a variety of problem behaviors in a 7-year-old hyperactive boy. In a group situation, seeing a model punished for exhibiting the behavior generally results in a decrease in the behavior. The second phase in the differential reinforcement procedure consists of establishing the desired behavior. If this behavior is already a part of the child's behavioral repertoire, then reinforcement procedures are an effective way of strengthening it. However, if the child does not possess or emit the response, modeling procedures should be used to transmit the response. Once the response has been established the child should be given a variety of situational tests to determine the stability of the response and the extent to which it generalizes to new settings. The extrinsic reinforcers must eventually be withdrawn and in the normal course of events the naturalistic social reinforcement that occurs, coupled with the child's own satisfaction, should maintain the behavior. Better results will accrue, however, if the child is also taught self-evaluative skills, and when these are mastered, self-reinforcement procedures (Bandura, 1969).

Differential reinforcement was used successfully (Ross, 1967) to modify the impulsivity of a 6-year-old hyperactive boy and to facilitate his acquisition of reflective tendencies. The child's problem was not attentional, he was able to maintain attention; rather it was that his responses in school, games, and choice situations were consistently hasty, impetuous, and lacking in forethought. His parents were concerned that his impulsivity was becoming increasingly costly for him in terms of failure on academic tasks, missed opportunities, and disappointment. The first phase of the procedure was conducted at home and involved a series of choice situations in which the child was punished through negative consequences whenever he responded without thinking. Because he was so quick to respond, he frequently accepted the first alternative offered, without even waiting to hear the second. His parents were instructed to offer him a reasonably attractive opportunity, for example, "Would you like a Coke or . . ." and, when he accepted without waiting to hear the alternative, to give him what was offered. When he was actively engaged with the chosen alternative, they offered the same choice to one of his siblings, all of whom were highly reflective by comparison. The second alternative was always more attractive and consequently was chosen. When the child saw his sibling enjoying the more attractive choice, he was invariably indignant and disappointed. At this point one of his parents explained that he had accepted without stopping to think and the consequence was disappointing. His parents were also instructed to use modeling procedures to enhance these demonstrations on the folly of impulsivity. At intervals one parent would make a hasty choice and complain about the consequences, chastizing himself all the while for not stopping to think. Occasionally, the child did spontaneously stop and think, and he received strong positive reinforcement for such action. Sometimes his parents urged him to think, helped him weigh the alternatives, and arranged situations so that when he did act reflectively he received both social and situational reinforcement. In addition to choice situations, small-group games were used in which one adult monitored the game so that impulsive moves could be punished and reflective actions rewarded. With this combination of differential reinforcement and modeling the child became more reflective in the home. As he began to show improvement, school-type games were included in the training program. One particularly effective game was *Quiz Program,* in which points were given for the best answer, additional points were awarded for the fastest best answer, and points were lost for incorrect or inadequate answers. This procedure constituted a genuine conflict situation for this impulsive child because his tendency was to raise his hand immediately, but when he did he was usually punished. In this game the only other players were his parents and older brother, and the procedure used was for them to model impulsivity with consequent punishment and reflectivity with positive reinforcement, and to demonstrate to him that he could take the time to stop and think and still win. Because of its similarity to the school situation, *Quiz Program* was used frequently. When the child demonstrated marked improvement as a function of the home training, his therapist enlisted the cooperation of his teacher and the differential reinforcement procedure was extended to the school situation with considerable success. The child was encouraged to recount his school experiences and appropriate positive and negative social reinforcement was provided for evidence of reflectivity and impulsivity, respectively. After the procedure had been incorporated into the school routine, the parents were then instructed to use a series of situational tests of the child's ability to respond reflectively, and to compile a weekly score. Within 6 months of the initiation of the program the child was sufficiently improved so that his teacher described him as a "good thinker." She was so impressed with the effectiveness of the procedure that she also began using it with several other impulsive children, thereby providing peer modeling for all concerned.

Operant conditioning procedures have been enthusiastically endorsed by proponents as the answer to behavior problems and denounced by critics as superficial techniques that are not fully understood, with at best transient and, in some instances, detrimental effects. There is some truth in both of these viewpoints. When correctly used operant conditioning procedures have proven highly successful with a variety of discrete operants. Sometimes the effects of these procedures are dramatic in terms of amount and speed of improvement and, for reasons that are not fully understood, are accompanied by widespread improvement in the child's general behavior. One major criticism is that the procedures do not get to the underlying cause of the behavior, the danger being that an untreated cause will manifest itself in some other misbehavior, that is, that *symptom substitution* will occur. There is no evidence that symptom substitution does occur following the successful modification of an operant, whereas there is some evidence that it does *not* occur (Nolan, Mattis, & Holliday, 1970). What sometimes happens is that the new behavior elicits rewards from the social environment and, as a result, a small cluster of related good behaviors develops. Sometimes already existing but lesser problems assume greater prominence when a major problem behavior is removed. It is unfortunate that the symptom substitution issue does not lend itself to empirical test (Bandura, 1969, p. 49):

. . . the symptom substitution hypothesis could never be satisfactorily tested because it fails to specify precisely what constitutes a "symptom", when the substitution should occur, the social conditions under which it is most likely to arise, and the form that the substitute symptom will take.

In some cases operant conditioning is detrimental. We are not referring here to outright abuse or careless use of the procedures but rather to the kinds of abuses that Ney (1975) has cited, for example, promoting control of the child from without rather than from within, an outcome that occurs when the child concentrates completely on the therapist and makes no decisions himself, or when the child makes value judgments as to "good" and "bad" behaviors solely in terms of response cost to himself. Any professional who is contemplating using operant conditioning himself or training nonprofessionals in its use should read Ney's article (1975) and the discussion by Greenspan (1974) of some of the complex issues in the clinical use of the procedures.

The lack of data on the long-term effects of operant conditioning, as well as on transfer and generalization, makes evaluation of the procedures difficult. O'Leary and Drabman (1971) have specified *procedures* for achieving generalization, but with few exceptions the research to date is limited to short-term studies in single settings. There is no real reason why situational tests of transfer and generalization, and long-term retention measures could not *routinely* be included in operant conditioning studies. At the current point in research on operant conditioning the state of the field would be considerably advanced if studies lacking these data were rejected for publication. Where appropriate, measures should also be obtained of the duration and generalization of changes in parents' behavior, since one major goal of a behavior modification procedure should be the transmission of understanding and retention of behavioral principles by parents and other socialization agents (Patterson, 1971).

Operant conditioning is a *potentially* valuable method for controlling and modifying behavior. Its effectiveness for behaviors other than discrete operants has not yet been proven, nor has it been shown to be superior to other forms of intervention in immediate outcome, duration of effect, or therapist time. Exaggerated claims, misuse, and abuse have resulted from the apparent simplicity of the method (Stein, 1975). A baseline of information has been established on the use of the procedure with *simple* behavior problems. What is needed now are systematic investigations of the efficacy of the procedure for *complex* behavior problems, in addition to the transfer and generalization data discussed above (Patterson, 1971).

## Modeling

There is extensive evidence that the behavior of an observer may be modified as a function of his discriminative observation of a live or symbolic model. Modeling has proven to be a particularly efficient method for teaching children new responses, with research (Bandura, 1969) demonstrating that almost any response that can be transmitted through intentional training procedures can also be acquired on a vicarious basis. Modeling procedures have also proven highly effective in eliminating fears and inhibitions, and in facilitating the expression of response patterns already in the child's behavioral repertoire. Providing an appropriate model may accelerate learning in some instances and be a critical requirement for learning in others. For example, when severe behavioral deficits prevent a child from functioning effectively, the provision of a model is often essential for developing the requisite competencies (Bandura, 1969).

There has been relatively little systematic use of modeling procedures with hyperactive children, possibly due to the established success of the operant conditioning procedures or to the fact that certain of the behavioral attributes characteristic of the hyperactive child (e.g., short attention span, impulsivity, distractibility, and relative lack of verbal ability) appear to make him inadequate as an observational learner. None of these characteristics constitutes a real obstacle to the effective use of modeling procedures. Most hyperactive children are attentive in a one-to-one situation with an adult; modeling therapy can be conducted in a setting in which distractions are controlled; and there is unequivocal evidence from studies of children of average (Meichenbaum, 1974) and below average intelligence (Ross & Ross, 1972; Ross, Ross, & Downing, 1973) that the verbal and imaginal mediational skills needed for observational learning can be taught.

Furthermore, hyperactive children typically are characterized by attributes that are known to make observers attentive to the behavior of models, including high dependency and a lack of self-esteem (Bandura, 1969).

### Modeling with Guided Participation

There are several ways in which modeling procedures can be used to help the hyperactive child; one of these concerns the use of the *modeling with guided participation procedure* (Bandura, 1968; Bandura, Blanchard, & Ritter, 1969; Ritter, 1968) that was developed for use with phobic subjects. In this procedure the model leads the subject up a hierarchy of increasingly difficult tasks with the subject first observing the model engage in the feared activity, next participating minimally in it himself with the model's help, and then proceeding on to more challenging variations involving the feared activity. All of these steps are conducted under optimal conditions of help and reassurance until the subject can perform the response without fear. This procedure has been used successfully with other behavior problems, including extreme social withdrawal (Ross, Ross, & Evans, 1971). The modeling with guided participation procedure is particularly appropriate for one of the hyperactive child's major problems, his inability to inhibit his motor behavior, a deficit in control that typically creates serious interpersonal difficulties. The negative effects of this problem are heightened by the child's lack of awareness of the consequences of this facet of his behavior; he is often genuinely surprised and outraged upon being reprimanded. One hyperactive 7-year-old boy, whose potential for accidents and breakage far exceeded that of any pupil that the school staff had seen in 25 years, told one of the authors, "I opened the door for her like she says boys should and she gave me two bad marks just because she fell down and when Maxie opened it for her she gave *him* a star." His mother reported that in his enthusiasm about helping the teacher he jigged about and inadvertently tripped her. He was genuinely baffled at the teacher's punitive reaction to the behavior sequence that he saw only as socially desirable.

There are no reports in the literature of the experimental use of the modeling with guided participation procedure with hyperactive children. However, the authors developed a two-phase program that combined modeling with guided participation with other modeling and reinforcement procedures. The program was designed for individual training in the inhibition of unnecessary touching behavior and was used successfully with a 6-year-old hyperactive boy who was virtually unable to interact with another child or adult, or look at an object, without taking hold of the person or object. Since the boy was also strong, aggressive, and clumsy, his need to establish tactual contact with other people and objects frequently resulted in negative consequences. In Phase One, extensive training was provided in the home in the inhibition of touching or handling. This training focused in part on teaching the child to discriminate between situations when tactual contact was *mandatory*, such as shaking hands or holding an object for someone; *optional,* such as being offered a helping hand or an object, but being under no obligation to accept; *unnecessary and undesirable,* as, for example, when requested to give a message to another person; and *forbidden*. The training was also designed to give practice in not touching in a wide variety of everyday situations. In the early sessions modeling with guided participation was provided by his parents and an older brother first demonstrating appropriate responses and then providing as much physical contact and direction as necessary to ensure success. Incompatible responses, such as keeping one's hands in one's pockets, physical barriers, stop lines on the floor, and other procedures, were also used to provide boundaries that made it impossible for the child to make tactual contact. These practice sessions also included role-play demonstrations by other members of the family, verbal modeling, discussions, and stories, all designed to teach the child the undesirability of unnecessary tactual contact. As the training progressed, situational tests with immediate feedback were used. Score cards, which when filled could be exchanged for small prizes or privileges, were used to maintain a high level of motivation. When, after 4 weeks of training the child demonstrated some proficiency at inhibiting tactual contact, Phase Two was begun. In this phase the cooperation of the child's teacher was enlisted and some of the training procedures that had been used in the home were used with appropriate changes in the school. In addition, self-evaluative training was begun. The child was asked to keep track of his own behavior, to notice the reaction of others to it, to report incidents to his mother, and also to notice what happened when other children engaged in inappropriate tactual contact. No blame or stigma was involved in this procedure, its sole purpose being to develop increasing awareness of the effects of inappropriate behaviors on others. At the same time, the child began to take lessons in swimming and motor training to develop physical skills to offset his clumsiness. In this second phase the child also learned to play a table game called *No Hands,* which contained a large number of variations that provided additional training in not touching. By the end of Phase Two, which required 7 weeks, the child could successfully inhibit tactual contact to an extent that made him indistinguishable from his first-grade peers.

*Role Play*

Modeling procedures can also be used to help the hyperactive child understand why other people, particularly adults in the school setting, do not react favorably to him. Many hyperactive children feel bitterness about the negative reactions that their hyperactive behavior elicits from others and feel strongly that they are being unjustly treated. *Psychodrama* (Sturm, 1965) is a highly effective method for transmitting understanding, and *behavior rehearsal* (Lazarus, 1966) and *role play* can provide practice in using the new behaviors in naturalistic settings. In one case (Ross & Ross, 1972) the authors enlisted a group of sixth graders and had them put on a series of skits demonstrating various problem behaviors, including three skits that showed the adverse effect of a hyperactive child on a classroom activity, in a small-group game, and at a birthday party. Following the performance an adult discussed the skits with an 8-year-old hyperactive boy whose horrified reaction indicated clearly that he had not previously recognized the impact of his behavior on others. The next step consisted of setting up behavior rehearsal activities with adults, followed by role play with peers, in which the boy practiced more appropriate behaviors for everyday situations. He was then encouraged to report and discuss how he and others had behaved in various naturalistic settings; the goal in this procedure was to develop his ability to evaluate his own and others' behavior and to increase his skill at observational learning. Additional psychodrama and role play procedures were used as necessary. The boy subsequently was judged by his parents and teachers to be markedly improved.

These informal trials of the modeling with guided participation and psychodrama procedures were successful and are consistent with empirical evidence of the efficacy of modeling procedures; unfortunately, there have been no systematic attempts to apply these procedures experimentally to the problems of the hyperactive child. Research is needed to establish the efficacy of such procedures, and to determine the extent to which they generalize to real-life settings.

## Fixed-Role Therapy

Fixed-role therapy is a role enactment form of therapy originally developed by Kelly (1955) for use with adults who want to develop new personality characteristics; but it could also be used effectively with the hyperactive child who is highly motivated to change, and who is able to specify some of the characteristics that he would like to acquire. With this treatment approach the therapist first constructs a description of the kind of person the client would like to be. The client is provided with this personality sketch, given a demonstration of the desired behavior along with opportunities to practice the new pattern in a protected therapeutic situation, and then is encouraged to act for a considerable period of time (e.g., several weeks), as he goes about his everyday life, as if he were that person. In this phase of the program the client is encouraged to feel as if he were trying out the new role rather than permanently adopting it, the purpose of this experimental orientation being to overcome any feelings of strangeness or unease at the magnitude of the changes. To maximize the value of the role prescription in naturalistic situations, treatment sessions are usually scheduled several times a week to provide the client with intensive practice in the new role in the context of situations that occur frequently in his everyday life. The therapist regularly assumes the role himself while the client acts as "the other" person or persons in the situation. This procedure serves the dual purpose of allowing the therapist to demonstrate appropriate and inappropriate ways of relating to others, and showing the client how other people might react. If the role proves effective and the client wishes to adopt it, behavior rehearsals and consultation are continued until the client is both adept at the new role and comfortable with it. A major advantage of fixed-role therapy over operant conditioning concerns the opportunities for feedback and the capacity for flexibility in altering the goals of the patient while the therapeutic program is underway. The client who enters fixed-role therapy with the goal of being $X$ may upon trial of this role decide that some other role would suit him better. This therapeutic approach permits a continuing reevaluation of goals, with a built-in feedback procedure that allows goals to be reassessed and changed after each role trial. By contrast, in operant conditioning the client is often on a relatively unchangeable course: once the problem behavior has been identified and reinforcers to elicit and maintain the desired behavior have been chosen, the client has little opportunity to change his goals, even in the unlikely event that he was the one who initiated the change program, and no opportunity to change them if the program was put into action without his knowledge (Bandura, 1971).

Hyperactive children are usually very aware of being different, and are almost desperately eager to be like their peers. With most of these children the desire to be like others is not diffused and unspecified or vague; usually there are one or two peers whom they would like to emulate, and occasionally they do spontaneously imitate the behavior of a greatly admired peer. The yearnings to be like other children are evident in the following excerpts from the answers given by hyperactive children in an out-patient clinic to the question, What would you like most?

Boy, 8 years, 6 months: What I would like best of all would be to be like Jimmy Markhall. When *he* says the wrong answer the other kids all laugh but not like mean laughs and when *he* drops something or knocks things down our teacher says, "Oh, Jimmy," but not being real cross and I would like that most of all.

Boy, 6 years, 11 months: Anything at all? Like are you maybe going to *do* what I say? Well, I'll tell you. First, I would like it a lot if Mrs. Miller (teacher) would just once in a while, even once in the whole of second grade, say, "Here's a boy who's really moving up fast" to me like she did to Stu and Jackie . . . And I also would like to do some things good like Elliot (older brother) does right from the start. Elliot hit a baseball right off, and he just catches good, and my dad says, "That boy is a natural," and I would like it if I was natural at something.

Boy, 8 years, 4 months: I just wish I could be just an *ordinary boy*, like I mean OK in school but not all A's and have the other kids ask me to play ball, and most of all I wish I could not cry when I get mad. It's really terrible when you can't stop crying and everyone's looking.

Boy, 6 years, 11 months: Well, can this be anything I'd like? OK here goes. I am very tired of everything always being wrong and having to go for tests and my mom and dad look awful worried and soon I might have to go to another school. And what I would like a lot would be if I could just sit still and be the way the other kids are and not have all these things happen. And most of all I wish I did not break that mirror at Teddy Work's birthday party.

For fixed-role therapy to be used effectively with a hyperactive child the complete cooperation of the child's family would be mandatory. The therapeutic team should include a same-sex assistant, such as a college student, with access to the school, home, and neighborhood environments. The functions of this assistant would be to assess the status and skills of the child in relation to his neighborhood and school peer groups, provide training in motor skills and other play behaviors to facilitate effective participation in the peer group, and provide intensive role play practice. Within the context of this change program he would also teach self-evaluative and self-reinforcement skills.

The therapeutic process should begin with the specification and discussion of the changes the hyperactive child would like to make. From the beginning the child should be helped to value his own positive attributes and skills rather than being allowed to think of himself as a uniformly inferior being; and selectivity in his choice of desirable attributes should be fostered by emphasizing that all aspects of the chosen model might not be completely desirable. It should be established with care and tact that some skills and attributes may be difficult or impossible for any one individual to acquire, so that the extent to which the goal of being like another person can be realized is invariably limited by this fact. Changes should be made first in single, clearly-defined behaviors that are potentially amenable to change, and a subskill training approach should be used in which complex skills or games are broken down into more easily grasped small-step divisions. As the child learns to evaluate and reinforce his own performance he is likely to become more perceptive and aware of others' behavior: as a result he should benefit more from opportunities for incidental learning and be more discriminating in his blanket judgments of others' behavior as always superior to his own behavior. As therapy progresses, he should acquire a feeling of competence based on concrete improvement in his own performance. He should also develop a sense of being in control of his own behavior rather than being a victim of it.

## Use of Multiple Procedures

The behavior modification procedures discussed in the preceding sections have been described as separate and discrete approaches to the problems of the hyperactive child. However, the efficacy of any one of these procedures can often be enhanced if it is used in conjunction with one or more of the other procedures. For example, if the goal for the hyperactive child is the acquisition of a new response, initially modeling would be the most appropriate way to transmit the new behavior. Once the behavior is acquired, operant conditioning could be used to strengthen it. There is considerable evidence that the efficacy of change procedures can be heightened with a combination of behavior therapies; and the results of such intervention could then be more strongly entrenched if some self-evaluative and self-reinforcing training procedures were introduced (Bandura, 1969).

## Ethical Considerations

The established effectiveness of these behavior modification techniques has been tempered by the issue of the ethical implications of reinforcement procedures such as operant conditioning. (See Bandura [1969] and Bergin [1971] for thoughtful discussions of the ethics issue.) The use of tangible rewards, particularly in the school setting, is almost guaranteed to elicit strong disapproval from parents on several counts: that such rewards constitute a form of bribery, good behavior should be rewarding in itself, the child who is frequently rewarded will soon be unwilling to perform unless he is rewarded, and the child becomes so reward-oriented that he stops thinking for himself and in the process becomes less creative. In a recent series of cognitive training programs with mentally retarded children (Ross & Ross, 1972) all of the foregoing objections were raised, mostly by parents whose life styles were governed by reward-oriented activities, but who were outraged at the suggestion that they might be reluctant to maintain their somewhat frenetic work routines if there suddenly were no rewards. However, if a reinforcement procedure is to be used with a child, it is important to allay parental anxieties. It should be emphasized to parents that behavior is strongly influenced by its consequences and the use of appropriate incentives has proven to be an effective method for the establishment of new responses, particularly when the new response must replace a well-established maladaptive response. The behavioral effects of reinforcement procedures are a function of their appropriateness in the situation and the skill with which they are used. Evidence from behavior modification studies has shown that with skillful use, reinforcement procedures can be used to effect enduring changes in a variety of social behaviors and can facilitate the acquisition of self-evaluative and self-reinforcement systems. Furthermore, as Bandura (1969) has pointed out, a behavior modification program is not a discrete experience, instead, it represents a continuum of psychological experiences in which the reinforcement regulating behavior gradually changes so that the original reinforcers can be expected to differ markedly from the stimulus events that ultimately serve to reinforce and control the behavior. Reinforcement procedures typically are required for only a relatively short time because, in most cases, once the desired response is established it will be maintained to a considerable extent by the child's own feelings of accomplishment and the social reinforcement he receives. Unequivocal evidence of this phenomenon occurred in an experiment in which tangible rewards were used to facilitate the acquisition of mediational skills in young mentally retarded children (Ross & Ross, 1972; Ross, Ross, & Downing, 1973). Initially, interest was focused almost entirely on the rewards, but as the children became proficient at the mediational task and were able to use their newly acquired skills to win games, the value of the tangible rewards diminished: the children naturally were still pleased with the rewards, but success in the game had become the primary reward.

Much of the controversy over behavior modification procedures in general, but particularly reinforcement procedures, stems from distorted accounts in the media that have associated behavior modification procedures with an undesirable kind of behavioral control and coercion, and from well-documented accounts of the misuse of these procedures by unskilled and, in some cases, unethical individuals. In addition, speculations, such as the following excerpt from an article on ways in which reinforcement procedures can be used to control behavior (McConnell, 1970, p. 74), have elicited anxiety and attached negative associations to behavior modification procedures:

I believe that the day has come when we can combine sensory deprivation with drugs, hypnosis and astute manipulation of reward and punishment to gain almost absolute control over an individual's behavior. It should be possible then to achieve a very rapid and highly effective type of positive brainwashing that would allow us to make dramatic changes in a person's behavior and personality. I foresee the day when we could convert the worst criminal into a decent, respectable citizen in a matter of a few months — or perhaps even less time than that. The danger is, of course, that we could also do the opposite: we could change any decent, respectable citizen into a criminal . . . The techniques of behavioral control make even the hydrogen bomb look like a child's toy, and, of course, they can be used for good or evil.

## Training of Nonprofessionals

Considerable attention has been given in recent years to the idea of training nonprofessionals to implement therapeutic procedures. This idea has gained impetus from the national shortage of therapists, from research that questions whether intensive specialized training and experience increase the incidence of favorable outcomes in therapy, and the growing recognition of the undermining effect on treatment of discontinuity between the locus of treatment and the patient's daily environment. Rioch, Elkes, Flint, Usdansky, Newman, and Silber (1963) found that married women who were given part-time practical training, over a 2-year period, in the application of psychotherapeutic methods performed as well as their professional counterparts. Poser (1966) compared the amount of improvement that occurred in the psychological functioning of psychotic patients over a 5-month period under four conditions: treatment in group psychotherapy by psychiatrists, group psychotherapy by psychiatric social workers, group discussions with undergraduate students, and no special treatment. The undergraduates were applicants who responded to an advertisement for summer employment. They were selected without any additional requisites, had had no training in psychotherapy or experience with it, and were given no suggestions as to how they should conduct their sessions. The psychotic patients who participated in the undergraduate group discussions made greater gains in behavior than any of the other groups. Undergraduates were also used effectively by Matefy, Solanch, and Humphrey (1975) as cotherapists in a home setting, and several studies have attested to the potential of young children in modifying the behavior of their peers (Patterson, 1971) and siblings (Cash & Evans, 1975). Further evidence of the efficacy of the nonprofessional in helping people with problems comes from Bergin's (1963) finding that one reason why disturbed *control* group subjects in psychotherapy experiments often show marked improvement with the passage of time is that many of these disturbed persons seek and obtain help from various nontherapeutic professionals, such as friends, teachers, clergymen, and casual acquaintances. This finding is consistent with Schofield's (1964) conception of the friend as a therapist. The clarity of the behavior modification procedures, coupled with demonstrations that many people with no professional training and of diverse background and experience have little difficulty using them effectively to modify clearly-delineated, single-problem behaviors also has provided support for the idea of training nonprofessionals in their use. This is not to suggest that once trained the nonprofessional should proceed without supervision. In a discussion of the potential value of the nonprofessional, Bandura and Walters (1963, pp. 258–259) state:

> Perhaps greater progress would be made in resolving these problems if more attention were devoted to establishing the principles whereby behavioral changes may be brought about and to utilizing the large pool of competent persons who are already available to apply those of the principles that have been convincingly established. In fact, some of the illustrative cases cited in this chapter indicate that nurses, teachers, and parents can serve as effective therapeutic agents under the guidance of well-informed behavioral scientists. Indeed, the primary tasks of the professionally qualified clinician should be to develop effective therapeutic procedures based on social learning principles, and set up programs which these persons may implement under his guidance and direction. In this way, more people would receive more help than they do under current professional practices.

One basic question in the issue of training nonprofessionals to implement therapeutic procedures concerns the efficacy of parents as therapists for their own children. Guerney (1964) has extended Rogerian approaches to the training of parents in group sessions for treatment of children with behavioral disturbances. His technique, which is called *filial therapy,* consists primarily of teaching mothers how to develop an empathic relationship with their children, the rationale being that once established, this relationship will facilitate improved communication and interpersonal relationships. Guerney (1964) and his colleagues (Guerney & Guerney, 1964; Guerney, Guerney, & Andronico, 1966) believe that once the parent acquires the essentials of the therapist role several factors combine to make him potentially more effective than the professional: he is psychologically more important to the child; a strong parent-child relationship has already been established; he has extended exposure to the child so that many learning trials occur in a day; the behavior to be modified was learned in his presence and can therefore be more effectively unlearned in the same setting; and he can help the child gain accurate expectations concerning interpersonal relations by first helping him to distinguish his own acceptable from unacceptable behavior. Some evidence for the effectiveness of filial therapy is presented in Stover and Guerney (1967). However, Levitt (1971) has suggested that training parents as therapists may not be practical (p. 482):

> Unlike other approaches to training nonprofessional therapists, filial therapy does not seem to save much time for the professional involved, and may, in fact, be

more time-consuming than traditional techniques. Its practicality in a world of professional scarcity, as well as its efficacy, remains to be demonstrated.

Although there is as yet little empirical support for the efficacy of parents as filial therapists, there is extensive positive evidence for their use of behavior modification procedures at very little investment of professional time. Williams (1959) trained parents to discontinue providing social reinforcers for their child's temper tantrums; Bernal, Duryee, Pruett, and Burns (1968) taught a mother how to modify her 8-year-old son's temper tantrums, aggressiveness, and bizarre verbal behavior by reducing her own verbal output, selectively ignoring her son's behaviors, and establishing certain maternal behaviors as conditioned negative reinforcers by associating them with physical punishment; Daniels (1973) used a combination of behavior modification techniques for increasing attending behavior and decreasing hyperactivity in a 6-year-old boy: the parents were instructed in the use of a conditioning procedure for the child and, because they were quite overactive themselves, were instructed to model an acceptable level of activity; and Hall and Broden (1967) also taught parents how to use operant conditioning procedures to modify hyperactive behavior.

The successful use of behavior modification procedures in all of the above examples was achieved with relatively small investments of professional time, a feature that in itself is a strong endorsement for the use of parents as therapists. In addition, there is great continuity between the "treatment" and the child's ongoing daily routine because the intervention occurs in the naturalistic setting of the home, with its many opportunities for practicing the new responses. When intervention has been initiated at school, maximum benefits will result only if there is continuity between the new school demands and the child's behavior at home, and this can best be achieved by actively involving the parents. However, the greatest advantage of training parents in behavior modification techniques concerns the long-term effects on the parent-child relationship. With the use of these techniques the parent comes to see that he is often the one who has been maintaining the child's misbehavior. When he sees how the situation improves as a result of changes in responses *he* makes to the child's misbehavior, the whole situation generally improves markedly. The parent feels a mastery of the situation, and at the same time recognizes his contribution to it. Once the parent grasps the principles guiding the responses he should make, only minimal professional help should be needed. A good example is a study reported by Barnard and Collar (1973) in which a mother appealed in desperation to a school nurse for help with her 8-year-old daughter's temper tantrums, crying, and disobedience. The child was hyperactive, aggressive, markedly uncooperative, easily frustrated, and excessively attention-seeking. Discussion with the mother suggested that the child's disruptive behaviors were being maintained by their attention-getting value: the tantrums usually resulted from some disciplinary measure, and the tantrum then served as a reason for attention from the mother in the form of argument and verbal persuasion. The mother was then instructed in the methods of behavior management and data collection procedures and she proceeded to gather baseline data over a 6-day period on the following behaviors: mother's positive comments to the child, mother's negative comments to the child, child's positive comments to the mother and other members of the family, child's negative comments to the mother and other members of the family, and child's aggression. The baseline data in Figure 7 show a high correlation between the mother's and child's comments in the positive and negative categories. Next, the mother was instructed in a time-out procedure and in management programs to modify the child's negative comments. Time-out procedures consist of the removal of the opportunity to obtain reinforcement contingent upon the emission of undesired behavior. In this case the child was sent to her room, contingent upon emitting negative comments. The graphic results show clearly that there was a marked reduction in negative comments and marked gains in positive verbal interactions. The relatively high frequency of positive mother-child interaction in the latter part of the 6-week period suggests many more periods of agreement than disagreement. The study is notable for the fact that it was monitored by a school nurse and effectively carried out by a mother with no previous experience with reinforcement procedures.

With a capable, highly-motivated parent of the kind in the Barnard and Collar (1973) study, a relatively short period of training, supplemented by discussion and further meetings with the supervising professional, is usually sufficient to ensure an effective outcome for the therapeutic intervention. Similar short periods of parental training have proven sufficient in other behavior modification studies (Daniels, 1973; Patterson, 1971). However, sometimes the qualitative and quantitative changes that must be effected in the parent's behavior require more than discussion and brief demonstration. Seitz and Terdal (1972) report a case in which a mother brought her 4-year-old son to a clinic with the presenting complaints being hyperactivity, temper tantrums, and disobedience. Observations of the mother-child interaction indicated that the mother's behavior evoked and reinforced the child's misbehaviors, a finding which suggested that a treatment program involving only the child would be inappropriate because his behaviors were manifestations of a mother-generated maladaptive interaction. A modeling approach to changing the parent-child interactions was used in which one therapist interacted with the child while the mother and a second therapist observed the interaction from an observation booth, and the mother subsequently interacted with the child while the therapists observed her. The modeling approach was particularly effective here because initially the mother did not have the appropriate responses in her behavior repertoire. For example, at the beginning of the program she did not use praise following compliance. Over a 3-month period the mother exhibited a marked increase in interaction skills with a consequent significant improvement in the misbehaviors that had prompted her to seek help. Straughan (1964) and Goodman (1975) have also successfully used modeling procedures to teach parents how to interact with their children.

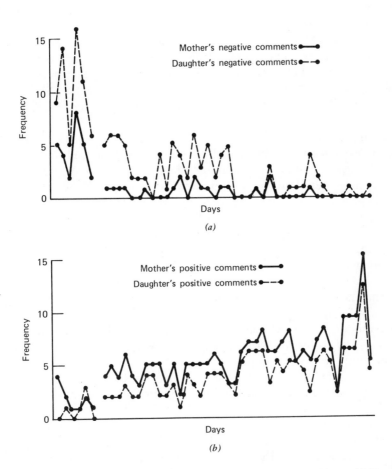

**Figure 7.** (a) Correlation between mother's and child's negative comments, and (b) correlation between mother's and child's positive comments. (Reprinted, by permission, from Barnard, K., & Collar, B. S. Early diagnosis, interpretation, and intervention: A commentary on the nurse's role. *Annals of the New York Academy of Sciences*, 1973, **205**, 373–382.)

Although modeling appropriate adult-child interactions is clearly an effective training procedure, some clinicians have preferred to use intensive laboratory training of parents with children with problems, and to observe parent-child interactions in the laboratory setting. Kaswan, Love, and Rodnick (1968) emphasized training the parent to attend more carefully to his own behavior as well as that of his child. In 15 hours of what these clinicians call "precision training" in the laboratory, they produced marked improvement in family interaction, and data collected in the school setting provided unequivocal evidence of the generalization of improvement in the child's behavior. Further evidence of the efficacy of this approach to parental training is contained in studies by Martin (1967) and his colleagues (Martin, Burkholder, Rosenthal, Tharp, & Thorne, 1968). Other investigators have trained parents successfully in their homes, but in most of these studies the children were of preschool age, therefore only a limited range of problems was covered (Hawkins, Peterson, Schweid, & Bijou, 1966; Patterson, Ray, & Shaw, 1968; Zeilberger, Sampen, & Sloane, 1968).

A unique approach to the training of parents as therapists involves the use of residence units. Wiltz and Gordon (1974) proposed that the ideal parental training situation should combine feedback, modeling, and instructional materials *in the child's natural environment*. To test the efficacy of this proposal these investigators had the entire family of a 9-year-old hyperactive aggressive boy live in a 3-bedroom experimental apartment for 5 consecutive days. During this period the father went to work in the daytime, and the mother was home all day. Both parents were observed and given extensive training in behavioral recording and control. A marked improvement occurred in the child's deviant behaviors. The family then returned home, maintained contact by telephone, and recorded the child's behavior for 30 days. The results showed significant reductions in deviant behaviors ($p < .01$). Although the procedure sounds time-consuming, in fact the *total professional time* spent by the two investigators on all phases of the study was 33-1/2 hours.

Some parents have benefited markedly from the use of an audiovisual feedback taping system in which short segments of parent-child interaction are recorded and playback sessions are used to instruct the parents in the modification of their children's behavior (Furman & Feighner, 1973). The specific advantages of this type of therapeutic approach are that the parents can see themselves as their child sees them, an interaction recorded on videotape can be played back as many times as is necessary for adequate discussion of the sequence, and sequences taped early in the course of therapy can be kept for comparison later in the therapy program to demonstrate improvement to the parents. Using a combination of parental counseling, video-taped parent-child interaction, and therapist observation of the parents in live action, Furman and Feighner (1973) report impressive results, which they attribute to the problem-oriented approach, the efficacy of the whole videotape procedure, the intensive training provided for the parents, their receptive attitude, and the fact that they were highly motivated to effect change in their difficult relationships with their children. The case report presented here was of one of the first children to participate in the program (Furman & Feighner, 1973, p. 794):

Larry, age 13, had been treated with methylphenidate by his family doctor for about one and one-half years when he was referred to this center. His history of hyperkinesis was typical, with the additional factor of a severe educational lag . . . He was gradually catching up in school and his hyperactivity had improved, but the tensions in the family, due to years of poor communication, persisted. Larry was described as stubborn, refusing to talk to his parents, lying, having temper flare-ups, and isolating himself from the family or doing bad things just to get attention. Although the parents were intelligent and reasonable people, their approach to Larry was inconsistent . . . The first session revealed the father was excessively critical and offering no positive reinforcement for good behavior, which he took for granted. The father noted this trait himself and reduced his harshness considerably. A schedule of rules to be strictly enforced was worked out that permitted many of the minor misbehaviors to be ignored. Because of the parents' life-long tendency to respond only to negative behavior, they were asked to keep a written diary of Larry's positive behaviors, thus heightening their awareness. Subsequent interviews showed a gradual reversal of parental response patterns and the placement of emphasis on the child's assets rather than on his faults. A four-month follow-up showed that both the parents and the child were pleased with themselves and each other.

Berkowitz and Graziano (1972) have presented an excellent comprehensive review of the theoretical, empirical, and ethical aspects of training parents as behavior therapists for their own children. The review categorizes studies in terms of the nature and extent of parental involvement and level of methodological sophistication, with research ranging from single case studies to large-scale multi-family training programs. The review would be of considerable value to any professional who is interested in the problem of training parents as therapists.

## THERAPEUTIC APPROACHES CONCEPTUALLY CLOSER TO TRADITIONAL PSYCHOTHERAPY

The previous therapeutic approaches, with their emphasis on reinforcement and modeling principles, fall largely within the realm of behavior therapy. However, approaches that are conceptually closer to traditional psychotherapy also have potential for the treatment of the hyperactive child. Although there has been a regrettable tendency in the literature to downgrade the contribution of such psychotherapies, especially individual psychotherapy of a traditional nature, the sole empirical support for this belief is the methodologically weak study by Eisenberg, Gilbert, Cytryn, and Molling (1961). In fact, the effectiveness of the more traditional psychotherapies with hyperactive children has neither been empirically proven nor disproven. However, one therapeutic approach that has proven effective in the clinical treatment of hyperactive children is brief therapy. The field of brief therapy has grown rapidly in the last decade and the specific technique selected for inclusion here is one of several approaches (Barten, 1971; Boszormenyi-Nagy & Framo, 1965; Ferber, Mendellsohn & Napier, 1972) for the treatment of hyperactivity.

### Brief Therapy

Weakland and his associates (Watzlawick, Weakland, & Fisch, 1974; Weakland, Fisch, Watzlawick, & Bodin, 1974) have developed a brief therapy procedure that focuses on present observable behavioral interaction and uses intervention to change the ongoing system. In this model the client's problem is viewed as a social phenomenon that reflects some dysfunction within the system of interaction and is best treated by effecting some change in that system. Treatment is limited to 10 sessions and a 3-month follow up.

The general view of problems and treatment underlying this approach is based on assumptions that are different from those often held about hyperactivity. The most fundamental assumption is that all one can ever have in attempting to understand and deal with human problems is a *view*, that is, a conception, rather than "the truth." The particular view held by the therapist is of great importance, because of its very real consequences. The view taken largely determines not only what one attends to and how one organizes what is observed in examining a problem, but also how one acts to handle it and what will result. For example, if hyperactivity is conceived to be a physiological problem, physical means of treatment, usually drugs, will naturally be utilized. If hyperactivity is considered a psychological problem in the usual sense, namely something related to a person's mental structure or functioning, some form of exploratory individual psychotherapy naturally follows as treatment. Weakland et al.'s view of the nature of human problems, different from both of these, is interactional. Unless there is clearly evident and relevant organic pathology, they consider the kinds of problems people bring to psychotherapists or often to physicians, including hyperactivity, to be matters of difficult, deviant, or symptomatic behavior. The two elements involved here are: first, the observable behavior, and second, how it is labeled and judged by the patient or others involved with him. All behavior is viewed as being primarily maintained and structured by interaction between people, especially in the family system, but also in other systems, such as the school for children and work situations for adults. Within this view the question "What is wrong with a particular individual?" is largely irrelevant, as is the search for the root cause of the problem, which presumes a linear idea of causality that is not relevant to this approach. Problems are regarded primarily as outcomes of everyday difficulties, usually involving adaptation to an ordinary life change or transition, that have been mishandled by the parties involved. Such mishandling may range from ignoring or denying difficulties on which action should be taken to attempts to actively resolve difficulties that need not or cannot be resolved, with a wide area in between where action is needed but the wrong kind is taken. When such ordinary difficulties are handled badly, things tend to snowball: bad handling increases the difficulty, soon relabeled as a "problem," then is usually followed by more of the same inappropriate handling, leading to exacerbation or spread of the difficulty, so that originally minor or common life difficulties may readily lead on to serious symptomatology.

Accordingly, the central question in this approach is "What behaviors in the ongoing system of interaction are functioning to maintain the behavior seen as constituting the problem?" The resolution of problems is seen as primarily requiring a change of the problem-maintaining behaviors so that the destructive spiralling effect is interrupted. The general treatment procedure stems directly from these basic principles. First the therapist inquires about the main problem or presenting complaint and attempts to get a clear statement of this in terms of specific concrete behavior. Next he inquires about what the patient and others who are involved are doing to try to handle the problem, because these problem-handling efforts are most likely to comprise the behaviors central to maintaining the problem. Then those who are involved are asked to state their *minimum* goal for treatment, that is, what observable behavioral change would signify some success in the treatment. This important question is a difficult one for most patients, but change can be most easily effected if the goal is clearly stated and, while significant, is small. If a small but definite change is made in a major but seemingly hopeless problem, this is likely to initiate a beneficial circular effect and lead on to more progress, whereas pursuing vague or global goals is apt to lead only to uncertainty and frustration. From the outset, an attempt is made through attentive observation and listening to grasp each client's "language," the ideas and values that are central to him, because the therapist must perceive and make use of existing motivations and beliefs if he is to change behavior that the patient already considers is right and logical. When all these inquiries and observations have been made, the therapist plans a treatment strategy based on his own summarization of the problem. He concisely formulates the main presenting problem, identifies the behaviors that are central in maintaining it, decides on a goal of treatment, and estimates what concrete behavior would be the best sign of positive change. In general, the therapist will want to prevent the occurrence of the behaviors seen as crucial to maintaining the problem, and often does this by substituting opposite behaviors for them. This latter step is generally done by reframing or redefining the problem situation in such a way that the original motives and beliefs of the persons involved will now lead to very different behavior. The following case study (Weakland & Fisch, 1975) illustrates the brief therapy procedure with two boys who had been diagnosed as hyperactive and who had both been on medication for several years. The case also serves as an excellent example of the damage that can ensue when labels that parents do not understand are arbitrarily attached to children, and no adequate follow-up procedures are provided to determine how the parents react to the diagnostic information they are given.*

The family was referred by the Juvenile Probation Department. The father and mother were both in their early forties, their sons, Roy and Dennis, were 13 and 11. The father was rather quiet although he followed all of the discussions with lively interest; the mother, a rather nervous, bird-like woman who came armed with copious notes on the boys' behaviors and histories, was much more active during sessions than her husband. The boys were rather well-mannered and listened attentively, at times indicating quiet amusement at their parents' tales of woe and mischief.

The mother immediately went into great detail about the boys' long history of behavioral problems. Dennis and Roy had consistently posed problems for their teachers, were inclined to be obstreperous in class, their attention lagged, and schoolwork was done shoddily or incompletely. By

---

* This case study is printed by permission from Weakland & Fisch, personal communication, 1975.

the time they reached the fourth and fifth grades the school psychologist had defined their behavior as "hyperactivity" and possible "minimal brain dysfunction," and had urged the parents to seek medical evaluation. A physician agreed that they were suffering from "hyperactivity," placed them both on Ritalin, and, in later years, prescribed Thorazine.

The medication made some improvement, but not enough to let matters rest there. Further psychological evaluation showed that both boys were also psychologically handicapped, having "poor impulse control." The parents, highly conscientious, conventional and unimaginative people who were impressed by all these determinations, regarded the boys as seriously disturbed and saw their sons' "lack of impulse control" as placing them constantly on the brink of explosive catastrophe. In addition to cooperating with medical and school regimens, they set about to exert *continuous* surveillance of the children, setting aside their own social and personal needs to implement this task, which resulted in considerable social isolation for them.

The precipitating event for Probation Department intervention occurred in mid-January when Dennis took the family car for a half-hour joy-ride. The parents alerted police who waited at the home for the boy's return. When he appeared unscathed, the policemen simply left. But the incident left the parents panicked, they regarded the taking of the car as "impulsive out-of-control behavior," and a situation that called for immediate and extreme measures. They took Dennis to the Juvenile Hall, demanded his immediate admission, and requested that he remain there.

When the family was referred to us it was mid-April and Dennis was still detained in the Juvenile Hall. The family was seen for 10 sessions, spaced weekly; the parents were present for all interviews, the boys for only the first four. From the start, both parents stressed the severity of the boys' disabilities, minutely detailing the history of their troubles, the need for medications, the failure of all previous measures to "control" them and the utter hopelessness of the situation. In keeping with our treatment view of "speaking the client's language," the therapist earnestly agreed with their pessimism. This had the desired effect of reassuring the parents that, at last, they had found someone who really understood the seriousness of their plight, and they relaxed enough to agree, by the end of the third session, to take Dennis home from Juvenile Hall. The therapist was careful to frame that step, not as any improvement in Dennis, but as a necessity to see how really bad he was when all special controls were removed. He explained that, since our treatment program was a brief one, we had to get to the heart of the matter right away. As a concomitant step, he asked the parents to discontinue both boys' medications for the week since the Thoraz' ̯e would also obscure the "illness." He then turned to the boys and pointedly instructed them that in the ensuing week they were to "be themselves" and not worry about getting into trouble since they had just heard their parents told to expect the worst. As was hoped, the parents reported in the following session that the week went much better than they had expected — enough better to convince them that neither boy required medication. The parents subsequently discontinued the medication.

In the fifth session the parents were seen alone and the therapist took a slightly divergent tack: the father had mentioned a problem with Roy, who was inclined to be aggressively defiant and, during one confrontation, had knocked his father down. The father simply took it and felt that he had handled it rather badly, but was at a loss as to what to do about such situations. He raised all kinds of objections to using force himself, to which the therapist rejoindered by redefining force as "therapeutic," stating, "If I were a son and felt my father couldn't protect himself, even against me, I would be fearful that he therefore couldn't protect me." This seemed to sit rather well with the father and the therapist added that such forceful action was well within the proper domain of an authority. Within the week, the father successfully put to use this new "therapeutic" permission with Roy.

After the sixth session, the therapist assessed the situation. Dennis was now back home, both boys were off medication and the parents were more relaxed. However, it was obvious that their feeling of control within the home was tenuous and the therapist felt that some additional step was needed to solidify their confidence. He probed for some everyday situation that, while in itself no major problem, signified to them their lack of control over the boys. The parents described such a situation. Either boy might be sent on some errand and instead of returning right away would "wander off." That these "wanderings off" were harmless meant little because to the parents it was a clear sign of a "lack of impulse control." Because they viewed it this way, the parents, on sending the boys on an errand, would give them overly detailed instructions regarding the errand, conveying great anxiety about "wandering off." Their very attempts to prevent the "wandering" were actually invitations to do so.

In the seventh session the mother suddenly announced, "This week there isn't anything I wouldn't trust Dennis with. I know he is in perfect control." When asked to explain this puzzling certitude, she said that she relied on her intuition. The therapist regarded her "intuition" as a serious obstacle to treatment that, if allowed to persist, could sabotage gains by bringing about a self-fulfilling prophecy. He suggested that such power to intuit could be converted into a sort of "sending set" to *project* thoughts, not only pick up another's thoughts. She was intrigued and expressed some interest in seeing what she could do about it. The therapist suggested that she attempt such an exercise when sending either of the boys on an errand, but it was emphasized that she would need to give the boys the most *minimal* instructions, otherwise, should they carry out the task successfully, she would have no way of knowing whether it was her fully detailed instructions or the new-found use of her "intuition." In the following session, the eighth, the mother reported two successful trials. In one instance, she had received a call from the school that Dennis was hanging around the bike racks and had failed to heed the bell signalling a new class. She then concentrated her thinking on him saying in her mind that he was to go right back into class, and a few minutes later received a call from school that Dennis had just returned to class. (This also illustrated the elaborate surveillance system the parents had set up, getting the school to call her at the slightest transgressions of the boys.) The other opportunity consisted of sending Roy on an errand and this trial went equally well. She acknowledged that this could be coincidence and the therapist agreed.*

Termination of treatment was anticipated in the ninth session when they indicated quite clearly a higher level of confidence in their ability to control the children and expressed satisfaction with the boys both at home and at school. Treatment was terminated in the tenth session and in a follow-up evaluation three months later the parents reported that they were having no difficulties. The mother had tried using her "intuition" a couple of times after terminating treatment but had not done so since because they could trust the boys. More significantly, the parents reported they were finally resuming their social lives — going to a movie without the boys, inviting friends into the home and accepting invitations.

In summarizing this case, we might say that the "problem" was not the boys' misbehaviors but the attempted solution, chief of which was to originally define their misbehavior as "hyperactivity," "minimal brain dysfunction," and "lacking impulse control." This "solution" set the course for further medical, school, and parental "solutions" which produced an escalating and elaborate structure of anxious mishandling. There-

---

* Procedures such as the therapist's use of the mother's belief in her intuitive powers have been criticized as "manipulative" and "deceitful." It is our opinion that the main criterion for the use of a therapeutic technique in medicine or psychiatry should be the immediate and/or long-term well-being of the patient. With this criterion it is also the therapist's responsibility to treat aftereffects of such a treatment procedure. In the case cited here it is unlikely that directing the mother to stop belaboring her sons with instructions would have been as effective as the approach chosen. The procedure described here was successful in terminating this tendency, the mother did not continue to rely on her intuition, and the therapist checked on this point at the 3-month follow up. It is interesting that critics of this general approach seldom question the clinical and experimental use of procedures such as placebos.

fore, we saw treatment as requiring the cessation of these "solutions." The parents were indicating the enormity of the burden required to maintain the view that the boys' difficulties were those of "hyperactivity," "minimal brain dysfunction," or "lack of impulse control." But they were overwhelmed and confused as to how to back off from that limb. It necessitated using their own "language" — concepts that were logical to them — but in a way that could allow them to redirect their efforts and bring about the putting to rest of a nonexistent "disease" and treat the boys as normal, albeit obstreperous, children.

## Transactional Analysis

Transactional Analysis is a system of individual and social psychiatry developed by Berne (1961, 1964, 1972) and recommended by Wolf (1974) for use with hyperactive children. Wolf believes that if teachers and parents understood this theory they would see that many of their interactions with the child serve to maintain and exacerbate his hyperactivity, and this understanding would, in turn, enable them to structure their time with the hyperactive child in a way that would facilitate his optimum psychological growth. Although it is our opinion that far more could be accomplished for hyperactive children with other methods, such as the brief therapy of Weakland, Fisch, Watzlawick, and Bodin (1974), Transactional Analysis is described briefly here because it is receiving increasing attention in the literature as a therapeutic approach for behavior problems in childhood.

Transactional Analysis is a system for examining the interaction between people and determining why the participants behave as they do. The basic unit is the *transaction,* in which two people interact, and a basic premise is that an individual has three potential ways of expressing himself in an interaction: as *Parent, Adult,* or *Child.* The Parent dimension reflects the viewpoints of psychologically important authority figures; the Adult dimension is often compared to a computer because its function is to evaluate facts, make decisions, and control the Parent and Child; and the Child dimension is fun-loving, involved with enjoyment and the present, and having neither worries about the past nor concern for the future.

Early parent-child interactions are of considerable importance in determining the immediate and long-term outcomes for the individual. Positive interaction patterns are called *strokes;* in the preschool years they generally result in a happy, confident child, whereas negative interactions of the kind a hyperactive child might experience produce a child with a potential for failure. On the basis of these interactions and input from other psychologically important individuals in the young child's environment, a *script* is written; the child and the adult he becomes live out the script in a way that verifies their early impressions of themselves. In one method of verification the individual plays games whose purpose is to have a bad feeling *(racket)* and thus verify his early feelings of inferiority. Wolf (1974) has noted that adults who were hyperactive as children exhibit behavior patterns that suggest their childhood experiences left a permanent residue of distress and malfunctioning. Ernst (1971) has stated that most learning disabilities are based on games resulting from the child's early conclusion that he is an inferior being. (According to Ernst, *Uproar* is a game that is frequently played by hyperactive children.)

In his interactions with socialization agents the child receives two kinds of messages: *counter injunctions* from important adults are usually verbal and instruct him on how to be a success in life, and *injunctions* provide verbal and nonverbal interference with normal psychological growth and development. Since the hyperactive child usually receives many injunctions, all indicating that he is in many respects an inferior being, he soon acquires a view of his worth in comparison to that of other people that is described in Transactional Analysis as the I'M NOT OK — YOU'RE OK position. When the NOT OK position is strongly established, the hyperactive child is caught in a downward spiral of events, reactions from others, and feelings about himself that exacerbate his problems. The goal of Transactional Analysis is to help the child shift from the I'M NOT OK — YOU'RE OK position, which summarizes all of his negative feelings about himself, to the I'M OK — YOU'RE OK position.

No empirical evidence exists of the efficacy of the Transactional Analysis procedure (Wolf, 1974). However, its application to understanding the problems of normal, mentally retarded, adoptive children, and children with problems has been discussed in several texts (Harris, 1969; James, 1973; Schiff, 1971) that document in detail the dynamics of the various problems and difficulties of the children, but unfortunately fail to include clear and precise descriptions of the specific course of action that interested adults could follow. It is difficult to see what advantage accrues to parents from advice such as (Harris, 1969, p. 189):

The parents of a youngster who is having difficulty in school . . . must always keep in mind the primary influence of the NOT OK. The rule is: When in doubt, stroke.

Also, we have serious doubts about the feasibility, value, and effects of presenting the Parent-Adult-Child concept to children with problems and expecting them to be able to "easily respond to the imageries of plugging in the Adult and turning off the frightened Child or the accusing Parent as one would a TV set." (Harris, 1969, p. 203.) The discussions in these texts of relevance to children with problem behavior offer very little that is new, and in most cases what has been discussed has been covered in greater depth by others in this field (see, for example, Bergin & Garfield, 1971).

Most of the therapeutic techniques described in this chapter have in common an explicitness of underlying rationale and a specificity of procedure that makes them readily comprehensible to the layman. One result of reducing the complexity of traditional psychotherapy to more specific operations has been the elimination of much of the mystique that has surrounded psychotherapy. This effect has been heightened by several factors: the view that behavior problems are social phenomena that are causally related to identifiable environmental events, the fact that nonprofessionals can be trained, often with a minimum of professional time, to use some of these therapeutic modes of intervention, and the explicit do-it-yourself descriptions of operant conditioning procedures that appear so regularly in the mass media and invariably predict optimistic outcomes. In considering the scope of treatment required and prognostic outcome, it is important to distinguish between clearly-delineated single-problem behaviors of a social nature in which a child possesses the requisite behaviors in his repertoire, problems that occur because of deficiencies in socialization training and therefore present more difficulty in modification, and complex multiple-problem behavior that includes primary, secondary, and sometimes even subsets of tertiary problems. It is our opinion that by the time most hyperactive children reach the referral stage, the problem of hyperactivity has been so complicated and exacerbated by a variety of social and nonsocial factors that it comprises a complex, multiple-problem behavior that must be approached within the framework of the entire social organization of the child and cannot be easily modified, for example, by a simple operant conditioning procedure. Certainly, such procedures should be a part of the therapeutic approach to the child's hyperactivity, and instruction in their use would have both the immediate value of reducing behavioral irritants that make day-to-day functioning with the hyperactive child difficult, and also the long-term value of improving parent-child interaction. However, the successful modification of the hyperactivity or of some of the related behaviors can rarely be viewed as a "cure." It is essential to remember that hyperactivity is a *symptom* and that the underlying cause must be effectively treated (and that cause may be parental mishandling of behavior, or school-related causes, or other causes internal or external to the child). Discussions of the management of the hyperactive child typically advocate multimodality treatment, the three major modes being pharmacological, psychotherapeutic, and environmental manipulation. It is our opinion that the prognosis is best when the psychotherapeutic intervention program itself includes *multiple* forms of treatment that involve both parent and child in varying degrees.

# CHAPTER 6

# *Educational Intervention*

Although hyperactive children have always presented problems in the classroom that were impossible for school personnel to ignore, the development of special school programs for these children has lagged far behind those for children with intellectual deficits and sensory handicaps. Prior to World War II special school programs for hyperactive children were virtually nonexistent in the public school system in this country. The hyperactive child who was judged too disruptive to remain in school was subjected to a variety of measures, none of which was likely to improve his classroom behavior. Some schools isolated him; others punished him severely, suspended him with the provision that he could return to school when he could demonstrate that he was capable of appropriate behavior in the classroom, or simply expelled him. Expulsion was rarely questioned or criticized, partly as a result of the explicit provisions concerning misconduct in most school by-laws, but primarily because in the period prior to World War II a large segment of the population viewed education as a privilege rather than a right. It was therefore considered completely justifiable to exclude from the classroom a child whose disruptive behavior prevented others from benefiting from the educational process. Often the only alternatives available to the parent determined to provide an education for his hyperactive child were to arrange home tutoring or to enroll him in a private school.

The paucity of special public school programs for the hyperactive child prior to World War II can be attributed primarily to the fact that at that time hyperactivity was viewed as a *medical* rather than as an *educational* problem, a viewpoint that has had a profound and lasting effect on many facets of the management of the hyperactive child. There were also other reasons for the lack of special programs: the field of special education was in the early stages of development; federal and state funds available for school facilities for children with special school needs were limited; hyperactive children were a heterogeneous group without the clearly defined and serious symptoms characteristic of groups such as the sensory handicapped; and the symptoms characteristic of the hyperactive child syndrome were viewed by many educators as variants of normal behavior that did not merit any form of intervention other than discipline.

185

The tendency to view hyperactivity as a medical problem was particularly apparent in the clinical descriptions of the syndrome published in the first quarter of this century. Still (1902) described the behavioral symptoms of a group of hyperactive children, stated that he knew of no medical reason for their behavior, but nevertheless recommended medical treatment. He made no suggestions concerning educational practices or socialization procedures that the teachers and parents might use, despite his belief that one of the causes of the behavior was "deficient training" in the home, and was unconcerned about the probability of lengthy absenteeism from school. The same strong medical orientation to the problem of hyperactivity was apparent in the clinical descriptions of children who were stricken with acute epidemic encephalitis during the 1918 outbreak (Ebaugh, 1923; Hohman, 1922; Grossman, 1921; Leahly & Sands, 1921). With the exception of Ebaugh (1923), these reports all treated the catastrophic changes in behavior that occurred in the children as an exclusively medical problem. Although the main emphasis in Ebaugh's treatment approach was on medical procedures, he expressed great concern about the failure of clinicians to show any active interest in the remediation of the disruptive behaviors of the children, and advocated a multifaceted interdisciplinary treatment plan that included psychotherapy, occupational therapy, and a period of observation in a psychiatric ward to provide the patient with a change of environment. The fact that his treatment procedures proved ineffective is of relatively little importance. What is important is that Ebaugh recognized that hyperactivity was a complex problem requiring long-term interdisciplinary intervention. His attempt to develop a comprehensive treatment approach was all the more impressive in view of the unequivocal medical basis for the behavior problems of postencephalitic children.

Although at this time there were almost no special public school programs for the hyperactive child, there were many private day and residential schools specifically for children whose hyperactivity and other behavior problems made it impossible for them to remain in the public schools. Many of these schools were administered by medical personnel, in keeping with the well-established view of hyperactivity as a medical problem. One of the best programs was that of the Franklin School of the Pennsylvania Hospital, a residential school program that has been described in detail by Bond and Appel (1931). The program evolved over a 10-year period during which the directors of the school, many of whom were in medicine or nursing, experimented with different hospital and boarding school regimens. They finally decided upon a "constructive, restrictive boarding school routine" (Bond & Smith, 1935) in which the emphasis was on individualized teaching, short periods of instruction alternated with periods of intensive motor activity, and extensive social training. The behavioral demands were firm and reasonable, the staff was noted for its tolerance and understanding of the children's behavior problems, and comprehensive medical care and individual psychotherapy were available to every child. The program was remarkable for its use of contemporary behavior control methods such as time-out, fading, schedules of reinforcement, modeling, and peer reinforcement. Despite the many good features of the program, the long-term results were disappointing, with less than one-quarter of the children showing lasting improvement. The failure to maintain the gains achieved in the school program was due in part to the deplorable home conditions of some of the children, but also to a lack of continuity between the school's practices and those used in the home. The school apparently failed to recognize that when a child has been in a special school environment, particularly a residential school, it is essential to instruct his parents in procedures to be used at home. In the account of the Franklin School (Bond & Smith, 1935), it is not clear if the school personnel regarded the parents as incompetent to carry out the school practices in the home, or if they simply did not know how to transmit their procedures to the parents. In a discussion of the school program, Bond stated that he had "no suggestions as to how a child who was unbearable because of constant restlessness could be managed at home" (Bond & Smith, 1935, p. 33).

The failure of the Franklin School program to demonstrate long-term improvement was interpreted by public school administrators as proof that special school programs were of little real benefit to the hyperactive child. The administrators, who were faced with parental pressures for special classes on the one hand, and the financial burdens of the Depression on the other, were thus provided with justification for making no special school arrangements for the hyperactive child. In effect, the Franklin School findings (Bond & Appel, 1931) served to maintain the management of the hyperactive child as a medical problem.

The period following World War II was notable for the rapid burgeoning of special educational programs and facilities at all levels of the educational hierarchy. Universities offered advanced degrees in the administration of special educational programs, established institutes for research in special school program development, and expanded their training programs for teachers of the handicapped. The number of textbooks in special education tripled and new journals were established. Public school systems allocated more funds for classrooms and other special educational resources, and community programs were developed to complement the special educational facilities in the schools. As educational intervention for the child with special needs became the rule rather than the exception, the attention of special education administrators shifted from children with severe abnormalities, such as blindness, deafness, and mental retardation, to those with less serious problems, particularly hyperactive children. Some states made no special school arrangements for the hyperactive child; however, others offered a variety of procedures ranging from special full-time classes in which 10 or 12 children worked with a specially trained teacher, to resource rooms where the child spent a part of each day working with a remedial teacher and the remainder of the day in the regular classroom, to itinerant services in which a remedial specialist consulted with the child's regular teacher and did some individual tutorial work with the child. Unfortunately, program development did not match the increase in special education facilities. Often the hyperactive child in a room labeled "special class" was not participating in a program geared to his special needs. Instead, he was being taught with a watered-down version of the regular curriculum, with any gains in his performance or improvement in his behavior being the result of an improved classroom environment rather than of specific course content.

Relatively few intervention programs for the hyperactive child have been developed in the last three decades and only a fraction of these has been subjected to rigorous experimental test. The paucity of research in this area can be attributed in part to the success of two powerful forms of intervention, drug treatment and behavior modification procedures. The dramatic and often immediate improvement effected in the hyperactive child with stimulant drugs frequently results in the child being able to function in the regular classroom and, as far as opponents of special class placement for the hyperactive child are concerned, eliminates the need for the development of special school programs. A second factor contributing to the lack of research and development in special school programs is the success of behavior modification procedures in eliminating the behavior problems of the hyperactive child and facilitating his cognitive growth. Behavior modification procedures constitute an attractive alternative to the special class program because they require a minimum of training, can be used in the regular classroom, and can be applied equally well to the problems of an individual child or an entire class. Furthermore, there is unequivocal empirical evidence of their short-term efficacy at least, and the improvement demonstrated is typically dramatic both in the amount of change and the shortness of the treatment interval.

The views of two powerful subgroups further reduce the likelihood that special programs will be developed. One group consists of educators who advocate the mainstreaming of almost all children with special learning needs, on the grounds that segregation in special classes deprives the child of the day-to-day opportunity for intensive social learning experiences from normal peers and exposes him to the stigma associated with special class placement. The other group is made up of the parents of hyperactive children of normal or above-normal intelligence who are reluctant to accept special class placement, particularly since the hyperactive child often functions effectively enough on stimulant medication to remain in the regular classroom. The willingness of parents of hyperactive children to accept drug intervention reduces the probability of research and development of special school programs for hyperactive children by decreasing the number who require special class placement, and eliminates a potentially strong source of pressure on the schools to develop programs to replace or supplement drug intervention. A report by Schaefer, Palkes, and Stewart (1974) suggests that once a child is on drugs and apparently functioning adequately, his parents tend to be disinterested in other forms of intervention. Another factor that has tended to discourage research and development is the belief that institutions should be changed to fit the individual, rather than the individual having to conform to the demands of the institution. This philosophy of education has its roots in prison reform, individual rights, and other issues basic to the changes currently underway in our society; and it has the support of a number of critics (Glasser, 1968; Holt, 1964) who have steadfastly maintained that altering the sedentary nature of the classroom and modifying the rigidity of present school requirements would eliminate many of the existing behavioral and achievement problems. The idea of changing the school to fit the child has gained the unqualified support of many parents who are convinced that their children's hyperactivity stems from the pressures of conforming to rigid classroom procedures. Some support for this view is contained in accounts of "open classrooms" (Kohl, 1967), although, in fact, these are anecdotal accounts that offer no empirical evidence of the efficacy of changing the classroom to suit the child.

The lack of systematic research on special school programs is also due to the disinterest that educators traditionally have shown in research of any kind. Programs frequently are established on an intuitive basis rather than on firm empirical evidence of their efficacy. Educational journals show this tendency to intuitive acceptance particularly in the field of special education: innovative procedures reported as successful by their proponents usually fail to produce the claimed results when they are subjected to objective assessment. In no other profession concerned with the problems of children is there such a lack of concern for establishing an empirical basis for new management techniques.

Programs for the hyperactive child that have been experimentally studied, or at least subjected to some attempt at objective assessment, can be grouped into the following categories:

1. Minimal stimulation programs in which the emphasis is on the reduction of extraneous social and nonsocial environmental stimulation.

2. Engineered classroom design programs with an emphasis on methodology, teacher manipulation of the classroom environment, the specification of the behavioral objectives necessary for the acquisition of fundamental learning competence, and the planning of school programs on an individual basis.

3. Programs in which educational and psychotherapeutic intervention have been systematically combined to modify the behavior of the parents as well as the child.

4. Behavior modification of deficient and maladaptive behaviors in the classroom.

5. Short-term intensive training programs designed to equip the child with a specific skill or modify a particular response pattern that is detrimental to his functioning in the classroom.

Programs in each of these categories will be described in some detail along with research findings relevant to the procedures and assumptions of the programs.

## MINIMAL STIMULATION PROGRAMS

In the post World War II era one of the first systematic attempts to design a comprehensive classroom program to modify hyperactive behavior in the school setting was developed by Strauss and Lehtinen and described in detail in their book, *Psychopathology and education of the brain-injured child* (1947). They viewed the hyperactive child as *brain-injured* and considered his central problem to be his distractibility, that is, his unusually high responsivity to environmental stimulation. The distractibility in turn resulted in a chain of maladaptive behavior responses that made it impossible for the child to function effectively under ordinary classroom conditions. In a learning situation he was unable to focus on the central part of a task for more than a few seconds, and instead was distracted by stimuli that were peripheral to the task context, but which for him had the same attention-directing value as the central stimuli. Strauss and Lehtinen reasoned that the child's ability to attend to the central stimuli would be improved by sharply reducing the number of stimulus elements in the environment. One major feature of their program was a *stimulus reduction strategy* that required the removal of visual distractors such as pictures and bulletin boards, elimination of patterned parts of the visual field by frosting the lower parts of windows, reduction of auditory stimulation, neutralization of parts of the environment that could not be removed (such as walls and ceilings) by painting them in neutral tones, and reduction of social stimulation by requiring teachers to dress inconspicuously with no attention-directing ornaments and by increasing the space between desks. To further minimize the unusual responsivity to stimulation, the desks of the most distractible children were sometimes placed in corners facing the wall. It is important to note that no stigma was associated with this procedure; both teachers and children viewed it as a constructive, helpful procedure and often the child was the one who decided when he was ready to rejoin the group. In this program the ratio of pupils to teachers was low, in order to increase the amount of individual attention, and lesson activities were designed to provide frequent activity breaks.

Strauss and Lehtinen (1947, pp. 132–133) described the behavioral response of children in these classrooms as "immediate" and provided impressive examples of the changes that occurred and of the responses of the children to the procedures used:

Loud talking, running in the room, attacks on other children diminish and often disappear in a matter of days; the formerly unmanageable child becomes quite tractable. A first grade pupil whom the teacher finally refused to keep in her class ran about the room, sang, laughed out loud, removed shoes and stockings, and completely disrupted any organized group activity. After a week behind the screen in the special class, this behavior disappeared so completely that the screen was no longer necessary; the behavior described has recurred only in moods of exaltation or in situations of relatively unusual excitement. The children often recognize the transformation in themselves and verbalize their reactions to the change in environment. A brain-injured child who was transferred to the special class from a sight-saving classroom because of inability to control loud talking, laughing, and wandering about the room remarked after a brief period of adjustment, "I'm glad I'm not in that other room any more; there were just too many kids in there; I couldn't stand it." (In reality the number of children in the sight-saving classroom at one time was no greater than in the special methods class.) The response to facing the wall or sitting behind the screen is similar. The children recognize the purpose of the separation and become aware of the feeling of well-being it produces. On some days children will spontaneously request permission to sit away from other members of the group or behind the screen. It is not unusual for a child whose desk has been replaced within the group after a period of separation to request a return to the old arrangement, explaining that he "feels better" or he "gets more work done."*

The work of Strauss and Lehtinen has been subject to much legitimate criticism particularly in respect to their failure to use adequate statistical control procedures in the evaluation of their results, and the lack of rigorous control in the procedures used to diagnose a child as brain-injured (see,

* Reprinted by permission, from Strauss, A. A., & Lehtinen, L. E. *Psychopathology and education of the brain-injured child.* New York: Grune & Stratton, 1947.

for example, Sarason, 1949). The methodological shortcomings should not, however, detract from the contribution that Strauss and Lehtinen made to the field of special education. They were important pioneers not for their specific educational approach but for the catalytic action they had upon the entire field of special education. Their conception of the problems of the brain-injured child served as a stimulus for research on psychoeducational problems, and the educational procedures they devised provided guidelines for subsequent remediation techniques. Their concept of the special classroom was of particular value in that the emphasis was on *adapting the classroom to the needs of the children,* a viewpoint now held by many present-day authorities who believe that the school should be changed to fit the child. To Strauss and Lehtinen, a special classroom was much more than just a room with a low pupil:teacher ratio; it was in itself a teaching instrument and they made maximum use of it.

## The Cruickshank Experiment

An experimental test of the Strauss and Lehtinen approach was conducted by Cruickshank and his associates (Cruickshank, Bentzen, Ratzeburg, & Tannhauser, 1961). The classroom program used was a modification of the procedures developed by Strauss and Lehtinen and incorporated five basic principles:

1. Environmental space should be reduced through the use of cubicles: Cruickshank believed that the child's learning activities should take place in the smallest possible space, the area required for a desk and chair, because reduced space is accompanied by a reduction in number of stimuli. To this end he recommended that each child have a 3-sided cubicle approximately 3 feet square, painted the same neutral color as the walls of the room, and with no pictures on its walls. The desk, which was fastened to the floor, faced away from the open side of the cubicle and contained only the basic materials needed to complete the immediate task.

2. Nonessential visual and auditory stimulation should be eliminated by optimal location of the experimental classroom and by reduction of extraneous social and nonsocial stimulation within the classroom.

3. A structured approach should be used in lessons, classroom procedures, and nonsocial classroom events: Emphasis was on heightening predictability throughout the school day, the initial elimination of choice situations, and the almost complete elimination of failure experiences.

4. Attention-directing teaching materials should be combined with minimal background distraction to focus the child's attention on the task.

5. Specialized teaching materials and techniques such as a multisensory teaching approach should be used.

The experiment was conducted in four classrooms in three public elementary schools. Two of the classes were designated as the Experimental classes and used the Cruickshank program, the remaining two classes served as the Control classes. The subjects were 40 children (M = 37, F = 3) selected from 460 children with learning and behavior problems who either had been in special classes or had been referred for special class placement. The 40 children were all educationally retarded and had emotional difficulties reflected in hyperactive aggressive behavior. A specific requirement of the research design was that half of the sample have unequivocal medical and neurological evidence of injury to the central nervous system, and the other half have no gross evidence of central nervous system damage. This requirement was made so that each class of 10 children would have an equal number of brain-injured and nonbrain-injured children. The four groups of 10 children each were matched in terms of chronological and mental age, achievement level, school experience, diagnostic evidence of central nervous system damage, and degree of hyperactivity and perseveration. The mean chronological age was 8 years, 1 month, and the mean IQ was 80.3.

Each classroom had an experienced teacher and a teacher aide. All four teachers and aides were given a 6-week intensive training program that consisted of theory, methods, and supervised practice teaching including the preparation of teaching materials with increased stimulus value. The Control group teachers and aides were free to use any traditional teaching methods and any aspects of the experimental program.

A pre- and posttest design was used with measures obtained with the Stanford-Binet, Form L, Goodenough Intelligence Test, Stanford Achievement Test, Bender-Gestalt, Vineland Scale of Social Maturity, and Syracuse Visual Figure-Background Test. *The major finding was that there was no convincing evidence for the efficacy of the minimal stimulation classroom.* With the exception of the Experimental group's gains on the Bender-Gestalt, the pattern of test gains was highly similar for both the Experimental and Control groups. Both showed significant improvement on the Vineland Scale of Social Maturity, the Stanford Achievement Test, and the Syracuse Visual Figure-Background Test, and neither group improved on the Stanford-Binet and the Goodenough Intelligence Test. One Experimental class showed a significant drop on the latter test. Since the Experimental and Control groups generally did not differ on their posttest gains, the results suggest that some variable other than the minimal stimulation component was operating in the classrooms to contribute to the gains that were made by both groups. The variable may have been a combination of the low student:teacher ratio and the excellence of the teaching personnel. The results do provide support for the efficacy of small classes with enough teachers to provide intensive instruction and individualized help.

Follow-up data were collected 1 year after the experimental test to determine how the children performed when they returned to classes having no special program or room arrangements. The groups showed no improvement in IQ, the differences favoring the Experimental group on the Bender-Gestalt disappeared, and both groups had significantly lower social quotients on the Vineland Scale of Social Maturity. Both groups improved on the Syracuse Visual Figure-Background Test.

Criticisms have been raised concerning the analysis and use of the test data and the failure to provide information generated by the data. When comparisons are made of posttest results for experimental and control groups, the assumption is that the two groups performed at an equal level on the pretest. In Cruickshank's data this assumption is not always met. When one or the other group performed better on the pretest no correction for this difference was made on the posttest analysis. This failure makes it difficult to determine the real meaning of inter-group posttest differences. Considerable emphasis was placed on establishing a balance in each class between children diagnosed as having unequivocal medical evidence of injury to the central nervous system and those having no such diagnosis. However, no comparisons were reported and no information provided on the performance of these subgroups. It would have been of value to determine whether the subgroups were affected differentially by either the experimental classroom or the control classroom environment and procedures. Including the control group teachers in the 6-week intensive teaching program for the experimental group teachers was a questionable practice when the purpose of the experiment was to evaluate the relative effectiveness of the new *method* of teaching. It would have been preferable to provide the control teachers with a list of the teaching *content* in the experimental classes and provide no information on the method to be used in teaching that content. No intercorrelations were computed among the various test measures. Such information would have permitted a comparison between the structure of abilities of the two groups of children and those of normal children, and indicated whether patterns of cognitive abilities were influenced by the two kinds of classroom intervention.


**Research on Cubicles**

Several of the procedures and underlying assumptions of the Cruickshank method have been subjected to experimental evaluation by other researchers. Rost and Charles (1967), in evaluating the use of cubicles, had brain-injured and hyperactive mentally retarded children ($n = 10$) sit together for lessons that required teacher explanation or group participation, but work in cubicles for silent reading and workbook assignments. The children worked in the cubicles for 1-1/2 to 2 hours a day for one semester. A matched control group ($n = 11$) followed the same general program but did not use the cubicles. Pre- and posttesting of academic performance with the Wide Range Achievement Test (WRAT) showed that both groups made substantial progress over the semester, but there were no differences between the two groups in either total WRAT scores or any of the three subtest scores. The authors concluded (Rost & Charles, 1967, p. 125):

. . . isolation in a booth in the classroom is not beneficial . . . there was no evidence to suggest that having a brain-injured or hyperactive child spend his study time in a separate booth has any effect whatever on his achievement.

It should be noted that neither Strauss and Lehtinen (1947) nor Cruickshank, Bentzen, Ratzeburg, and Tannhauser (1961) ever suggested that the use of isolated desk placement or cubicles would, in itself, result in an improvement in achievement. In their work these procedures were only one of a number of social and nonsocial environmental variables whose purpose was to reduce distracting stimulation; the multivariable nature of the Cruickshank study would have made it impossible to isolate the specific effect of the cubicles.

Stephens (1967) has stated that general achievement tests (such as those used by Rost and Charles, 1967) are insensitive to most materials, procedures, and administrative arrangements in the classroom. Several studies have used the less general and more sensitive measure, amount of work accomplished, as the dependent variable. Shores and Haubrich (1969) evaluated cubicles with a single-subject design in which individual daily records of reading rate, arithmetic rate, and measurements of attending behavior were collected while hyperactive elementary school children ($n = 3$) of normal intelligence performed under two conditions. In the control condition the children performed independent work in arithmetic and reading for 2 hours a day for two 8-day periods while seated at their desks. In the experimental condition the only change in the above procedure was having the children work in cubicles that were enclosed on three sides. The results showed that academic rate was not affected by the cubicles, but that attending behavior was increased for each child by 10 percent or more. Jenkins, Gorrafa, and Griffiths (1972) also used amount of work accomplished to assess the efficacy of cubicles. Their subjects were 6- to 11-year-old educable mentally retarded children ($n = 8$) with poor attention spans and other learning problems. They used a single-subject time-series design with counterbalancing to compare the amount of assigned reading accomplished in cubicles (small study rooms adjacent to the classrooms and under surveillance of a one-way mirror) with that accomplished under regular classroom conditions. With median pages completed as the dependent variable, all subjects completed more pages on cubicle days than on corresponding classroom days.

Further evidence for the positive effect of cubicles comes from a study by Scott (1970), which measured hyperactive children's ($n = 4$) level of productivity in completing academic assignments under a variety of classroom conditions. In the two conditions of relevance here the children either sat at their desks and worked under normal classroom conditions, or worked in three-sided booths. Statistical comparisons were not made because of the limited sample size. However, inspection of the data suggests that the use of a booth resulted in a marked increase in productivity over the normal classroom situation, the mean number of arithmetic problems accurately completed being 27.3 for the booth condition and 18.4 for the classroom condition.

Taken together these results suggest that children who are easily distracted or have poor attention spans may attend better or accomplish more work in a cubicle than under normal classroom conditions. The efficacy of cubicles in these studies may not be due solely to the reduction in extraneous auditory and visual stimulation, however. In classrooms that we have observed, a strong novelty effect was associated with the cubicles that did not appear to diminish over time, and this could have enhanced performance. Also, the children genuinely liked going to their cubicles, often referring to them as their "offices."

## Research on Distractibility

The belief of Strauss and Lehtinen and Cruickshank that distractibility was often the most obvious difficulty of the brain-injured child has been questioned by recent research. The major work on distractibility comes from the McGill University laboratory of Douglas and her associates (Douglas, 1972, 1974). In one study they introduced distracting and competing stimuli while hyperactive and normal children were performing a choice reaction time task and a continuous performance test. On the choice reaction time task conflicting color cues were used on one series of trials, and on the continuous performance test noise of 80 decibels intensity was intermittently piped into the room at random intervals. These distracting conditions disrupted the performance of the two groups equally. The same results were obtained in a more recent study (Douglas, personal communication) that included an incidental memory task, a new naming task, and a dichotic listening task. Further investigations using distracting and competing stimuli with the Color Distractor Test (Santostefano & Paley, 1964) and the Stroop Color-Word Interference Test (Stroop, 1935) have also provided evidence negating the assumption that hyperactive children are more distractible than are normal children. Additional support for Douglas' findings comes from a study by Browning (1967). In a discrimination task in which correct responses were rewarded, irrelevant peripheral visual stimulation had a more adverse effect on the learning of normal children than on that of hyperactive children. In a third study, Worland, North-Jones, and Stern (1973) compared hyperactive and normal boys on three performance tasks (coding, tone discrimination, and connecting dots) in nondistracting and highly distracting settings. They concluded that distraction did not have a more detrimental effect on the performance of the hyperactive boys than on the controls. Instead, what *appeared* to be lower performance by the hyperactive boys under distracting conditions was actually a function of their uniformly inferior performance, regardless of degree of distraction.

On the basis of the research conducted in her laboratories Douglas (1974) has specified some learning conditions and training methods that are likely to facilitate effective school task performance in the hyperactive child. These procedures include making provision for self-pacing on learning tasks, breaking down tasks into subtasks and reorienting the child's attention to each subtask by verbal instructions, using attention-directing materials, scheduling rewards carefully to reduce dependency on extrinsic reinforcement, manipulating failure experiences skillfully to develop tolerance for failure, and making graduated use of feedback to help the child acquire self-reinforcement skills.

The stimulus-reduction strategy of Strauss and Lehtinen and Cruickshank was a logical offshoot of their belief that distractibility was often the most obvious difficulty of the brain-injured child. Underlying this strategy was the assumption that the elimination of extraneous visual, auditory, and tactual stimulation would result in an improvement in attention, with a concomitant decrease in activity level. The validity of the stimulus-reduction strategy has been seriously questioned in recent discussions (Douglas, 1972; Dykman, Ackerman, Clements, & Peters, 1971; Satterfield & Dawson, 1971). Research on activity level suggests that the hyperactive child needs as much or more environmental stimulation than does the normal child; and Dykman and his associates (1971) have suggested that reducing stimulation may *increase* restlessness. Cleland (1961) reported a reduction in activity level under conditions of increased stimulation in hyperactive mentally retarded boys in a residential setting. He used bagpipe music and a drum and cymbal record at three different levels of volume and, at the loudest volume, noted a sharp reduction in activity level accompanied by an improvement in attention. In the same setting the redecoration of a playroom in a manner guaranteed to produce maximum visual stimulation resulted in a significant decrease in level of activity and considerable interest in visual stimulation. Cleland commented that levels of auditory and visual stimulation of this magnitude would have had an excitatory effect on the average child.

Scott (1970) reported that the introduction of background music served to decrease the activity level of hyperactive normal boys ($n = 4$) in a classroom setting. At the same time their level of productivity, as measured by the number of arithmetic problems completed in a 10-minute period, increased. Furthermore, comparisons of productivity under regular classroom conditions with increased auditory stimulation in the form of background music, and cubicle conditions with identical increased auditory stimulation revealed that the more stimulating environment of the regular classroom was superior. Similar findings have been reported by Turnure (1970, 1971) with distractible preschool children of normal and above-normal intelligence, and by Cromwell, Baumeister, and Hawkins (1963) and Gardner, Cromwell, and Foshee (1959) with hyperactive mentally retarded children.

## Concept of Optimal Stimulation

Leuba's (1955) theoretical formulations offer one explanation for the finding that decreased environmental stimulation may result in increased restlessness. According to Leuba, each individual requires a particular level of total stimulation for effective physiological and psychological comfort. The organism strives for a state of optimum stimulation and learns to adjust his own level of activity to changes in stimulation in the environment. When exteroceptive stimulation is sharply reduced, as it is in a minimal stimulation situation, the organism can increase the total stimulation to a level acceptable to his own needs by increasing his motor activity, thus providing proprioceptive stimulation. Similarly, when the exteroceptive stimulation is at a level too high for the organism, he can reduce the level of total stimulation by decreasing his motor activity, thus minimizing the amount of proprioceptive stimulation in the total stimulation of the environment. If the level of optimal stimulation for some hyperactive children is higher than that of children of normal activity level, in a stimulus-reduction situation one would expect that the hyperactive child might need to increase his level of activity to his point of optimal stimulation. Similarly, when the level of environmental stimulation is increased, as in the case of Scott's (1970) background music, then a decrease in the activity level of the individual would be expected.

Empirical support for a relationship between level of stimulation and activity is contained in a study by Forehand and Baumeister (1970), which examined the effects of variations in auditory and/or visual stimulation on the activity level of severely retarded adult males in a residential setting. Increased audio-visual stimulation (relative to a baseline measurement under conditions of moderate stimulation) was associated with a decrease in activity level, and reduced audio-visual stimulation was associated with an increase in activity. Furthermore, when the effects of each mode of stimulation were evaluated separately, the same relationships were demonstrated. Additional support comes from research on sensory deprivation (Solomon, 1961), which showed that subjects were unable to tolerate conditions of almost total stimulus reduction and sought to reduce their discomfort by proprioceptive and tactual stimulation. Increased internal stimulation, such as awareness of heartbeat, was also reported, which suggests that under limited opportunities for exteroceptive and proprioceptive stimulation there is an increased tendency to register stimulation that ordinarily passes almost unnoticed.

In both the Strauss and Lehtinen (1947) and Cruickshank, Bentzen, Ratzeburg, and Tannhauser (1961) classrooms, structure was an integral part of the school program. There are numerous clinical recommendations in the literature on hyperactivity that emphasize firm, consistent handling (O'Malley & Eisenberg, 1973; Stewart & Olds, 1973; Wender, 1973) and some accounts (Kauffman & Hallahan, 1973) in which highly structured programs have been credited with effecting positive change in the hyperactive child. Structure in a school program suggests order and predictability, definite but not inflexible classroom routines, consistency of demands and consequences, and a logical step-sequence of academic tasks and behavioral demands. *Structure* should not be confused with *rigidity*. A school program characterized as rigid is one that is fixed and inflexible in its procedures, makes no allowances for fluctuations in behavior, and cannot be modified in the case of unusual events. Accounts of some military academies suggest a pervasive rigidity.

## ENGINEERED CLASSROOMS

Hewett, Taylor, and Artuso (1969) have developed a comprehensive teaching program known as the Engineered Classroom. The emphasis is on giving the child tasks that are well within his capabilities so that he can readily handle them and thus experience some success right from the beginning. Task difficulty is systematically and gradually increased. Each child's program is based on an analysis of his developmental deficits and the identification of behaviors that disrupt or prevent his learning. The ultimate goal is to enable the child to return to the mainstream of education and function effectively at his own grade level.

In each classroom there is a teacher, an aide, and a maximum of 12 children. The children sit at double-sized desks in three rows; there are also cubicles along one wall to provide a postural change and allow the children to work without visual distractions. The lessons are 15 to 20 minutes in length. At the end of each period, check marks are given to each child on his Work Record Card, a behavior modification technique. The child is given checkmarks depending on his progress and behavior in each lesson period, with a maximum of 10 checkmarks per period. Completed cards are exchanged for tangible rewards during the initial phase of the program and for permission to pursue special self-selected activities during later phases. The emphasis throughout is on attaching positive reward value to school and learning. To this end, a child who becomes disruptive, stops working, or becomes inattentive, is not reprimanded. Instead, the teacher provides a more attention-directing assignment, which is selected on the basis of high interest value rather than grade level appropriateness. As long as the child works productively on the new assignment he is not seriously penalized in terms of the number of checkmarks that he could earn for that period. Morning periods are spent on basic academic subjects, with an assignment wheel at the front of the room denoting assignments for each of the three rows. The wheel encourages independent work, without the need for continual directions from the teacher. Afternoon periods are spent with the class divided into two groups, each with the teacher or the aide. The groups rotate at activities at four centers in the room: art, science, communications, and order (order tasks may include sorting objects on the basis of size and color, puzzles, or map coloring and labeling).

Most children remain in the Engineered Classroom for 6 months, although some may stay for as little as 6 weeks or as much as 2 or 3 years. When it becomes apparent that a child will soon be capable of full-time participation in a regular classroom, he begins to spend an hour or two in that classroom on a transition basis to become oriented to the new classroom's routines. The strong points of the program are the carefully controlled learning environment in the form of a step-by-step presentation of tasks for individual children, flexibility of the assignment procedure, immediate reinforcement with the checkmark reward system, and the usual benefits of any special class set-up: low pupil-teacher ratio and individual help. The weak points involve omissions in the program. Most serious is the lack of parental involvement: No systematic use is made of the parents as agents contributing to the desired changes, which suggests that there may be considerable discontinuity between the demands and procedures at school and those at home. A second omission concerns the lack of intensive training in social skills, particularly those interaction skills that facilitate entry into and acceptance by the peer group. Although some social behavior problems are modified by means of the checkmark system, as they occur throughout the day, no formal lessons on social behavior are provided in this system. This is a serious omission because one reason for the hyperactive child's failure in the peer group and alienation from it is his deficit in social skills.

## PARENT-INVOLVEMENT PROGRAMS

The Medical College School Program (MCSP) is a treatment-oriented day-school program for 7- to 12-year-old children of normal intelligence, whose behavior problems are so severe that they are unable to function effectively in regular classrooms. The majority of problems are characteristic of the hyperactive child, including hyperactivity, poor attention span, excessive talkativeness, teasing, and fighting (Zupnick, 1974). This Program represents a unique and effective three-pronged attack on the problems of the hyperactive child and his family. A structured classroom setting based on behavior modification principles is used to promote behavior change in the child. To extend the gains achieved through the school program into the family setting, the parents are required to participate in two kinds of intervention: An *insight-oriented therapy group* is designed to help the parents understand their feelings about the problem, and facilitate change in behaviors and family structure that may be maintaining or exacerbating the child's problems; a course in the *use of behavior modification techniques* teaches the parents how to apply these principles in the home, thus ensuring continuity between the school and home environments. Previous attempts (see, for example, Cantrell, Cantrell, Huddleston, & Wooldridge, 1969) to make systematic and simultaneous use of both home and school in modifying behavior problems have focused almost exclusively on the treatment of the child. The MCSP is unique in using psychotherapeutic techniques to bring about change and understanding in the parents, while concurrently instructing them in techniques of contingency management for the child.

Because the primary difficulty for children admitted to the MCSP is poor behavioral control, the children are grouped according to their behavior patterns and problems, rather than on the basis of academic standing. The classes are divided into three levels: Incoming (Level 1), Intermediate

(Level 2), and Outgoing (Level 3). All children are placed in Level 1 when they enter the program and baselines of their behavioral and academic strengths are determined. As a child progresses he moves to Level 2 and then to Level 3. A point system is used to determine rate of advancement and daily privileges, with points being earned for good behavior and completion of class assignments. The maximum number of points that can be earned per day in either category is 50, with the maximum weekly total being 500 points. Good behavior is defined according to each child's specific problems, for example, a child who is characterized by excessive talkativeness would earn points for being quiet. The children are required to reach a specified point level within a designated time period. If they are so badly behaved that they cannot meet this requirement, they are returned to the public school system to a more appropriate special class or are provided with home tutoring. The point system provides an objective method of feedback information to the parents as well as to the children, and allows the parents to set up a reward system in the home contingent on behavior in school.

In all three levels there are six children in each class. A child is expected to function more independently as he moves from level to level. On reaching Level 3 he is expected to function as he would in a regular classroom with a minimum of individual attention. Because of their presumed shorter attention span, children in Level 1 work on a point reinforcement schedule of 15-minute periods, while Level 2 children receive point feedback every 30 minutes, and Level 3 children every 60 minutes. Point totals are charted at the end of each period to ensure immediate knowledge of results. Social and free-time reinforcement activities are built into each day, with participation in them being determined by points earned. The total points required to participate in a special activity, as well as the desirability of the activity, increase at each level. During the 1 to 2 academic years that children spend in the program, there is an emphasis on academic advancement as well as behavioral improvement. Upon completion of Level 3, a child is returned to a regular classroom appropriate for his academic level. Children who have completed the program show significant advancement in the core subjects and continue to function effectively in the regular classroom.

The procedures described above can best be illustrated with an actual account of one child's program. The case of Robert (Zupnick, 1974, pp. 81–83) demonstrates clearly how well the MCSP program lends itself to carryover in the home. It also shows how continuous contact with the parents, and support from them, results in their being able to independently develop and successfully use reinforcement procedures in the home setting. The case study also underlines the importance of requiring the parents to participate in therapeutic sessions.

Robert S., a 10-year-old white male, was referred to the MCSP because of consistent behavioral disruption in his fourth grade classroom. Examples from the referral report indicate that he was "not able to sit still longer than 10–15 minutes; (is) constantly speaking out of turn, disrupts teachers and students; (is) disrespectful to the students and teachers; (is) constantly putting things in his mouth." Furthermore, "He reads well but functions below grade level because he will not complete an assignment." At home, according to Mrs. S., "Robert is constantly disrupting all games, talks loudly, yells, throws objects, and uses foul, horrible language. He makes odd noises with his mouth and nose, blinks his eyes and torments the dog. He voids on the bathroom floors on purpose and in general is a disruptive influence in the home." He had previously been labeled emotionally disturbed, hyperactive, and minimally brain damaged, and had been on medication since age four. Upon admission to the program, he was taking upwards of 300 mg. of Deaner per day.

Upon entrance into the program, Robert was continually provoking others, engaging in fights, leaving the classroom, and fighting so frequently in the cab, that the driver refused to transport him. He was constantly attempting to manipulate the environment by crying, and asking for his mother. He varied between charming and cursing the adults around him.

In line with the goals of the program, the treatment employed a two-fold approach. At first, Robert was given only minimal work but was provided with strict structure and behavioral guidelines. Classroom disruption resulted in spending "time out" sessions in an isolated carrel in the hallway with a corresponding loss of opportunity to earn points. During this period, there were a number of incidents of flooded toilets and complaints by other children in regard to Robert's teasing and hitting. He had few children with whom he could play or socialize. It soon became apparent, however, that this was Robert's method of "adjusting" to a new situation based upon previous negative experiences. Thus, as he became more acclimated to the setting, structure, and children, he was able to complete longer and more difficult assignments. More importantly, he began to interact in a meaningful fashion with other children. The frequent trips to the bathroom, sniffling, hitting and teasing, all but disappeared. In addition, his medication was gradually decreased so that by the end of the school year it was totally discontinued. Table 3 shows Robert's combined academic and behavioral point totals for his initial two quarters on Level 1. It points out the increase in positive behavior as he progressed through the weeks such that from the sixth week on, he was able to meet the weekly criterion of 350 points.

Table 3.   Robert's Level I Point Totals

| Quarter 1 | WEEKS | | | | | | | |
|---|---|---|---|---|---|---|---|---|
| | 1 | 2 | 3 | 4 | 5 | 6 | 7 | 8 |
| | 250 | 215 | 190 | 327 | 305 | 355* | 395 | 355 |

| Quarter 2 | WEEKS | | | | | | | | |
|---|---|---|---|---|---|---|---|---|---|
| | 9 | 10 | 11 | 12 | 13 | 14 | 15 | 16 | 17 |
| | 360 | 370 | 377 | 411 | 371 | 373 | 382 | 375 | 425 |

Despite Robert's general improvement, he continued to display much difficulty in the area of verbal self-control. He was constantly losing behavioral points for swearing, and quite often the other children would complain about his language—a sure indication that it was well out of hand. Near the end of the final school quarter, a specific program of extinction was designed to reduce this behavior. Every time Robert's teacher or two classmates heard him swear, he was made to stand in a corner of the hall and in a loud voice, repeat the word for a three-minute period. This technique resulted in the rapid reduction and frequency of classroom swearing in a little over a week's time (Table 4).

Table 4.   Robert's Frequency of Classroom Swearing

| Days | 1† | 2 | 3 | 4 | 5 | 6 | 7 | 8 | 9 | 10 |
|---|---|---|---|---|---|---|---|---|---|---|
| Frequency | 11 | 10 | 12 | 8 | 5 | 3 | 1 | 3 | 0 | 0 |

Concurrent with Robert's treatment program within the school, Mr. and Mrs. S. were seen on a continuing basis in an effort to produce changes within the home. Initially, their attitudes regarding Robert, and his effect upon the family structure, were discussed. Since he was one of five siblings, it was pointed out that certainly, he was not the sole cause of *all* the fighting and arguing occurring at home. Furthermore, an effort was made to bring Mr. S. back into the family (as an insurance agent, he frequently was conveniently not available in the evenings). Finally, Mrs. S.'s feelings concerning her reluctance to punish Robert, and her habit of immediately defending him in family squabbles, were discussed. She became aware of

*Criterion reached for the first time. At the time of Robert's entrance into the program, the distribution of time within Level I was one of two quarters.
†Days 1–3 were baseline days.

how these actions fostered Robert's extreme dependency and how they might have arisen in defense against her negative feelings toward him.

Following the initial sessions of insight therapy, specific behavioral plans, designed to extinguish Robert's annoying behaviors at home and school, were discussed and implemented. It had been noted in the classroom that Robert would often work to his minimum — i.e., once his daily points were earned, he would begin to disrupt the other children. To counter this, two simultaneous plans were inaugurated. On the one hand, Mr. and Mrs. S., on their own initiative, hired a local university student as a "Big Brother" for Robert. He visited the home twice weekly and on the weekends. The length of his stay became contingent upon Robert's behavioral points on two successive school days.

Mrs. S. also inaugurated a plan so that when Robert earned his minimum number of daily points he was taken to his favorite local restaurant. What he could order depended upon the number of points earned beyond the minimum. Both plans were inaugurated shortly after Robert began the program, and they began to take effect concurrent with his upward surge of weekly points (Table 3). The visits to the restaurant were quite significant in that the family had stopped taking him to any restaurant because of his "atrocious manner." Furthermore, the frequency of noisemaking, blinking, and excessive urination previously noted at home all began to dissipate during the same time period. Other plans designed to regulate Robert's temper tantrums at home and utilizing a time-out procedure were initiated and met with similar success. These tantrums, which involved screaming, banging walls and swearing, decreased in frequency from an average of four to two times per day.*

## BEHAVIOR MODIFICATION PROCEDURES

Behavior modification procedures have been used successfully in the school setting to change a variety of inappropriate behaviors. Their efficacy is incontrovertible in the case of simple misbehaviors such as talking out and out-of-seat behavior. The topic of behavior modification has already been covered in some detail, so the coverage here will be limited to research on training teachers in the use of the procedures, classroom use with individuals and groups, vicarious reinforcement effects, and types of effective reinforcers for classroom use.

* Reprinted, by permission, from Zupnick, S. A new approach to disturbed children: The Medical College School Program. *Psychiatric Quarterly* (N.Y. State Dept. of Mental Hygiene), 1974, 48, No. 1, 76–85.

## Teacher Training in Behavior Modification

Most teachers assume that maladaptive classroom behavior is indicative of problems in the child or his home environment. In fact, an increasing body of research evidence has shown that much of the disruptive behavior that occurs in the classroom is a function of the teacher's responses. For this reason, it would be of considerable value to the child, school, and community for the teacher to understand behavior modification principles and be capable of using the related procedures. Although there is unequivocal evidence that the systematic variation of teacher behavior can result in the production or elimination of disruptive classroom behavior (Becker, Madsen, Arnold, & Thomas, 1967; Thomas, Becker, & Armstrong, 1968), relatively little attention has been given to the question of the kind of training that might result in competence in this facet of classroom control. To determine what mode of instruction would facilitate both the acquisition *and* application of behavior modification principles by elementary school teachers, McKeown, Adams, and Forehand (1975) compared the effectiveness of four instructional conditions: participation in a laboratory group in which a written manual was provided, participation in a laboratory group but with no manual, provision of a manual to be read with promise of group instruction, and a no-treatment control condition. Teachers in the two laboratory groups were given lectures, participated in discussion groups, and used role-play to increase their skill in the use of behavior modification techniques; those in the group given only the manual were assigned readings in the manual and were asked to begin to apply the principles in the manual in their classrooms. Teachers in the control condition were not given any information. The dependent measures were knowledge of behavior principles assessed by a written test and change in the frequency of classroom disruption measured by trained observers. The results showed that teachers who participated in the laboratory groups demonstrated a significantly greater increase in knowledge, and decrease in disruptive behavior in their classrooms, than those who were given a written manual only or no instruction of any kind. The efficacy of the laboratory training method was attributed to the availability of immediate feedback and reinforcement in the laboratory situation, and to the "shaping" of the teachers' behavior in the training situation through the use of a variety of procedures including the modeling of appropriate teacher behavior to assure exposure to excellent demonstrations on using behavior modification techniques. It would have been interesting to have a fifth group with training identical to the laboratory and written manual condition, but given the option of participating. This condition would approximate the reality of most in-service training, in that a selective factor operates because participation is voluntary.

## Behavior Modification with Individual Class Members

Kauffman and Hallahan (1973) used novel contingencies and directive teaching to control the rough physical behavior exhibited by an unruly, hyperactive, 6-year-old boy. The novel contingencies included a variety of tangible and activity reinforcers that were determined by card selection whenever the boy had played in a socially desirable way; the directive teaching method made use of the Distar program which, because of its use of explicit rules, modeling, and vicarious reinforcement, proved to be an excellent adjunct to the reinforcement procedures. Patterson, Jones, Whittier, and Wright (1965) increased attending behavior in a hyperactive boy by rewarding him with a buzzer sound for every 10-second interval in which he maintained attention to task; the back-up reinforcers were pieces of candy, which he could share with his peers. The modification procedure was used first in an isolated room and then in the classroom. Classroom modification programs have also made use of nonreward and punishment techniques. By ignoring a hyperactive boy until he returned to a discontinued activity, Wahler, Sperling, Thomas, Teeter, and Luper (1970) succeeded in reducing the number of activity shifts that occurred. Although their time-out and differential attention procedures were aimed at a single behavior, a second important behavioral effect that occurred was a reduction in the boy's stuttering. Zimmerman and Zimmerman (1962) ignored a child's temper tantrums and presented highly desirable stimuli contingent upon the cessation of tantrum and related disruptive behaviors. Sachs (1973) used a time-out procedure in which a 10-year-old hyperactive boy was placed in isolation in a room and required to remain there quietly for 5 minutes whenever he engaged in any of a group of specified disruptive behaviors. A prompting and differential reinforcement procedure was used by Twardosz and Sajwaj (1972) to increase sitting behavior in a hyperactive retarded boy in a remedial preschool setting. This procedure not only increased sitting behavior, it also generated positive collateral changes in other social and nonsocial behaviors. The fact that such multiple behavioral effects have been reported in a number of single-subject studies suggests that behavior modification procedures could be used to treat several target behaviors simultaneously.

In a four-phase study of three hyperactive elementary school children Ayllon, Layman, and Kandel (1975) compared the relative efficacy of stimulant medication and token reinforcement, the dependent variables being effect on academic progress and hyperactivity. The first two phases provided baseline data on math and reading performance, and time-sampling observational data on level of activity during math and reading. In Phase 1 the children were on medication for 17 days during which time their math and reading performance averaged 12 percent correct and level of hyperactivity was about 20 percent. A 3-day wash-out period followed in which medication was discontinued. In Phase 2, a 3-day period in which no drugs were administered, hyperactivity rose sharply from the previous drug-controlled level of 20 percent to 80 percent, accompanied by a slight improvement in math and reading. Phase 3 was a 6-day period, again without drugs, but with token reinforcement for math only. During math periods hyperactivity dropped to approximately the same level as Phase 1 and math performance rose to about 65 percent correct. However reading performance and hyperactivity during reading remained unchanged, with performance low and hyperactivity high. In Phase 4, a 6-day period without drugs, token reinforcement was given for both math and reading. Level of hyperactivity was comparable to that under the drug condition of Phase 1, but math and reading jumped from the 12 percent correct level of Phase 1 to 85 percent correct.

This study represents a genuine contribution to the literature on classroom control of hyperactivity, both for its comparison of drugs with a behavioral technique as methods for controlling hyperactivity, and for its focus on *actual academic progress* rather than the component skills of learning, such as attention. However, it is our opinion that a successful 12-day demonstration on 3 children does not merit the conclusions voiced by Ayllon et al. (1975, pp. 144–145):

> The present results suggest that the continued use of Ritalin and possibly other drugs to control hyperactivity may result in compliant but academically incompetent students. Surely, the goal of school is not to make children into docile robots either by behavioral techniques or by medication. Rather, the goal should be one of providing children with the social and academic tools required to become successful in their social interactions and competent in their academic performance. Judging from the reactions and comments of both parents and teacher, this goal was achieved during the reinforcement period of the study. The parents were particularly relieved that their children, who had been dependent on Ritalin for years, could now function normally in school without the drug. Similarly, the teacher was excited over the fact that she could now build the social and academic skills of the children because they were more attentive and responsive to her than when they were under medication . . . This study offers a behavioral and educationally justifiable alternative to the use of medication for hyperactive children. The control of hyperactivity by medication, while effective, may be too costly to the child, in that it may retard his academic and social growth, a human cost that schools and society can ill afford.

What is needed to justify the foregoing conclusions is a *long-term* demonstration, on a larger group of subjects, of the efficacy of this behavioral intervention for academic progress and the suppression of hyperactivity.

The results in the Ayllon et al. study could have been due in part to a novelty effect that would diminish in time, and, in the absence of follow-up data, this possibility is a valid one.

## Behavior Modification with Classroom Groups

Several investigators have applied a common set of modification procedures to an entire class. Pihl (1967) reinforced sitting behavior in hyperactive boys with no demonstrable brain damage who had been unable to benefit from drug therapy. The boys were given primary reinforcers for each 25 seconds of sitting behavior, and after 8 hours of training were able to double their sitting time. It is interesting that Pihl was unable to effect significant gains in the sitting behavior of *brain-injured* hyperactive boys. Madsen, Becker, Thomas, Koser, and Plager (1968) showed that sitting-down behavior increased when primary grade teachers intermittently praised children who were remaining seated and ignored those who were out of their seats. In this study the effect of continual sit-down commands was to increase the overall rate of standing up. The management of out-of-seat behavior was handled by Wolf, Hanley, King, and Giles (1970) with a variable interval contingency procedure in which a kitchen timer was set to ring at various intervals. Those children who were seated when the timer rang received tokens, and those who were out of their seats were fined tokens. After 6 hours of training, out-of-seat behavior decreased from a class average of 8-1/2 minutes per hour to an average of only 1 minute. MacPherson, Candee, and Hohman (1974) used a counterbalanced design to compare three methods for eliminating disruptive lunchroom behavior in an elementary school setting: basic operant conditioning procedures alone, and in combination with either punishment essays or mediation essays. The punishment essays were written assignments unrelated to the misbehavior, whereas the mediation essays were directly related in that the child was required to copy descriptions of the consequences of appropriate and inappropriate lunchroom behavior at the time he was tempted to misbehave. This use of mediated self-control training was based on research by Blackwood (1972). The results indicated that the operant conditioning-mediation essay combination was by far the most effective of the three methods, and almost totally eliminated the target misbehaviors. Operant conditioning combined with punishment essays was more effective than operant conditioning alone. The use of operant conditioning procedures combined with mediational training to help the child gain control of his own behavior is a potentially powerful method of effecting behavior change. Additional empirical investigations should be conducted to determine whether this mediational component increases the duration of effect and whether generalization occurs.

Whereas the procedures in the above studies were self-contained within the school setting, a study by O'Leary, Pelham, Rosenbaum, and Price (1974) provided continuity between the school and home by involving parents in the reinforcement procedures. O'Leary et al. treated hyperactive children in regular classroom settings using a program involving the following components: specification of daily goals for the child, teacher praise for goal-directed efforts, end-of-day evaluations of goal achievement, clear specification of reward contingencies to the child, communication to each parent via a *daily* report card of the child's progress, and rewards given by the parent at home. In the examples given, it is our opinion that food rewards figure too prominently, although we agree with O'Leary et al.'s emphasis on the importance of daily and weekly rewards that are "maximally motivating." The methodology in this study is impressive in that it provides good school-home continuity similar to that in the Medical College School Program (Zupnick, 1974). It is also effective: the results showed a substantial decrease in hyperactivity and other classroom problem behaviors. Unfortunately, no long-term follow-up data are available, and this lack is a characteristic of all of the other studies reported here.

The technique used by O'Leary et al. (1974) of specifying the reward procedures to the child is called *contingency contracting*. It has been used with a variety of school problems and appears to have considerable potential for the modification of hyperactivity. Briefly, the procedure involves analyzing teacher (or parental) reports of problem behaviors in the child, determining what is maintaining the problem behavior, identifying events that could serve as positive reinforcers to strengthen the desired behavior and negative reinforcers to weaken the problem behavior, and then writing a contract for the child specifying the desired behaviors and reinforcers. Receipt of positive reinforcers is contingent on adaptive behaviors that in most instances are incompatible with the problem behavior. To facilitate acquisition of the desired behavior, it is often broken down into sequential steps with reinforcement for each successfully accomplished step. For example, if coming into the classroom and starting work without disturbing others is one goal for a hyperactive child, the steps might be opening the door quietly, going to his seat, putting his books away quietly, getting out the new work, and starting to work on it. When the desired behavior is strongly established, a fading procedure can be used to wean the child away from the contract system. The strengths of the contract system lie in the child's knowledge of the reward contingencies, the immediate feedback, and the opportunities for continuity between home and school. For a detailed discussion of this technique see Cantrell, Cantrell, Huddleston, and Wooldridge (1969).

## Vicarious Reinforcement Effects

The results of an extensive body of research on vicarious reinforcement have established that observers tend to reproduce the behaviors of models who are positively rewarded and to inhibit behaviors that they see punished in others; and that when an observer perceives the model as similar to himself, the probability of such modeling effects increases (Bandura, 1969). Several investigators have demonstrated the effect of vicarious reinforcement on the behavior of peers, the assumption here being that the behavior of the peer observers will change in the same direction as that of the reinforced model. Kounin and Gump (1958) showed that by disciplining target students, adjacent students who were not directly disciplined were clearly affected; the spread of effect was described by these investigators as a "ripple effect." Broden, Bruce, Mitchell, Carter, and Hall (1970) demonstrated that reinforcing a target student's attending behavior increased attention in a peer who was seated nearby. However, the fact that there was a slight concomitant increase in contingent teacher verbal attention and proximity may have contributed to the effect of the specific reinforcement. Kazdin (1973) controlled for the amount of reinforcement and proximity of the reinforcing agent and demonstrated a clear effect of vicarious reinforcement for attention on the attentional responses of adjacent peers. However, his results showed that positive reinforcement of *inattentive* behavior of target students also increased the *attentive* behavior of adjacent peers, which suggests that the effects of vicarious reinforcement in the classroom are more complex than would be expected on the basis of the laboratory modeling findings of Bandura (1969). A good example of the complexity of effect of vicarious reinforcement in naturalistic settings is Sechrest's (1963) finding that explicit and direct positive reinforcement of one child under certain circumstances serves as implicit punishment for a partner.

## Types of Reinforcers Used

Intermediate stimuli, such as tokens, counters, tones, and lights, have been used in classrooms to signal students that positive or negative primary reinforcement has been earned. The efficacy of these procedures has been demonstrated by Ramp, Ulrich, and Dulaney (1971): to reduce disruptive classroom behavior a time-out delayed reinforcement procedure was used in which a red light signaled an infraction. An intriguing finding of relevance to the signal procedure is that signals alone, without reward or punishment exchange value, can reduce disruptive behavior; for example, tokens without exchange value (Drabman, 1973) and a red light with neither reward nor punishment contingent on it (Medland & Stachnik, 1972) both reduced disruptive behavior, although in each case there was a possibility that the signals had acquired reward value. Lobitz (1974) controlled for this effect and demonstrated that a red light, which had no specific consequences attached, substantially reduced talking-out and out-of-seat behaviors in elementary school children, a finding that suggests that specific back-up reinforcers may not be necessary in some circumstances.

A recent series of studies on reinforcement procedures by Douglas and her associates (Douglas, 1975; Firestone, 1974; Parry & Douglas, in press) has important implications for the use of behavior modification procedures with hyperactive children. These investigators have demonstrated that reactions to reinforcement contingencies in hyperactive children differ from those of normal children. For example, when praise was contingent on performance of a reaction-time task, the performance of both hyperactive and normal children improved (Parry & Douglas, in press). However, when noncontingent praise was used, the normal children's performance improved, but that of the hyperactive children deteriorated. Partial positive reinforcement also resulted in deterioration of performance on a variety of tasks for hyperactive children, who became more upset when rewards ceased than did normal controls. On the other hand, mild negative reinforcement seemed to enhance performance by decreasing the hyperactive child's tendency to respond impulsively. On the basis of the foregoing results, Douglas (1975) has suggested that for the hyperactive child praise should be response specific, methods of coping with partial reinforcement should be taught, self-reinforcement procedures should be valuable, withdrawal of reward should be a gradual process, and mild negative reinforcement can be effective if used judiciously. Douglas (1975, p. 206) concludes with a note of caution that users of behavior modification procedures with hyperactive children would do well to note:

. . . the above findings have made us reluctant to place too heavy reliance on some of the more common techniques employed in reinforcement programs. It is clear that we need to know a great deal more about the impact of the various kinds of positive and negative reinforcement on these children before we can design behavior-modification programs tailored to their special needs.

Operant conditioning, modeling, and other behavior modification procedures are not difficult to use; they require careful planning and a realistic approach to the question of how much actual recording is practical in view of the teacher's other responsibilities. These procedures do not require expensive equipment, nor do they require costly reinforcers. There is unequivocal evidence that elementary students can be trained as data recorders (McLaughlin & Malaby, 1972) and that under some circumstances self-recording of behavior offers major benefits (Bolstad & Johnson, 1972). The apparent simplicity of these procedures, however, often results in their being misused. The teacher who is interested in using behavior modification techniques should first familiarize herself with some of the excellent review articles (Patterson, 1971), texts (O'Leary & O'Leary, 1972), and manuals (Buckley & Walker, 1970; Homme, 1971) on the use of these procedures in the classroom, then conduct a series of dry runs to acquire skill in recording baseline and other data and practice in providing reinforcement. The teacher should then find a consultant who is qualified in the use of these techniques in the classroom milieu because, when properly used, these procedures can markedly improve the functioning of the classroom.

Behavior modification procedures should be viewed as procedures to be used to establish the skills and behaviors that are prerequisite to effective learning in the hyperactive child. They should not be seen as a simple solution to the problem of hyperactivity in the classroom, and they are not a substitute for individualized teaching. The teacher must still determine how the hyperactive child can best learn and find a way to teach to his strengths.

## SPECIFIC SKILL PROGRAMS

Short-term intensive training programs have been developed with the goal of equipping the hyperactive child with a specific skill needed for effective functioning in the classroom, or modifying a response pattern that represents a serious detriment to his ability to function effectively. Research in this area has focused on self-instructional training and inhibitory motor training.

### Self-Instructional Training

Keogh (1971) has suggested that the hyperactive child makes many errors on academic and nonacademic tasks even though he may have the information or skills necessary for a correct response; he responds so quickly that his efforts can best be described as guesses or chance stabs at the task. Strauss and Lehtinen (1947) recognized this difficulty and used slowing-down devices. A remedial strategy would involve training the child to delay his response long enough to consider the alternatives.

Palkes, Stewart, and Kahana (1968) hypothesized that training a hyperactive child to use self-directed verbal commands in the performance of a task would result in an improvement in performance. The impetus for this intervention strategy stems from the work of the Russian psychologist, Luria (1961), who contends that the critical step in the child's development of voluntary control over his own behavior is the internalization of self-directed verbal commands, and hyperactive children typically have not acquired this type of self-regulation of behavior. On the basis of extensive work with children, Luria (1961) has distinguished three stages by which the initiation and inhibition of voluntary behavior come under verbal control. In the first stage, the child's behavior is controlled and directed by the speech of others, usually adults; in the second stage, the child begins to use overt speech to regulate his behavior effectively; and in the third stage his covert or inner speech comes to govern his voluntary actions. Palkes and her colleagues (1968) were concerned with the second stage, the use of overt speech in the self-regulation of behavior. The purpose of their study was to determine if two half-hour training sessions in the use of self-directed overt verbal commands, such as "stop," "look," "listen," and "think," would effect an improvement in performance on the Porteus Maze Test. The subjects were 20 hyperactive boys whose mean age was 9 years 3 months, and who were of normal intelligence. Subjects in the Experimental group were given individual training in the use of self-directed verbal commands to govern their performance on tasks such as matching familiar figures, finding simple geometric figures embedded in more complex figures, and joining irregularly spaced dots in the correct order without lifting the pencil from the paper. They learned to verbalize a set of self-directed commands before responding to any task or subpart of a task. Subjects in the Control group were required only to perform the same tasks. The Porteus Maze Test Revision Series was used as a pretraining measure of impulsivity and the Porteus Extension Series was used for the posttraining measure. Posttraining scores for the Experimental group on both the Porteus IQ (Porteus Test Quotient) and the Porteus Qualitative Scores were significantly higher than those of the Control group. The investigators noted that some of the most striking changes occurred in those error categories which reflect the characteristic work habits of the hyperactive child. The self-directed command training group cut fewer corners, crossed over fewer lines, lifted their pencils less often, and threaded the maze with fewer irregular lines than did the Control group. The fact that these behaviors had not been specifically taught suggests that the hyperactive children generally were performing more carefully and behaving less impulsively during the testing. A second study by Palkes, Stewart, and Freedman (1972) provided further evidence of the efficacy of this verbal training procedure.

The training procedure used by Palkes and her colleagues effected an improvement in the use of *overt* self-directed verbal commands. Meichenbaum and Goodman (1971) extended this procedure to encompass the third stage in the development of voluntary control of one's own behavior, the internalization of self-directed verbal commands (Luria, 1961). They developed a treatment program that has been used successfully in teaching children to use *covert* self-instructions followed by self-reinforcement, on a variety of tasks ranging from simple sensorimotor activities, such as finger mazes, to more complex problem solving tasks. The training in self-instruction developed by Meichenbaum and Goodman was conducted in a one-to-one situation and followed the same three-stage developmental sequence that Luria (1961) described. In the first stage of training the overt verbalizations of an adult were used to control and direct the child's behavior: The child observed an adult perform a task such as the finger-maze task and, as the adult worked, he engaged in explicit self-directive verbalizations. The child then performed the same task with the adult providing step-by-step directions. Note that this procedure is similar to the modeling with guided participation procedure of Bandura (1969). In the second stage, the child was instructed to use overtly the same adult verbalizations to guide his performance of the task. In the third and final stage of training, he was instructed to use covertly the verbalizations that the adult had modeled and that he himself had used effectively overtly. Thus within the context of the training situation, the child's covert speech became an effective regulator of his task behavior. The verbalizations initially used by the adult varied with the nature of the task but, in general, included questions that encouraged planning, self-encouragement and self-guidance, strategies for coping with difficulty and failure, and self-reinforcement. The following is an example of the adult's verbalizations on a sensorimotor task, copying line patterns (Meichenbaum & Goodman, 1971, p. 117.):

Okay, what is it I have to do? You want me to copy the picture with the different lines. I have to go slow and be careful. Okay, draw the line down, down, good; then to the right, that's it; now down some more and to the left. Good, I'm doing fine so far. Remember go slow. Now back up again. No, I was supposed to go down. That's okay. Just erase the line carefully . . . Good. Even if I make an error I can go on slowly and carefully. Okay, I have to go down now. Finished. I did it.

Of relevance here is a procedure used by Patterson and Mischel (1975) in which normal preschool children were provided with strategies for resisting distraction in a self-control situation. In two well-designed studies these investigators demonstrated that young children can be helped to achieve better control of their own behavior if they are provided with verbal strategies designed to help them sustain attention to the task at hand. This procedure could be used to equip the hyperactive child to resist distraction in naturalistic settings such as the classroom. However, we would strongly recommend that great care be taken in selecting the materials to be used in such training, to avoid the strong fear reaction that some of the preschool children later exhibited to stimuli similar to those that had been used in the study.

### Inhibitory Motor Training

The possibility that motor inhibition can be directly taught to hyperactive children is consistent with existing empirical data from children with average activity levels. For example, Feldstone (1969) demonstrated that primary, elementary, and junior high school children who were rewarded for low-amplitude responding, such as turning a hand crank slowly and squeezing a dynamometer weakly, were better able to inhibit their responses on these tasks than were yoked control children. Inhibitory motor training has great potential for the management of hyperactivity, but to date there has been little research interest in it.

Flynn and Hopson (1972) have proposed that hyperactivity can be reduced by providing the child with an inhibitory motor training program. Their basic assumption is that hyperactivity is an imbalance of the excitatory and inhibitory processes. With this imbalance the child reacts indiscriminately and receives negative feedback; his behavior becomes increasingly random, disorganized, and hyperactive. If the inhibitory processes can be trained to work more effectively, the imbalance will be corrected with a consequent reduction in the episodes of hyperactive behavior exhibited by the child. Flynn and Hopson have developed a program of sequential motor exercises to train and develop the inhibitory functions of the hyperactive child. The exercises use inhibition at the levels of the innate response system, such as the tonic neck response, general motor system, such as bilateral abilities, and special motor system, such as eye-hand coordination. The exercises go from simple to more complex tasks. The training is designed to follow the natural development of the child and to be used in classroom settings with groups of children. The suggested time period is about 15 minutes a day. The training is presented within the context of activities having appeal for young children, for example, animal actions, parades, role play, and competitions such as races. Many of the activities used are well-established physical education activities.

Although the idea of training for motor inhibition has considerable potential, Flynn and Hopson's training program has several serious weaknesses. The demands on the teacher are unrealistic. Flynn and Hopson state that inhibitory motor training activities can be used with an entire class but they also say that children differ in the area and level of lowered inhibition. They urge the teacher to be specific in her observations so that she may train children in the specific area level needed. It is difficult to see how a teacher could handle all this effectively. The teacher is also expected to interpret the program to any child who needs the training. It is our opinion that the training should accomplish its goals without a lot of explanation. Perhaps most important, the inhibitory motor training program has not been subjected to controlled study, the reason given being the difficulties of finding similar groups and teachers, and the multiplicity of the training. These are inadequate reasons for failing to progress to the evaluation phase, having completed the development phase. Pre- and posttests could be quite simple and sequences of clearly described exercises for specific inhibition profiles could be developed.

A multisensory approach to inhibitory motor training developed by the authors (Ross & Ross, 1971) was based on the premise that the hyperactive child needs to increase the *range* of his rate of response as well as to improve voluntary control of his motor behavior. The rationale underlying this approach is as follows. The hyperactive child typically is described in terms such as "tornado" or "speed artist," the implication being that his rate of movement is significantly faster than that of the normal child of the same sex and age. In fact, this is not the case. Timed observations of hyperactive and normal elementary school boys in classroom settings, in competition, and under various incentive conditions revealed that when rapid response was required, the hyperactive boys were slower than the normal boys. However, when rapid response was inappropriate, as under classroom conditions, the hyperactive boys responded more quickly. In terms of motor behavior the hyperactive boys could best be described as being slower and having a more limited range of speed than their normal counterparts (Ross & Ross, 1971). Schematically, this relationship is shown in Figure 8.

These observations are consistent with the results of the Stevens, Stover, and Backus (1970) study described earlier, in which it was demonstrated that hyperactive elementary school boys had basically one response tempo, moderately fast, and functioned at this rate irrespective of the presence or absence of incentive conditions, with the result that under no-incentive conditions they performed faster on a tapping task than did the control subjects, but under high-incentive conditions they were unable to significantly improve their performance and tapped more slowly than the controls. It will be recalled from the previous discussion that Stevens,

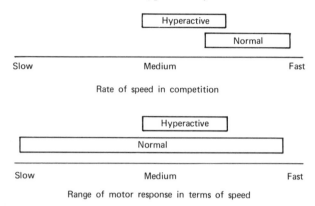

**Figure 8.** Rate and range of motor response of hyperactive versus normal boys.

Stover, and Backus attributed the inability of the hyperactive children to adjust effectively to the change in incentive conditions to a defect in the brain structures regulating arousal and concentration. The fact that hyperactive children can effectively use overt speech to regulate their behavior (Palkes, Stewart, & Kahana, 1968) suggests that the tendency to one response tempo is not irreversible.

The following training program was designed for a 5-year-old hyperactive boy. Its purpose was to increase his range and rate of speed of response and bring his motor activity under voluntary control. In Phase One, a multisensory approach was used with systematic exposure to a variety of experiences within each response area. Training was provided in the recognition of speed of response including *visual* experiences in which the child first observed attractive objects such as cars, bicycles, mechanical toys, balloons, balls, and arrows moving at different speeds, and then later identified, compared, and predicted speeds of objects; *auditory* experiences with music and common sounds such as passing footsteps and spoken words; *tactual* experiences in which the child felt moving objects in the absence of visual and auditory cues; and *proprioceptive* experiences, again with visual and auditory cues minimized, in which he was required to categorize movement experiences as fast, medium, or slow; for example, he rode blindfolded in vehicles moving at different speeds and identified by kinesthetic cues the "fastest and slowest rides." As soon as the child was proficient at these tasks, Phase Two was begun consisting of a series of games and movement activities where winning required specific levels of speed. Games offer several important advantages as a training medium for the hyperactive child. They provide him with an opportunity to acquire proficiency in social game skills; can be modified so that they are within his ability, thus he does not experience continual failure; can be used to teach him the meaning of winning and losing; can acquire reward value in themselves through association with prizes; can allow immediate feedback; can encourage planning; and can be adjusted to his attention span and used to extend it. Competitions were used in which the child tried to beat his own record, the clock, or the adult. This one-to-one procedure allowed the child to acquire the skills prerequisite to successful functioning in group games before he participated in them. The child first observed others competing in the activities, then participated in the same activities, first with graduated amounts of help and later, independently. Most of the activities were exciting and all of them were fun. Motivation was heightened and feelings of success enhanced through the use of score cards and prizes. The efficacy of the games was increased by suspense, colorful props including balloons and parachutes, and appealing game names such as *Stuntman, Creepy-crawler, Speed Limit*, and *Sneakup*. In this second phase attention was directed to gross as well as fine motor training. One of the activities that allowed varying degrees of guided participation in gross and fine movement was a game called *Three-Armed Bandit*, in which the child's dominant hand was tied to the adult's hand and the goal was to pick up as many objects as possible in the tied pair of hands, while at the same time obeying stop, go, and go-slow traffic signals. It is important to note that in the training procedures speed and voluntary control of movement were an intrinsic part of the activity. There was never any suggestion that the program was designed to overcome the motor deficits of the child. If the child commented on his inability to moderate his rate of speed or control his movements, the adult discussed individual differences with him. There was never any censure or any drill. After a total of 22 hours of individual training in Phase One and 14 hours of individual and small-group training in Phase Two, the child could successfully inhibit motor responses on command and was indistinguishable from his peers in this respect.

**Biofeedback Training**

Biofeedback is a relatively new behavior modification technique. It involves the use of electronic equipment to monitor physiological processes to which the individual normally does not pay much attention and then increases his awareness of these processes through the use of auditory or visual external stimulation such as a tone or light. The presentation of external information about internal processes such as heart rate, blood pressure, and muscle tension allows the individual to gain voluntary control over certain internal functions.

Two pilot studies have been conducted recently on the use of electromyographic feedback as a technique for the control of hyperactivity in children.

Simpson and Nelson (1974) have reported a pilot study in which respiration recordings were used to help hyperactive children ($n = 3$) gain control of their motor behavior. The method combined biofeedback and operant conditioning procedures to teach breathing control. During the training period the child's attention was expected to improve because he had to attend closely to his respiration recordings. An advantage of this procedure is that the child is required to focus on only one behavior, breathing, and the feedback system provides immediate knowledge of results. The rationale for this approach to the control of hyperactivity was as follows: Respiration is a higher-order behavior, so that once voluntary control of it is gained there should be an indirect effect on a group of lower-order behaviors. By learning to control his breathing the hyperactive child should be able to acquire self-control that encompasses disruptive motor behaviors. Braud, Lupin, and Braud (1975) used electromyographic biofeedback to teach a 6-year-old hyperactive boy to reduce his muscular activity and tension. In 11 sessions the child learned to turn off a tone that indicated the presence of muscular tension. With this procedure hyperactivity and muscular tension decreased both within and across sessions, and a seven-month follow-up showed retention of ability to control hyperactivity. The child showed improvement of hyperactivity in other settings, gains in achievement and other test scores, and increased self-confidence. This team of investigators is currently comparing the relative efficacy of biofeedback and relaxation procedures in the control of hyperactivity.


## THE OPTIMAL SCHOOL PROGRAM ISSUE

The question of providing an optimal school program for the hyperactive child has become a subject of considerable controversy. Central to this controversy are two basic issues: one concerns the widespread belief that inadequacies of the structure, demands, and content of the school program cause children to become hyperactive; and the other, a natural off-shoot of the first, concerns the problem of defining an optimal program for the hyperactive child. There is no evidence that inadequacies of the school program *cause* hyperactivity, although they may exacerbate existing tendencies. Critics of the schools frequently attribute hyperactivity to a diverse group of inadequacies in the schools, such as overcrowding. In a recent discussion of hyperactivity Feingold (1975, p. 798) stated:

In establishing data for the incidence of H-LD (Hyperactivity-Learning Disabilities) in schools, consideration must be given to the so-called "crowding syndrome" of experimental animal psychology. In these studies rats confined to a limited space were found to develop increased activity and aggression . . . Teachers have observed similar responses among children in a crowded classroom. With one or at the most two hyperkinetic and aggressive children in a classroom, not only do the normal children develop a higher level of activity and expression of aggression but even the teacher becomes hyperactive.

The effects that Feingold described are more likely to be modeling effects (Bandura, 1969) than overcrowding effects. In fact, there is no evidence with children in crowded classrooms (Price, 1971), or with adults in either short-term experimental crowding situations (Epstein & Karlin, 1975) or long-term naturalistic settings (Paulus, Cox, McCain, & Chandler, 1975), to support physical or social crowding as etiological factors in overactivity or in hyperactivity. In the Price study preschool and first-grade children were compared under crowded and uncrowded classroom conditions. The major findings were that crowding increased solitary, noninteractive behavior, decreased social interaction, and had no effect on level of aggression. It is our opinion that *in the majority of cases* a child does not become hyperactive as a result of the school program. Hyperactive tendencies are present in the preschool years or earlier (Nichamin, 1972; Stewart & Olds, 1973), and may pass unnoticed in unstructured play situations or be attributed to the natural exuberance of childhood. Entry into the new environment of school is a period of some stress for even the most able child; for the child with hyperactive tendencies the stressful aspects of the new environment are markedly heightened, with the result that the child's hyperactive tendencies stand out in sharp relief. The fact is that even an unstructured program makes demands on the hyperactive child that far exceed those of the preschool years, and the child is seldom able to cope with them. It is his distressed reaction to what is often his first major failure experience that is new, upsetting, and highly disconcerting for his parents, and it is this reaction that leads adults to identify the school as the cause of the problem. In the case of boys the distress reaction may be heightened by several factors. Boys in the preschool and early school years are less advanced than girls in verbal abilities, are less willing to conform to the demands of the school situation, and have less capacity for school tasks. Since the educational system rarely makes any allowance for these early sex differences, boys in general, and particularly those with hyperactive tendencies, tend to be at a serious disadvantage in this situation from the beginning. The consequent loss of self-confidence and self-esteem, with the concomitant lessening of motivation in the face of continued inadequacy, creates a downward spiral effect. The advantage that girls have is heightened by the fact that many of the demands of school and much of the task content have higher appeal for girls (Fagot & Patterson, 1969), the activities may be quite boring for boys, and may be in conflict with their cognitions about sex-appropriate behavior (McCandless, 1967). Furthermore, boys are rep-rimanded and punished more severely than girls for identical mis-behaviors (Serbin, O'Leary, Kent, & Tonick, 1973). It would be interesting to replicate this finding in the laboratory by having teachers rate videotaped sequences in which boys and girls exhibited the same misbehaviors, includ-ing hyperactivity and related behaviors. Although the foregoing factors clearly would not cause hyperactivity, they would almost certainly exacer-bate existing hyperactive tendencies. Segregating classes at least in the early years is one procedure that might make school a markedly more enjoyable and profitable experience for boys and result in fewer boys with hyperactive tendencies becoming full-blown problems. This procedure would permit more sex-appropriate curriculum content for boys and could significantly reduce failure experiences. A recent report by Wray (1975) on the early school system in China strongly suggests that some of our school problems are of our own making. Wray states (1975, p. 726):

Chinese children learn to read after the age of 7 . . . By waiting until the whole group is ready, the Chinese avoid the problems which arise when younger children are pushed to learn to read and those who simply are not ready are marked as failures — and may be haunted by this label, and live up (or down) to it for the rest of their school career . . . Physical punishment . . . is no longer acceptable in China, either in the home or in the school. Children must be persuaded, reasoned with, shown, and taught how to behave correctly. The behavior that we observed in schools was, in fact, quite remarkable. Fighting, scuffling, rough-housing, or dis-putes seemed to occur rarely or not at all among the children that we saw. Their ability to concentrate on their tasks, in the face of foreign visitors to their class-rooms, was most impressive. Yet it was clear that the children are by no means lacking in spirit or in energy.

Although the school does not *cause* hyperactivity, it may heighten an already existing hyperactivity problem. In many cases, particularly those in which the children are only mildly hyperactive, much of the trauma of school entry could be avoided if greater continuity existed between the experiences of the late preschool years and those of the beginning school years. At one time the function of kindergarten was to bridge the experien-tial gap between preschool and school, its main purpose being to prepare the child for the nonacademic and social demands of suddenly being away from home for long, consecutive blocks of time, in the company of a large number of other children, all of whom were expected to conform to the commands and rules of an adult stranger. In relation to the main goals of the kindergarten, academic training was of only secondary importance, and was introduced in the form of readiness training on a sporadic and informal basis as the teacher felt the children could handle new demands. This year-long transitional period was particularly beneficial to the child who, for whatever reason, was not quite ready to cope with the demands of school. The previous transitional function of kindergarten programs has currently given way in a number of states to a strong academic orientation, a shift that we believe has been detrimental to the subsequent school adjustment of the child who is not equipped to cope with the demands of school. It is probably not a coincidence that the prevalence of school problems reached an all-time high about a decade after the Russian Sputnik episode, with the related sharp increase in academic demands and standards in the American school system.

However, school stresses sometimes do elicit problem behaviors of a hyperactive type in children who either have borderline IQs or behavior tendencies that overlap to some extent with hyperactive characteristics. The borderline IQ child who is placed in a regular class may be genuinely incapable of meeting the academic demands of the class as the result of many factors (e.g., lack of persistence) interacting with his lower IQ. This child is constantly frustrated by his own feelings of failure heightened by the derogatory reactions of his peers, and may abruptly react with the behaviors that commonly characterize the hyperactive child. Such a child typically becomes restless and fidgety, is unable to maintain attention to material that is beyond his comprehension, often engages in negative-attention-getting behavior to gain approval from his peers, and makes desperate and disastrous bids for the teacher's approval. This child is thought of as a situational hyperactive or a reactive hyperactive, rather than as a true hyperactive child. To restore him to a more desirable state of equilibrium all that is usually required is class-placement appropriate to his abilities and some help for his battered self-esteem. A more serious problem is the child of average or above average intelligence who is not hyperactive but who would be described as "lively," and who has tendencies toward a high level of activity, impulsivity, distractibility, and kinds of nonconformity. A school program that fails to channel his behaviors in appropriate directions, and instead exacerbates the negative aspects of his personality, will result in the child being labeled a candidate for a special class due to his hyperactivity. The following case study is a good example of a school program creating a problem for this kind of child:

Stephen was a cheerful, energetic, enthusiastic 7-year-old boy, the oldest son of professional parents. He was in the second grade and had been labeled as hyperactive and "a probable candidate for special class placement." His pediatrician disagreed with this evaluation and arranged for an outside observer to assess the problem. Observations were made on the playground and in the classroom over a three-day period. The child's IQ was 117 on the Stanford-Binet, Form L-M, and his performance on the Stanford Achievement Tests indicated some difficulty with reading and spelling; this difficulty was possibly due to the fact that Stephen had spent the previous year in England, when his father had a sabbatical, in a class that used the International Teaching Alphabet.

On the playground Stephen had good peer relationships, was a reasonably popular member of the group, and was very agile and quick at games. However, in the classroom he became restless, easily distracted, and impulsive. The teacher treated him as inept, derogated his ideas, many of which were quite creative, and emphasized his reading and spelling weaknesses by constantly drawing attention to them. The observer cited several incidents indicating unfair treatment: During painting the children were told to paint a picture story about fish. When Stephen painted a picture of salmon going upstream to spawn and showed them using a series of watery overpasses and cloverleafs, the teacher made caustic comments about children who always had to be different and heaped lavish praise on less interesting paintings. In physical education the children were free to choose one of several activities, but when Stephen chose to work out on the bars, the teacher pressured him to play soccer (which he disliked) and suggested that he was afraid to play it. After stumbling through a passage in reading, he was told that he should go back to the first grade.

The physical organization of the classroom was a far from desirable environment for a distractible child. Class enrollment was overly large and the room was so cluttered with books, boxes, maps, special audio-visual equipment, and physical education materials that it was difficult to move about. The timetable was equally confusing: some children came an hour late (and left later at the end of the day) causing a sudden influx after school had started; some children went to other classes for certain subjects and others left the classroom for remedial help. The desks were arranged in pairs and Stephen was seated in the back corner next to a disruptive and noisy boy who was continually in trouble and often involved Stephen. The teacher frequently shouted and the classroom was usually noisy and chaotic.

On the basis of these observations it was decided that Stephen's behavior was largely a function of classroom confusion and teacher harassment. It was recommended that he complete the two months remaining in the school year and then transfer to a private school. The delay in transferring was recommended so that Stephen's attention would not be drawn to his inability to cope with the classroom problems, he would not be put into the position of having to explain why he was leaving, and he would enter the new school in September on an equal basis with other entering children. The new school offered considerable individual instruction, had smaller classes, an orderly atmosphere that was structured but not rigid, and offered extracurricular classes highly appropriate for a child with creative tendencies.

Three months after Stephen enrolled in the new school another observation was made. Stephen was well-behaved in class, happy, popular with the other children, and well-liked by his teacher. There was no evidence of behaviors that would justify labeling him as hyperactive and, with some special help in reading and spelling, he was making good progress in all areas.

## Characteristics of an Optimal Early School Program for the Hyperactive Child

A school program for hyperactive children must be flexible enough to be readily adaptable to the needs of the individual child and to the ways in which he can best learn. The principle of adaptation to individual needs is basic to all good special education programs, however, it is particularly relevant to hyperactive children because of the marked heterogeneity within this group of children. There is no one definitive school program for the hyperactive child any more than there is one kind of hyperactive child. Explanations vary for the learning problems of hyperactive children. Keogh (1971) has proposed three hypotheses: One attributes the behavioral and cognitive difficulties to some type of neurological impairment; a second views the high level of motor activity as a disruptor that interferes with the acquisition of learning; and a third assumes that hyperactive children make decisions too rapidly. All three hypotheses have some empirical support (Douglas, 1972; Keogh, 1971), so that it is likely that each applies to a different subgroup of hyperactive children. However, there are other possibilities in addition to those suggested by Keogh: One possibility basic to the program to be described here is that a major obstacle of great importance is the hyperactive child's deficit in the covert verbal skills needed for benefiting from group instruction in the classroom.

Keeping the necessity for flexibility in mind, the optimal school program for the young hyperactive child can best be described in terms of three components, *content, method,* and *personnel*. The program described here is for children in the primary grades who are of average or at least border-line intelligence, and have no major sensory, motor, or emotional pro-grams. An extensive series of experimental tests (Ross & Ross, 1972) has proven the efficacy of such a program for young, educable, mentally retarded children whose problems are, in some respects, remarkably simi-lar to those of the hyperactive child in that they have many of the same academic, cognitive, social, and motor problems, and typically have poor self-esteem. The program should not be regarded as remedial, but rather as a plan of action for the habilitation of the young hyperactive child, the assumption being that many of these children would make satisfactory progress in school if they were in a special program for a year or two in the early grades. One major goal of the program is to help the child enjoy school. Lindy (1967) reported that hyperactive kindergarten children had poorer school attendance than their normally active peers despite the fact that they did not differ in physical health. It is essential to prevent the hyperactive child from developing an avoidance reaction to school.

### Content

The course emphasis is on basic academic subjects, cognitive skills, social, and motor training. Reading, writing, and arithmetic are the only academic subjects taught at this level and each has a heavy loading of language skills. Cognitive skills include planning, problem solving, listening, remembering, and visual attending. Social training is directed toward the acquisition of the social skills needed in the informal activities of the peer group, more formal games and other peer group experiences, and adult-child interac-tion. Motor training consists of two kinds of activities, one directed to-wards increased skill in movement, the other to increased game skills. The object here is to help the child acquire the control and precision of move-ment that he needs to function effectively in routine motor movement situations, and also to impart proficiency in the skills basic to the individual and group games of childhood. Inhibitory motor training is an important part of this training.

### Method

The way in which the training is conducted is of vital importance for what is learned and also for the child's view of himself as a learner. Failure and derogation may have a disastrous effect on his self-esteem and can set the stage for later school difficulties. The general emphasis here is on teaching to the child's strengths, making reasonable allowance for his activity level, presenting work in ways that will allow him to learn best, and assuring a balance of success and failure that is consonant with his needs but at the same time is compatible with reality. Considerable care is taken to direct his attention to the task at hand; the procedures used here are ones that have previously proven highly effective with young mentally retarded children (Ross & Ross, 1972) and include the use of models, attention-directing techniques of a social and nonsocial nature, and reinforcement procedures. In previous work with children with attention difficulties, we have found that the use of small groups; peer models, particularly high-status peer models; novel and exciting activities, particularly small-group games; and individual competitions all provided excellent contexts for attention training as well as for presenting academic and other material. To ensure a reasonable degree of success, self-pacing and a subskill approach is used whenever possible. By *subskill* we mean the breaking down or simplifying of the component parts of an activity to a point where even the most inept child can succeed. For example, in throwing a ball, one basic subskill is the act of holding the ball in one hand. The transmission of cognitive skills lends itself well to game activities, one value of games being the amount of repetition that can occur while still maintaining the interest of the child. Many social behaviors are transmitted through role play, with the children themselves acting as participants on some occasions and as the audience on other occasions when high-status peer models, such as the sixth graders in an elementary school, serve as actors in short skits designed to teach peer interaction skills. Psychosocial feedback is provided in the form of role play, tape recordings, and ratings by peers of special activities. These children clearly need help, and it is our opinion that they benefit greatly from being made to take some responsibility for their own behavior; but before they can do this they must be shown how they are behaving and how they should behave. Another method of helping the child to take such responsibility requires the use of contracts, that is, written agreements with the teacher about work to be accomplished or progress to be made in a specified time period, in return for some kind of reward, such as a privilege.

A variety of motivational procedures is used, including a score card system with prizes or privileges as rewards, and reinforcement schedules such as variable ratio and variable interval reinforcement, which introduce an element of pleasurable uncertainty into the daily routine. Punishment is held to a minimum; in our experience reward procedures are quite effective. Although there are elements of surprise in the daily routine, the emphasis is on structure and predictability, neither of which should be confused with rigidity.

Small groups are used to teach the academic and cognitive content. The small-group formation serves to focus attention, and it can facilitate the development of covert language skills if the activity is carefully planned.

Young children typically need a lot of repetition; in the small group each child works individually with the teacher, then observes each of his peers interacting in the same way. In the process he is required to verbalize, then observe his peers verbalize. If a game is being used, and it is an exciting game, he will soon verbalize not only when it is his turn but also overtly and then covertly when it is another child's turn. Thus in the small group activity there can be a reciprocal interaction between the intentional training and observational learning of covert language skills that is valuable to any child, but particularly so to the hyperactive child, who often has a deficit in this area of language development.

*Personnel*

The teaching personnel consists of a qualified teacher and a teacher's aide who need not be trained but who must be capable and reasonably skilled with children. One requirement of enrollment in the class we are describing is a reasonable amount of parent cooperation, the point being that continuity between home and school is essential for progress. Volunteer help from the highest grade in the school can be of enormous help and is usually available since many schools regard volunteer experience as an essential part of the elementary school program.

# CHAPTER 7

# *Prevention*

The pediatrician's responsibility in the care of children can be conceptualized in terms of two main functions: the *prevention* of potential problems and the *management* of ongoing health. In the early part of the century the major portion of the pediatrician's time and energy was directed toward the management of incurable diseases, chronic conditions, injuries, and particularly the contagious and respiratory diseases. Preventive practices, consisting mainly of immunization procedures associated with contagious diseases and education in the area of family health, occupied little of his time. In the past 2 or 3 decades a major shift has occurred in the proportion of time allocated to prevention and management; now, significantly more time is spent on prevention. With advances in preventive procedures and improved chemotherapeutic agents, many conditions previously regarded as contagious, acute, chronic, or incurable have changed status. They are less severe or have almost been eliminated.

Associated with these improvements in medical practice is a change in the expectations of our society: Society today does not accept defects as inevitable, considers the attainment of health as an inalienable right of every child, equates health to a broader spectrum that includes psychological wellbeing rather than solely the absence of disease, and consequently expects pediatric care to encompass the entire continuum of growth and development including psychological development. The result is that the pediatrician now has the time and is also expected to turn his attention to the less clearly delineated function of prevention. In doing this he has been drawn inevitably into areas that previously were of little concern, primarily the home and school and their various effects on the whole child.

Most pediatricians are skilled in the prevention and management of *medical* diseases and problems, as a result of their extensive medical training and clinical experience. In addition, recent advances in pediatric science and technology have produced preventive strategies and management techniques that are well-defined, widely known, and often require only a minimum of intervention. Pediatricians generally are not as well-equipped to handle the prevention and management of *behavior disorders*, one reason being a deficiency in well-established knowledge and

**229**

techniques in the field. Prior to this century there was a minimum of scientific interest in the behavior disorders, which were not considered within the sphere of medical inquiry and consequently were not subjected to the intensive investigation accorded to most medical problems. Knowledge about the prevention of most behavior disorders is still in the embryo stage, and the management of behavior disorders is in a more primitive stage of development than almost any other problem in pediatrics. Furthermore, behavior problems are seldom amenable to the accurate measurement and precise definition possible with the easily quantifiable concepts in medicine, such as height, weight, calorie intake, and temperature. The behavior assessment procedures that are available lack the precision and ease of administration of most medical instruments, generally are not as well-standardized, are more open to multiple interpretation, more likely to have a substantial margin of error, and are likely to present difficulties in use. Consider a comparison of the procedures used to record electrical activity in the brain, the electroencephalogram (EEG), and in the heart, the electrocardiogram (ECG). The EEG is used in the study of behavior disorders, particularly those that are presumed or known to have an organic base. Some children who exhibit substantial evidence of organic damage have normal EEGs, whereas others with no evidence of behavior disorder and no known history of organic damage have abnormal EEGs. The meaning of different EEG patterns is a topic of considerable controversy; depending on the criteria used, between 10 and 55 percent of normal subjects show EEG abnormalities (Schulman, Kaspar, & Throne, 1965). The EEG is a time-consuming procedure that may be mildly painful, is expensive, and not without risk (Werry, 1968). In contrast, the ECG, which is considered a valuable and indispensable tool in the management of the cardiac patient, generally presents clear and unequivocal diagnostic information about the heart; the meaning of different patterns has been clearly established; and the procedure is quick, easy to administer, painless, safe, and relatively inexpensive (Nadas, 1963).

The pediatrician's relative lack of skill in the area of behavior problems is also due to his lack of psychological training and experience. A broad base of psychological knowledge is encompassed in the management of behavior problems and in most medical schools the teaching of the psychological aspects of these problems is neither as well-organized nor as intensive as the teaching of medical care, yet many behavior problems that confront the pediatrician are far more complex than medical problems. In dealing effectively with a behavior disorder the pediatrician cannot focus on a single aspect of the child, or even only on the child, as he often can with a medical problem. Instead, the nature of most behavior problems that the pediatrician is likely to encounter forces him to consider the interactive influences of biological, social, and psychological factors. Effective management is further complicated by the fact that the child and his parents are often the major determinants of the duration and outcome of the problem, with the child's behavioral symptoms being a cause as well as a result of his parents' behavior.

The foregoing deficits in knowledge and pediatric training are particularly apparent in the case of hyperactivity, a problem that comprises a substantial portion of the behavior problems that come to the pediatrician's attention. It is likely that these deficits are one reason why the pediatrician must be "pressured" (Solomons, 1973) into the care of the hyperactive child. It is our opinion that much of this reluctance would disappear if the pediatrician were familiar with and could apply the clinical and research findings that are directly or peripherally relevant to the problems of the hyperactive child. There is in progress an extensive and systematic attack on the problems presented by the hyperactive child, with many projects having relevance for prevention and management. In addition, there is a substantial amount of research in areas such as early stimulation, sensory deprivation, observational learning, and biofeedback, in which the focus of research interest is on other problems, but whose findings have important implications for the prevention and management of hyperactivity.

This chapter is concerned with the prevention of hyperactivity. The level of preventive effort that we are proposing here is *secondary prevention,* in which the preventive strategies used are focused on the early identification of infants at risk for hyperactivity and the prompt initiation of intervention procedures to modify the hyperactive tendencies of the infant and limit sequelae, particularly those of a psychological nature (Mausner & Bahn, 1974). At risk tendencies are often present and identifiable in the neonatal, infancy, or early preschool years (Nichamin, 1972; Schleifer, Weiss, Cohen, Elman, Cvejic, & Kruger, 1975; Stewart, Pitts, Craig, & Dieruf, 1966). The purpose of the chapter is to discuss the procedures for the early identification of the infant or young child at risk for hyperactivity, outline the grounds for making a decision of whether or not to initiate a preventive intervention program, and describe the procedures and professionals involved in such a program. The assumptions here are that the pediatrician will play a primary role in the development and implementation of the program, other professionals will be involved in the prevention strategy as well as in the diagnostic procedures, and the at risk period generally occurs in infancy or the early preschool period.

## PREVENTION

Prevention is a two-phase process involving the early detection of the cluster of symptoms and events that are indicative of a child at risk, followed by the active initiation and monitoring of procedures to eliminate the symptoms or prevent them from developing further. The pediatrician has an excellent opportunity to identify the infant or young child who is at risk for hyperactivity because he is experienced in the range of normal behavior and attributes of infants and children, he usually sees the infant at monthly intervals for the first 6 months because this is a period of rapid development and increased vulnerability, and then continues to see the child regularly through the early childhood years.

It is important to emphasize that in the first year there usually is no single sign or cluster of symptoms that can be regarded as *unequivocal* diagnostic evidence of hyperactivity. The signs of an infant at risk for hyperactivity are in his adaptation to the basic functions of sleeping, eating, and style of responding to the environment; patterns of deviation in these functions indicate a disturbance in the overall adaptation to the environment. One pattern of deviation that should cause the pediatrician to watch an infant closely is that of restlessness and irritability characterized by a light, uneasy sleep from which the infant can easily be aroused, crying of long duration that appears to be intensified by efforts to comfort him, a wild driven kind of physical activity that continues to a point of exhaustion, startle responses to a variety of mild sensory stimulants, and a tendency to be very easily distracted during feeding. Note that this pattern of behavior could be due to brain damage, poor maternal caretaking, temperament, or physical disorder; or it could be a precursor of hyperactivity. It would be very difficult to specify with certainty the cause of the behavior; however, it is essential that the pediatrician be alert to the presence of the behavior and note its development and duration. Pediatricians often dismiss such patterns of behavior lightly and assure the parents that the infant will grow out of it. In giving this advice they are committing two errors: they are implying that the difficult behavior is a normal variant and, more seriously, at a time that is optimum for intervention they are failing to initiate immediate action to help the parents cope with the management of their difficult child. In discussing the tendency to assume that difficult infants grow out of it, Berlin (1974, p. 1454) states:

> The aphorism of past generations that children "will grow out of their troubles" is not true. Children, especially those with troubles related to biologic rhythms — sleep, feeding, activity rate — discernible in the first year of life, *do not grow out of these problems*. They rather grow *into* them.

The following case study is a typical example of this pattern:

At 7 months he was described by his parents as a dynamo who never slept for long, cried all the time in a piercing, shrieking kind of way, seldom smiled except when he burped, and didn't act as if he knew anyone in the house. His mother reported that he was friendliest and nicest with strangers and almost invariably difficult when she wanted to feed, dress, or bathe him. The whole bath routine was exhausting for her and she had come to dread it. He could creep backwards and forwards at a remarkable rate of speed and he was always bumping into things or knocking over light objects in the creeping process. If his mother picked him up when he wanted to creep he had a real tantrum and he'd kick and flail at her with his arms and really create an uproar. Both parents agreed that this infant, their first-born, was exhausting, exasperating, and a great disappointment to both of them. The pediatrician attributed the infant's behavior to temperament, suggested to the parents that it was normal for new parents to take an exaggerated view of things with a first-born infant, and made no suggestions about how the behavior might be modified for the better.

The onset of patterns of deviation may occur as early as the first few days of extrauterine life and often occurs in the first year. Frequently, maternity nurses report that one neonate stands out from the group in the hospital nursery as being unusually difficult to handle in routine caretaking situations; he is characterized by a disturbance in sleep patterns and by a pervasive restlessness that is expressed in his waking hours as an unusually high level of general motor activity and in his resting periods as an inability to settle down. Empirical evidence of the early onset of these patterns of deviation comes from the excellent longitudinal study by Chess, Thomas, and Birch (1968) in which a behavior pattern was identified that included high activity, restlessness, and marked lability of mood similar to the behaviors described here, and was clearly discernible at the age of 2 months. Retrospective interviews with parents of hyperactive children (Anderson, 1963; Barnard & Collar, 1973; Stewart, Pitts, Craig, & Dieruf, 1966) showed that the parents were often aware in infancy that their child was different, and the differences they described were similar to those identified by Thomas, Chess, and Birch (1970). In mothers of hyperactive school-age children that we have interviewed, the mothers' recall of the early onset of patterns of deviation usually has been verified by the children's pediatric records, and the same mothers' reports of excessive fetal activity in the third trimester of pregnancy have been confirmed by their obstetrical records. Although retrospective accounts do have well-documented weaknesses (Robbins, 1963; Solomons, 1973), there is reason to believe that a mother would accurately recall her first awareness of her infant being different because of the trauma involved. The following is a verbatim quote from a mother discussing this point:

Even when I first had Petie, even on the second day in the hospital I knew *something* was wrong. He acted so different from all the other babies, at feeding time he didn't cry, he *screeched,* and all the nurses looked funny and he was so stiff and he kicked all the time same as he did when I was pregnant. But then I thought it was probably something wrong with how I handled him because I was an only child and I never had much to do with little babies and I thought I wasn't doing a good job and Petie knew it. Then when I got him home he'd have some real bad days so I almost went crazy and some days that were so great I'd think, "What could be wrong with a baby like this? It's all in your mind." And John (her husband) was away a lot so he didn't really know what Petie was like and I never *really* told the pediatrician. I'd say about Petie's bad days but not what it was really like and he'd say that they all have bad days the first year. And I didn't want to know, I know that now, I'd take Petie to the park on good days but on bad days I'd bake and clean and stay in so people wouldn't say anything. And when other babies screamed their lungs out I'd feel good and think that they all do it.

Then, one day my pediatrician was sick and the other doctor saw Petie and we had to wait and Petie was just terrible in the waiting room, the worst he'd ever been. It was *awful.* And when I saw the doctor he sat and asked me all about Petie and I started to tell him *really* how it had been for the whole 8 months and all of a sudden right in the middle of telling — I'll never forget it, it was St. Patrick's Day, and there were all of the doctor's certificates on the wall and a whole lot of cute really happy-looking baby pictures that I guessed he'd delivered and I was looking at them and all of a sudden I thought, "Petie is *not like them,* he's not like them *at all.* There's *something wrong* with Petie;" and I felt all shaky like getting flu and I felt like yelling and screaming and I thought "What'll I do, there's something wrong with Petie?" and I looked at the doctor and I could tell, *he* knew too.

The patterns of deviation, such as restlessness and irritability, often disappear spontaneously during the first year of life and the pediatrician is justified in suggesting this possibility to the parents (while also offering concrete suggestions for improving the immediate situation). Often the termination of these behaviors coincides with some normal developmental change, giving the impression that the disappearance of the difficult behavior is so abrupt that the mother may report that the behaviors "just disappeared overnight." More often, however, they disappear so gradually that the mother comes to wonder if her complaints were justified. However, sometimes they persist into the early years of childhood and become more clearly defined.

In the 2-year-old child the patterns of behavior indicative of a child at risk for hyperactivity typically are more defined than in infancy and are *qualitatively* similar but clearly *quantitatively* different from those of the average child. Many 2-year-olds are overactive, rebellious, easily upset, difficult, given to temper tantrums, distractible, impulsive, and irritable, and suffer minor injuries *at times.* Gesell and Ilg's (1943) term "the terrible twos" is often a very appropriate descriptor. When a young child exhibits these behaviors to a degree that seriously disrupts the household, has few quiet sunny periods, and generally seems very difficult to manage, the probability is high that the child is at risk for hyperactivity or some behavior disorder, or that the mother's mode of caretaking is seriously at fault, or that the child's behavior is a normal variant. We assume here that physical diseases and disorders that might be associated with hyperactivity have been ruled out. The following observation was made at age 2 years, 4 months of the same infant who was described on page 232. Although his behavior at that time was highly suggestive of an infant at risk for a behavior disorder, no intervention was introduced. Two years later his parents sought help for him. Having noted the existence of the at risk pattern in infancy, the pediatrician should have been alert to its subsequent development by his own observation of the child and by questioning the parents. Two years should not have gone by, particularly since there was evidence on the pediatric record that during this interval the mother had mentioned the problem, only to be told on several occasions that the child would "grow out of it." In this observation, which was part of the diagnostic workup, note that although the behaviors the child exhibits are more clearly defined and differentiated, the basic response modalities are the same as they were in infancy.

At the age of 2 years, 4 months this boy was clearly hyperactive. He darted about the playroom snatching toys from other children in a very aggressive manner, knocking over toys and children, screaming when the playroom supervisor tried to quieten him down, and throwing objects at other children most of whom were immediately terrified at his chaotic behavior. He dashed about and sometimes ran right into the wall, he seemed unable to stop. When it was time for the pediatrician to see him he refused to leave, lay on the floor screaming and kicking, and bit the nurse who helped his mother carry him in.

His mother reported that he had walked early, slept and ate poorly, and was prone to severe temper outbursts, rarely smiled, spoke only a few words, had ups and downs of mood that she called "manic," and had seriously disrupted the household for most of his life. Caretaking functions were extremely difficult and, as in the previous observation, both she and her husband were exhausted by the effort it took to care for their difficult child. Neither of them wished to have another infant and the mother commented bitterly that he was delightful on his rare good days but on any other day and every night when he woke them with his lengthy bouts of screaming, she would gladly give him away.

All infants and young children exhibit the behaviors in any of the patterns of deviation at times, but generally do not show them with any degree of consistency. When *consistent* deviations from the norm occur in the infant or young child's characteristic pattern of adaptation to the basic functions of activity, sleeping, and eating or in his individual style of responding to the environment, a style that is clearly discernible in the second month of life (Thomas, Chess, & Birch, 1970), then the pediatrician must decide if the deviations are chance fluctuations of little importance, a normal variant, the result of the maternal style of caretaking, or if, taken together, they comprise a basis for treating the infant or young child as at risk for hyperactivity. The individual behaviors themselves are easy to recognize. *The problem for the pediatrician lies in seeing that a group of behaviors forms a pattern that warrants a decision concerning intervention.*

## ASSESSMENT PROCEDURE

When an infant or young child is identified as possibly at risk for hyperactivity it is essential that a comprehensive investigation be conducted to confirm the at risk diagnosis and provide a basis for intervention. In such an evaluation a basic clinical history, physical examination, and some psychological testing should be regarded as mandatory.

### History

The purpose of the history is to obtain as complete and sequential a health and behavior record as possible, to assess the quality of the mother-child relationship and family relationships, and to identify any familial and environmental factors that might increase the probability of the occurrence of a behavior disorder. Knowledge of the family relationships is essential in determining the extent to which the family may be causing or contributing to the child's behavior problems, and in assessing the positive and negative potential that different members of the family have for participation in the intervention process. The optimal arrangement would be to see each parent separately and then, if it appears that some form of intervention would be required, to see them together, and then to see them with the child. The information sought in the parent interviews falls into two major categories, factual and affective, and both are of major importance in reaching a decision about the child.

Particular attention should be given to the following: Familial instances of hyperactivity, other behavior disturbances, and psychiatric disorders in the first or second degree relatives of the infant; stress factors in the prenatal (infectious or viral diseases or other problems during pregnancy) and perinatal periods (prematurity, respiratory or hemolytic complications) and beyond (Apgar rating, failure to thrive, illnesses and accidents); the birth and obstetrical records; noxious nonsocial or social events or influences that could be causally related to or might exacerbate the infant's state of disequilibrium (e.g., lead exposure, food additives, allergy, and tension in the household); and concern that the mother expresses about the infant particularly if this concern is stated in poorly defined terms or is quantitatively or qualitatively different from that of the average mother. For example, one mother frequently commented about the personality clash between her newborn son and her husband. With questioning, the pediatrician was able to elicit the fact that the infant's interactions with her and with the babysitter were also consistently negative. With some encouragement the mother then elaborated with a series of examples of other situations that left little doubt that a real problem existed.

In terms of stimulus input the nonworking mother typically has more information about the infant than has any other adult in his environment. It would be of great assistance to the pediatrician if this information could be retrieved in a form that would facilitate the early identification of problems. If the pediatrician is to make optimum use of the mother as a source of information, it is of critical importance for him to determine the accuracy of her information through methods such as the repetition of questions, the assessment of the degree to which the mother-child interaction in the office confirms her reports of her caretaking procedures, and checks on previous histories and other records. It is essential, for example, to be sure that the mother's complaints are based on fact rather than reflecting her delusions about her infant or her dissatisfaction with the demands of motherhood. There have been relatively few empirical attempts to determine the accuracy of maternal report. One of the most careful checking systems is that of Thomas, Chess, and Birch (1970) who found mothers in their sample to be quite accurate possibly, in part, as a result of the specificity and careful wording of their questions. Other accounts of the accuracy of maternal report are less positive. Minde, Webb, and Sykes (1968) found little agreement between birth histories and maternal report, and Solomons (1973, p. 335) stated that:

. . . a history given by parents concerning the behavior and activity level of their child is largely unreliable. Studies show little agreement between the parents, and they are unable to provide objective information concerning the maladaptive behavior of their own children. Not only does their lack of objectivity affect the accuracy of their perceptions, but it may also affect their willingness to report and their honesty in reporting. Compared with fathers, mothers are more defensive, distorting and censoring their information. A mother may describe with chronological precision the onset of a cough, rash, or temperature, or the duration and character of a pain; however, she may color her appraisal of the mental age of her child and the manifestations of his behavior and personality because of her fears of the evaluation and her unrealistic expectations for the child's future.

Clearly, the pediatrician should make every effort to check the accuracy of the information elicited in the interview and give careful thought to the mode and content of questioning. Ambiguous or vague questions can be expected to elicit inaccurate information.

The importance of knowing how to ask questions and what questions to ask has been emphasized by Thomas, Chess, and Birch (1970). The questions should be phrased in terms of common situations to elicit factual descriptions of the infant's or mother's behavior in specific situations. For example, in considering one of the areas of behavior relating to temperament, level of activity, the pediatrician might ask:

"If you were drying the baby after his bath and you had to get another towel from the other side of the room, would you feel safe in leaving him for a few seconds or would you be afraid that he'd fall off the counter?"

"If you put the baby to bed for his afternoon nap and he didn't go right to sleep would you have to go in and check that he was still covered or would you know that the blankets would still be in place?"

"If you are visiting friends and you put the baby down on a blanket on the floor with some toys to play with would he just stay on or near the blanket or would he wriggle off and be over on the other side of the room in a very short time?"

In taking the history there are three major questions that should be investigated as an aid in pinpointing the primary causative factor in the infant's behavior. Is there support for the behavior problem being a function of the child's difficult temperament, that is, his own individual style of responding to the environment? Is it the way the mother handles the infant in her interactions with him? Is there something in the environment affecting the child negatively? It is essential to try to pinpoint which of these three factors, that is, infant temperament, mother-child interaction, or environmental factors is the primary contributing cause or a major factor in the infant's problem behavior. The same problem behavior could result from any one or a combination of these factors, and the approach used to modify the problem behavior would differ markedly depending on the relative contributions of these factors.

In investigating *the question of temperament* the pediatrician would find it helpful to review the work of Thomas, Chess, and Birch (1970). These researchers have identified nine areas of behavior against which the child's characteristics can be scored to obtain a behavioral profile. Certain characteristics cluster together and define types of temperament ("easy children," "difficult children," "slow to warm up children") into which 65 percent of the children fell. The areas of behavior are (Thomas, Chess, & Birch, 1970, p. 102):

(1) level and extent of motor activity; (2) the rhythmicity, or degree of regularity, of functions such as eating, elimination, and the cycle of sleeping and wakefulness; (3) the response to a new object or person, in terms of whether the child accepts the new experience or withdraws from it; (4) the adaptability of behavior to changes in the environment; (5) the threshold, or sensitivity, to stimuli; (6) the intensity, or energy level, of responses; (7) the child's general mood or "disposition," whether cheerful or given to crying, pleasant or cranky, friendly or unfriendly; (8) the degree of the child's distractibility from what he is doing; (9) the span of the child's attention and his persistence in an activity.

Thomas, Chess, and Birch (1970) recommend that the pediatrician routinely familiarize himself with the infant's temperament to increase the probability of providing the parents with appropriate advice on basic care, weaning, toilet training, and so on. They also suggest that when a behavior disorder arises a knowledge of the child's temperament and the environmental demands that are conflicting with it is essential if the pediatrician is to guide the parents effectively in changing their handling of the child.

On *the question of the mother's handling of the infant,* the pediatrician should make the following kinds of observations. Is the mother relaxed? If her leg muscles are tense the infant is unlikely to rest peacefully on her knee. Are her movements as she holds him unhurried or are they jerky? While she is doing any caretaking does she carry on a quiet affectionate conversation with him? When does she respond to the infant? Does the infant appear to be warm and comfortable? Discuss in specific terms what happens in everyday caretaking that makes it difficult for the mother.

In determining whether there are *environmental factors* affecting the child negatively, obtain information about allergy, noxious substances in the environment such as lead, noxious forces in the environment such as noise and interpersonal tension, discomfort factors in the infant's immediate environment, and maternal psychological and physical wellbeing.

## Physical Examination

Although the hyperactive child is usually physically normal, the possibility of a medical disease or condition, such as a progressive or treatable disease of the central nervous system that presents as hyperactivity, must be investigated. A routine neurological examination should always be performed. An examination by a neurologist and the use of specialized neurological tests ordinarily are not required except to rule out seizures, growths, or degenerative brain disease. Clements and Peters (1962) have specified the complete set of procedures that should be included in a neurological examination of a child tentatively diagnosed as hyperactive. Descriptions of neurological examination procedures for the detection of soft signs are contained in Close (1973) and Werry, Minde, Guzman, Weiss, Dogan, and Hoy (1972), and a play neurological examination that can be conducted in conjunction with a psychiatric interview of the child is described by Goodman and Sours (1967). Careful attention should be given to the presence of minor physical anomalies such as head circumference out of the normal range, epicanthus, widely-spaced eyes, curved fifth finger, no ear lobes, and a wide gap between the first and second toes. Table 7 contains a list of the anomalies and the scoring weights assigned them by Waldrop and her associates (Waldrop, Pedersen, & Bell, 1968). These investigators have reported a high incidence of these anomalies in hyperactive children, particularly boys, and have attributed the anomalies and the hyperactive behavior to the *same* causative factors occurring early in the first trimester of pregnancy. The increased incidence of minor physical anomalies in hyperactive boys has been confirmed by Rapoport, Quinn, and Lamprecht (1974), and was associated in their sample with severity of hyperactivity and with either reported childhood hyperactivity in the father or a history of early obstetrical difficulty in the mother. The findings of these two groups of investigators suggest that hyperactive children with an increased incidence of anomalies may constitute an etiological subgroup. It follows that a high stigmata score might be an early indicator of an infant or young child at risk for hyperactivity. It will be apparent that the anomalies are not all applicable to all ages. For example, fine electric hair does not appear in infancy. It is important to emphasize that it is the presence of *multiple* minor physical anomalies that may be important. Many children who are clearly not at risk for hyperactivity and are not afflicted with Down's Syndrome, other major congenital defects, or any other problem, have one or two of these anomalies. During the physical examination, the pediatrician should take the opportunity to validate through direct observation the mother's reports of the child's behavior, particularly those categories of temperament that may show up in the examination setting, and should observe the way the mother handles and interacts with the infant.

To help determine if the child's physical growth and development and his intellectual development are progressing normally the pediatrician may decide to have developmental screening and/or intelligence tests adminis-

# Table 7. List of Anomalies and Scoring Weights

| Anomaly | Weight |
|---|---|

Head - Electric hair:
    Very fine hair that won't comb down . . . . . . . . . . . . 2
    Fine hair that is soon awry after combing . . . . . . . . . 1
Two or more whorls. . . . . . . . . . . . . . . . . . . . . 0

Eyes - Epicanthus:
    Where upper and lower lids join the nose, point of union is:
        Deeply covered. . . . . . . . . . . . . . . . . . . . . 2
        Partly covered. . . . . . . . . . . . . . . . . . . . . 1
    Hypertelorism:
    Approximate distance between tear ducts:
      $\geq$ 1.5 inches. . . . . . . . . . . . . . . . . . . . . . . 2
      $>$ 1.25 $<$ 1.5 inches . . . . . . . . . . . . . . . . . . . 1

Ears - Low seated:
    Bottom of ears in line with:
      Mouth (or lower). . . . . . . . . . . . . . . . . . . . 2
      Area between mouth and nose . . . . . . . . . . . . . . 1
    Adherent lobes:
    Lower edges of ears extend:
      Upward and back toward crown of head. . . . . . . . . . 2
      Straight back toward rear of neck . . . . . . . . . . . 1
    Malformed ears. . . . . . . . . . . . . . . . . . . . . . . 1
    Asymmetrical ears . . . . . . . . . . . . . . . . . . . . . 1
    Soft and pliable ears . . . . . . . . . . . . . . . . . . . 0

Mouth- High palate
    Roof of mouth:
      Definitely steepled . . . . . . . . . . . . . . . . . . 2
      Flat and narrow at the top. . . . . . . . . . . . . . . 1
    Furrowed tongue (one with deep ridges). . . . . . . . . . . 1
    Smooth-rough spots on tongue. . . . . . . . . . . . . . . . 0

Hands- Fifth finger:
    Markedly curved inward toward other fingers . . . . . . . 2
    Slightly curved inward toward other fingers . . . . . . . 1
    Single transverse palmar crease . . . . . . . . . . . . . . 1
    Index finger longer than middle finger. . . . . . . . . . . 0

Feet - Third toe:
    Definitely longer than second toe . . . . . . . . . . . . 2
    Appears equal in length to second toe . . . . . . . . . . 1
    Partial syndactylia of two middle toes. . . . . . . . . . . 1
    Gap between first and second toe (approximately $\geq$ 1/4 inch) . 1

tered, usually by a psychologist. An intelligence test will not establish whether or not an infant or young child is hyperactive. It is usually used to rule out the possibility that the restless or difficult behavior is related to gross intellectual abnormality. The sources of the following brief discussion on tests are Anastasi (1968) and Buros (1972).

## Developmental and Intelligence Tests

Infant tests, covering the period from birth to approximately 18 months, all require individual administration, with the infant either lying down or supported on someone's lap. The tests generally measure sensory and motor development, and involve little or no speech on either the infant or examiner's part. Motivation depends on rapport with the examiner, and this may be a problem if the infant has been adversely conditioned to the doctor's office. Several sessions are usually required because fatigue is a problem; distractibility is also a strong possibility.

In selecting tests, and also in basing treatment decisions on test results, the pediatrician should keep the following points in mind. Scoring is often very difficult and potentially unreliable because the child's responses are fleeting and immediate judgments are required by the examiner. Standardization procedures often use smaller and less representative normative samples than is the case for tests for older children. Longitudinal methods are generally used, with the children being tested at successive ages. Test reliability, particularly in the first 3 months, is generally lower than that of tests for older children. However, the split-half reliability method which is commonly used probably gives a lower reliability coefficient than would be obtained if comparable forms were available, because the test content is designed to cover a wide variety of functions and thus is very heterogeneous. To determine split-half reliability, a test is divided into two halves, one consisting of the odd-numbered items, the other, the even-numbered items. The two halves are then correlated. When the items are very heterogeneous, splitting the test in half in this way can result in the two halves measuring quite different behaviors, with a consequent low correlation between scores on each half and, therefore, a low split-half reliability coefficient.

Validity is difficult to establish because appropriate cirteria are scarce. The criterion that is most frequently used is age differentiation and in these terms good validity is usually shown with clear progressive changes in performance even over short periods of time. The criterion of prediction of subsequent intellectual status is difficult because items at an early level may be quite unlike items at a later age level, a change reflecting the rapid intellectual development of the infancy period. Long-term prediction from early test results is difficult because a very small proportion of the infant's total development has already occurred and many circumstances will influence his subsequent development.

Testing the preschool child presents many of the same problems in administration as infant tests do. The child usually has a short attention span, is susceptible to fatigue, and may be difficult to motivate. In addition, he is often shy, easily distracted, hard to understand, and quite negative about the test situation. Because the preschool child is much more aware of and responsive to the examiner, prior to the testing session the examiner should have one short session in which he and the child play simple games or engage in other interesting activities.

Norms for preschool tests generally are obtained through cross-sectional procedures (the Cattell Infant Intelligence Scale being an exception). Consequently, the normative samples are usually large and are representative of a clearly-defined population. These tests are generally used to evaluate the current status of the child, although the predictive value of the tests continues to be of interest. Before selecting a test, the pediatrician should review or obtain an expert opinion on the standardization procedures, including the description and selection of the normative sample, and consider the reliability and validity data. A brief description follows of two developmental tests and one intelligence test for infants and early preschool children.

## Bayley Infant Scales of Development

The purpose of this test is to establish the current developmental status of children ranging from 2 months to 30 months in relation to others of the same age. The Scales have three parts, with items arranged by age level. One group of 163 items, giving a Mental Score, measures responses to visual and auditory stimuli, manipulation and play with objects, social interaction responses, discrimination of shapes, simple problem solving, memory, naming objects, understanding prepositions, and having the concept of "one." A second group of items, giving a Motor Score, measures gross motor abilities such as sitting, standing, walking, and stair climbing, and fine motor coordination such as grasping objects. The third part of the Scales is a rating scale measuring such aspects as the child's emotional and social behaviors, activity level, response to objects, attention span, persistence, and endurance. Testing proceeds by first establishing a basal level. If any item is failed in a level, the next lower level is administered. This procedure is continued until the child passes all items at a level and this point becomes his basal level. Testing then proceeds upwards and the raw score consists of each item plus items below the basal level. Testing usually is done in several sessions. The Mental and Motor Scales take from 45 to 90 minutes. Excellent standardization procedures have been followed in developing the Scales and providing norms. The test reliabilities are satisfactory. Split-half reliability for the Mental Scale ranges from .81 to .93, and for the Motor Scale, .68 to .92. The Mental Scale validity coefficient (.57) was determined by correlating the scores of 2-year-old children with their Stanford-Binet scores over the 6-month age overlap of the two tests. There are no validity data on the Motor Scale. In reviewing the Bayley Scales, Collard (1972, pp. 728–729) states:

The value of the Bayley Scales as a research instrument lies in its careful standardization, high reliability, and broad coverage of many aspects of the behavior repertoire of infants . . . (It is) by far the best measure of infant development available today.

### Cattell Infant Intelligence Scale

This test is considered to be a highly satisfactory instrument for infant testing. It provides an extension of the Stanford-Binet Intelligence Test from 30 months down to 2 months and gives a mental age (MA) and ratio IQ computed in the same way as the Binet MA and IQ. The test items are grouped into age levels, with 5 items and 1 or 2 alternatives at each level. Age levels are at 1-month intervals for the first year, 2-month intervals for the second year, and 3-month intervals for the half of the third year covered by the Scale. The short time intervals between levels, and the relatively large number of items per level, provide a more precise measurement than is usually the case with infant tests. At the youngest level the tasks are largely perceptual (e.g., following a dangling ring with the eyes or looking at a spoon) with a few motor items (e.g., transferring an object from hand to hand). With increasing age, more complex manipulatory tasks are introduced using blocks, formboards, cups, dolls, and other toys, and increasing use is made of verbal functions. At the upper levels the child follows oral instructions with these objects and does more highly verbal tasks, such as naming pictures of objects. If a child passes any test at the 30-month level testing is continued with Level III of the Stanford-Binet. All of the materials are standardized. There are no time limits and the order of item administration can be modified to suit the child and the testing circumstances. Testing usually requires 20 to 30 minutes. The standardization sample came from lower middle-class families and the procedures were satisfactory. Split-half reliability is unsatisfactory only at the 3-month level; other level reliabilities are between .71 and .90. When Cattell IQs were correlated with Stanford-Binet Form L IQs for 3-year-old children in the standardization sample, the reliability coefficient was .87. The predictive correlations of Cattell IQs for children below the age of 12 months and the Stanford-Binet IQs of the same children at age three are little better than chance. However, after the 12-month age level the predictive correlations become increasingly high, ranging from .56 at 12 months to .83 at 30 months.

### Denver Developmental Screening Test

This test is intended as a screening device for the early detection of delayed development in children of 2 weeks to 6 years. It is fairly widely used although it is inferior to other well-known tests. It is included here to provide examples of characteristics that indicate an unsatisfactory test. The 105 items on the test form four categories covering behaviors similar to those of other infant and preschool tests. The categories are gross motor, fine motor-adaptive (e.g., reaches for an object), language, and personal-social. Many items are dependent on the mother's recall. The geographical selection of the standardization sample is very limited. The test has questionable reliability up to the 2-year level. The reported test-retest and scorer reliabilities were done on very small groups and are spuriously high, due in part to the large number of items showing no variation from session to session or scorer to scorer because they are dependent on the mother's recall (over a short test-retest interval). The validity data were obtained quite properly by correlating test scores against another test as a criterion. However, the data are doubtful because the criterion test, the Revised Yale Developmental Schedule, is *not* an independent criterion. The Yale is based on three other scales and the Denver Developmental Screening Test consists of items from the Yale as well as from the three scales on which the Yale is based. Consequently, in correlating the Denver and the Yale, identical items appear in both scales, resulting in a spuriously high validity coefficient. Even more serious is the fact that as a screening device for detecting delayed development, the Denver misses a high proportion of children identified by other superior tests such as the Bayley and Cattell.

### The At Risk Diagnosis

No absolute guidelines can be given for diagnosing an infant or young child as at risk. What is urgently needed is a scoring system analogous to the *optimality score* that Kalverboer, Touwen, and Prechtl (1973) used to provide a global measure of the integrity of the nervous functions in the newborn infant. Such a score would provide an objective basis for assigning *at risk* status to a specific infant. Instead, the diagnosis must depend in part on the global impression of the child yielded by the various assessment measures; although if a child is at risk for hyperactivity one would expect to find *some* supporting evidence in the history to eliminate medical, neurological, and intellectual bases for the behavior, and to see sometime during the assessment period some clear cut demonstrations of the behaviors that have prompted the investigation. It is unlikely that an infant or young child whose behavior has justified such a thorough investigation would remain serene and untroubled throughout this series of procedures. If psychological tests have been used as part of the assessment procedure the pediatrician should consider the psychologist's impressions of the mother and child in reaching a decision about the need for intervention. During the testing session the psychologist who is experienced with infants and young children will form impressions of the psychological status of the infant over and above his actual test performance; he will also notice characteristics of the mother's behavior and of the mother-child interaction that may be relevant to a decision about the need for intervention.

Since no *absolute* guidelines exist for identifying the infant or young child at risk for hyperactivity or most other behavior disorders, the possibility exists that a child will be incorrectly diagnosed as at risk and started on a preventive intervention program that is unnecessary because his difficulties will disappear spontaneously with time. The potential advantages of early preventive intervention far outweigh the disadvantage of false identification. There is little risk to the child or his parents in the preventive intervention approach to be described here *if* the pediatrician presents the intervention procedures as routine changes in caretaking that are likely to be better suited to the child's temperament, avoids labeling the child or using any anxiety-arousing terms, and is matter-of-fact about the difficult behavior of the infant. There is a substantial risk in a "wait and see" or "he'll grow out of it" approach.

## THE PREVENTIVE STRATEGY

If on the basis of the result of the above examination strategy the pediatrician decides to treat the child as at risk, it is important to be clear about what this decision implies. The kind of preventive intervention required would consist of modifications in caretaking and socialization routines that would not impose any undue hardships on the parents, seriously disrupt the household, or convey the impression of abnormality in the child. No label such as hyperactivity would be associated with the intervention procedures. Basically, what happens in a preventive program is as follows. The pediatrician and a team of professionals use the information already obtained and make further assessments of the infant or young child and his environment and decide what elements in the situation, such as maternal attitudes, factors in the mother-child relationship, infant behavior, and nonsocial factors, should be changed. Then the pediatrician outlines the plan to the parents, prescribes certain procedures to be followed, arranges for additional professional help to the parents in carrying out the procedures, and monitors the child's progress just as he would if the child had some medical problem.

## Preliminaries

Before initiating a preventive strategy for an infant or young child at risk for hyperactivity the pediatrician must first have gained the basic trust and confidence of the parents. Any intervention process for an infant at risk is likely to be of long duration and will require that the parents, particularly the mother, work closely with the pediatrician. It is of critical importance to the success of the intervention process that the mother feel that the pediatrician is a firm ally who understands and is genuinely sympathetic about her problem, is ready and qualified to discuss any aspect of it with her, and who receives without censure her sometimes negative confidences about her child. Only when this relationship is firmly established can the pediatrician set in motion the preliminary procedures, the most important one being a comprehensive assessment of the infant's social and nonsocial environment. The assessment is normally conducted by one or more professionals from other disciplines with the pediatrician contributing information on the basis of his own long-term experience with the family and the history he has just taken. The assumption here is that regardless of the primary cause of the at risk behavior, there are likely to be secondary factors that are maintaining or even exacerbating the behavior, and modification or elimination of some of these factors could result in a significant improvement in the problem behavior. The assessment procedure also provides information of critical importance for developing the prevention strategy, including parental attitudes to the infant, parental philosophy of child rearing, the quality of the mother-child interaction particularly during basic care routines, the tone of the household, the financial status of the family, and relevant information about siblings. The bulk of this information would be obtained by other professionals, such as a pediatric or developmental psychologist or a social worker, since the pediatrician has neither the time nor the expertise to obtain it. With this information the pediatrician and other professionals are ready to develop the preventive strategy.

In designing an intervention strategy the potential extent of the child's contribution to the problem should not be underestimated. In the household environment even the best behaved infant or young child is a powerful and active force who directly and indirectly affects the interpersonal relations of other members of the household. The effect of the child is even more powerful if he is an only child or if he has a difficult temperament. Because the infant and young child are relatively helpless in a number of areas the tendency is to view them as somewhat passive recipients who are acted upon by other forces in the environment. In fact, there is substantial evidence that in the early years the child shapes the responses of his caretakers to an astonishing degree (Bell, 1968). For example, in a study of the frequency of interaction sequences between infants and their mothers Moss and Robson (1968) found that 1-month-old infants initiated the exchange 80 percent of the time. The child at risk may create a network of interpersonal difficulties such as alienation, negative affect, and tension in the household, and one goal of the intervention program is to modify the response patterns of the infant and his parents and thus reduce the radiating network of difficulties.

Although the specific intervention procedures used in any particular case vary, most prevention programs require procedures that provide psychological support for the mother, instruct the mother in routine caretaking techniques that facilitate the handling of a difficult child, and modify the infant's behavior.

### Psychological Support for the Mother

Mothers of difficult infants and children are frequently characterized by incapacitating feelings of self-blame and guilt that sometimes lead to a disorganizing anxiety. In some cases these feelings are the result of critical and careless comments by harassed husbands or busy pediatricians implying that the mother has failed in the performance of her responsibility to the infant. The effect is to reduce the mother's already shaky confidence in her ability to care for her infant; thus the troubled mother-child relationship suffers further deterioration. Particularly in the case of the young infant, the mother must accept that in general the infant's behavior is largely independent of her child-rearing practices. Where the problem behavior appears to be a function of temperament, the pediatrician should emphasize that this is the child's own style of responding to the environment. The pediatrician and the mother will have to work within it; but at the same time changes can be made to improve the situation, and highly qualified help will be obtained to assist the mother in making changes.

The mother should enroll in a discussion group for the mothers of infants with problems. These groups are conducted regularly by public health agencies in most metropolitan areas, the purpose being to teach mothers ways of interacting with their children that will strengthen the mother-child relationship, provide an opportunity for the exchange of information, and reduce through group interaction the feeling of aloneness that besets almost every mother of a child with a problem (Berlin, 1974). The efficacy of such groups on the participants' morale and anxiety is well-documented (Bandura, 1969; Schacter, 1959). The report of a young, inexperienced, and very anxious mother to her pediatrician after several group meetings demonstrates another beneficial result, the development of a critical but not self-destructive assessment of the problem (Ross, 1973, p. 8):

I think that was the first time I realized that I wasn't the only mother in the world with a problem baby and in that group my problem was mild, really practically nothing, compared to what some of them had to contend with. I used to look around at them and think that they were all managing in spite of it, they all looked kind of attractive and even quite happy some of the time and not as if the end of the world had arrived and after a few meetings I thought if they can do it, I can do it too. And that day for the first time I began to think about how really awful the whole thing had been for Ed (her husband) and that maybe things had been pretty nasty for the baby too and I just gave myself a real hard talking-to about getting in there and starting to work on the problem. Then I went home and I really tried and there were still some pretty bad times but I began to feel a bit better. And I got to know some of the girls, we did exchange sitting because when you have a baby like mine it's not all that easy for a sitter who's used to a quiet baby and some of the girls had pretty good ideas about how to work out some of the problems around the house and after a while I began to think of some ideas too. I even started feeling better about the baby, not much better but a little better. . . .

## Arrangements and Instructions that Make the Child Rearing Task Easier

One major change perhaps initiated by the pediatrician but carried out by other professionals such as a public health nurse would be in basic care routines, an *ease routine*. With a difficult infant or young child there are almost always changes that can be made in basic care routines that will result in a more harmonious mother-child interaction. For example, the overactive infant typically is very difficult to handle in the bathing situation: he wriggles about, flails his arms, screams his protests, and generally prolongs the period required to complete the bath routine far beyond the time that should be needed. The mother should be shown how to set up the needed materials and impose restraints on the infant so that the bath routine does not leave the participants exhausted. One procedure that helps the mother keep control of the infant is to put a terry-cloth harness on that she can grasp if the infant wriggles away. One mother reported that she eliminated her son's tendency to flail about with his arms by having a box of small light-weight waterproof toys beside the bath. Whenever she picked one up he would grab it and as soon as he threw it away she handed him another. It is important that the overactive infant be protected from self-injury through such devices as a padded crib, a padded high-chair, and blunt play objects.

A basic change must usually be made in the mother's *behavior management techniques,* particularly in her reactions and responses to signs of distress or disruptive behavior in the child. Typically, the mother responds immediately to crying, screaming, and unrest, partly because the noise is disturbing to her but primarily because she thinks she can remedy the situation. When the baby is quiet she leaves him alone. According to reinforcement principles this behavior pattern will prolong the disruptive behavior and might even increase it because the mother is rewarding and thus strengthening the baby's distress behavior by responding to it, and not rewarding his quiet behavior and thus weakening any tendencies to be quiet. The fact is that with the really difficult child she often cannot directly stop the screaming and restlessness. What is important for both parents is that they have *planned responses* to the infant's difficult behavior. By this we mean that the parent decides in advance what his response will be if the infant responds in a particular way. This procedure has the effect of making the parent feel that he is in control of the situation and is ready to cope with any problems that arise. Psychologically, he feels ahead. The planned response strategy is also applicable to older hyperactive children. One effective response for the mother to use when the child screams is to check that he is comfortable and not hungry, thirsty, or wet, provide brief attention and, if he fails to respond, leave him, preferably with the door shut. Nothing will happen to the child if the mother does this and she will know by the volume that the child is alive and active. When he becomes quiet she should re-enter the room and talk to him and play with him for as long as is reasonable. Thus she can reward his quiet periods and nonreward his restlessness. The mother must be convinced that this is the correct procedure to follow; she should reassure the neighbors and have available a statement from the pediatrician because the publicity about battered children has had the commendable effect of increasing the tendency of neighbors and bystanders to call the police when a child sounds as if he is being mistreated.

An excellent example that could be used to show parents the way in which a mother's social behavior may function as a powerful reinforcer for such tantrum-type behaviors is contained in a study by Williams (1959). The subject was a 21-month-old boy who had been seriously ill for the first 18 months of life and had required special care and attention. When he had recovered from his illness he continued to demand attention by screaming and fussing when he was put to bed. The parents were instructed to put him to bed in a leisurely and relaxed fashion, shut the door, and not return no matter how long he screamed and raged. Figure 9 shows that the duration of screaming and crying after the door was closed was 45 minutes the first time this procedure was used, zero minutes the second time, possibly because he was exhausted, 10 minutes the third time, and by the tenth time he no longer fussed. The second extinction series was necessary because a week later when an aunt put him to bed he fussed and she reinforced the tantrum behavior by returning to the bedroom and remaining with him until he went to sleep. Following the two extinction series no further tantrums were

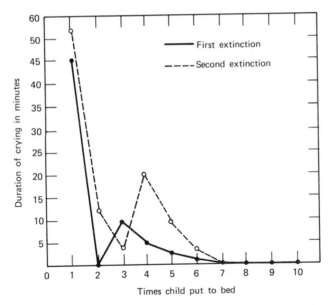

**Figure 9.** Length of crying in two extinction series as a function of successive occasions of being put to bed. (From Williams, C. D. The elimination of tantrum behavior by extinction procedures. *Journal of Abnormal and Social Psychology*, 1959, **59**, 269. Copyright 1959 by the American Psychological Association. Reprinted by permission.)

reported in the next 2 years. It is important to emphasize that no aversive punishment was used: all that was done was to remove the positive reinforcement of parental attention and proximity when the undesirable behaviors occurred.

Caring for the difficult infant or young child is an exhausting task. An essential component in any preventive strategy is the provision of some *regular child care arrangement* that will provide the mother with a breathing space and permit both parents to enjoy outside activities together. The infant's father will have a better picture of the difficulties the mother faces daily if he regularly acts as babysitter. The father's participation in the prevention program is likely to be limited, of necessity, by the demands of work. However, he should be included in some discussions with the pediatrician and should assume some of the caretaking responsibilities. The mother will be better able to cope with the infant if she knows that her husband is aware of the difficulty of the problem.

## Procedures that Modify the Infant's Behavior

### Sleep

If parents of hyperactive infants were asked to rank the infants' problem behaviors in terms of annoyance value, it is likely that sleep problems would rank highest. The hyperactive infant typically does not go to sleep easily and when he does the duration of sleep is much shorter than that of the average infant. Research by several investigators (Ambrose, 1969; Barnard & Collar, 1973; Freedman, 1969) has suggested that duration of quiet sleep may be increased through stimulation of the infant by rocking. In an ongoing study at the University of Washington, Barnard and Collar (1973) have used an isolette rocker that combines horizontal rocking movements with auditory stimulation in the form of heartbeat sounds at approximately 85 decibels. Automatic programming turns on this combination of stimulation for 15 minutes every hour. These investigators reported a marked increase in duration of quiet sleep in premature infants after 4 weeks in the rocker. Freedman (1969) used movement stimulation only, as did Ambrose (1969), and found that adaptation to the rocker was associated with increased fussing, but thereafter most infants tended to be hyperrelaxed and almost immediately drowsy. Although the rocker used in these studies would probably constitute a major expense for young parents, Stewart and Olds (1973) have suggested that a similar effect can be achieved with a set of four springs that can be attached to the legs of the infant's crib and an electronic gadget that simulates a heartbeat, both of which are available in department stores and are quite inexpensive. The sleep-inducing property of other types of continuous monotonous stimulation, such as continuous white noise, lullaby, and metronome, have also been demonstrated. Several research findings suggest that continuous stimulation can increase the total sleep time as well as the duration of quiet sleep without decreasing the duration of active sleep. This stimulation procedure can also reduce motor activity. For a comprehensive review of the present state of empirical knowledge of the effects of continuous monotonous stimulation on sleep in early infancy see Schmidt (1975).

## Waking Restlessness

Research by Denenberg (1969) and others (Scott, 1970; Van den Daele, 1970, 1971; Wolff, 1966) has shown that restlessness in young infants and children can often be reduced by introducing specific types of stimulation into the environment. Their findings suggest that *visual stimulation* in the form of patterning as opposed to plain colors, and visual movement such as mobiles; *auditory stimulation* in the form of talking, singing, and recorded music; and *tactual stimulation,* touching and holding, all serve to quieten the restless infant and young child.

When the daytime restlessness takes the form of steady crying that is not terminated by events suggestive of gastrointestinal discomfort, such as passing gas, spitting up, or being burped, there are several other interventions readily available to the mother that may serve to quieten the infant. Pacifier sucking is particularly effective early in life. Wolff (1969) has suggested that the pacifier sucking facilitates sleep by serving the protective function of inhibition of diffuse activity. The rationale for this statement is as follows: One prerequisite for sleep is a relative absence of variable stimulation, and this condition is not met in the motorically active infant because the proprioceptive feedback from his restless movements maintains a state of arousal. Furthermore, restlessness of the degree characteristic of a hyperactive infant tends to maintain itself in the same way that a temper tantrum does. Pacifier sucking inhibits competing motor behaviors including restlessness, thereby interrupting the self-perpetuating cycle of crying and restlessness and providing the essential conditions for sleep. According to Wolff's (1969) reasoning rocking is often successful in facilitating sleep because it substitutes a constant, rhythmical form of stimulation for the higher arousal proprioceptive stimulation from spontaneous restlessness and crying and this constant stimulation lowers the general arousal state, thus facilitating sleep or quietening the wide-awake infant.

## Swaddling

This procedure for restraining an infant by wrapping him firmly, almost tightly, with strips of cloth is one that has been used for centuries to quieten crying infants and is very effective providing it is skillfully done. If the swaddling only restricts the range of movement rather than immobilizing the infant, the result is an increased arousal effect as the infant forcefully resists and may elicit what is known as an angry cry. Incomplete swaddling increases *variable* proprioceptive feedback, whereas good swaddling provides *constant* tactile stimulation. Continuous stimulation in the form of white noise or white light well below the pain threshold has a similar effect, but neither of these methods is as available to parents as are pacifier sucking and swaddling. Tapping various parts of the body, particularly the spinal column, and rhythmically rubbing the infant's back may also stop crying.

## Positive Mother-Child Interaction

The most difficult change for the pediatrician to effect is to teach the mother to relax and enjoy her difficult child by interacting with him in a positive way. Such interactions occur less frequently between a mother and child at risk than in the normal mother-child relationship so that the child suffers a form of social deprivation the consequences of which add to his existing problems and future interpersonal difficulties. By the time a mother who has had no guidance seeks help for difficulties with her child, she has learned to feel one way about him, and typically these feelings are not loving. It is essential that the mother learn to enjoy the child. Participation in a discussion group for mothers with difficult children often facilitates this kind of learning in addition to its other benefits. The mother must learn how to interact with the infant in positive, loving, relaxed ways that will facilitate the development in the infant of basic trust. One such method, developed by Henderson and his associates and reported in Dahlin, Engelsing, and Henderson (1975), consists in part of increased amounts of gentle, loving, physical contact in the form of massage for relaxation of muscle tension and accompanied by talking in a soothing tone. The infant is held on the adult's lap throughout this interaction. Dahlin et al. note that the physical containment of holding ultimately comes to represent comfort and security to the infant. Most of all she must begin to play with him in a relaxed way. Play will reduce irritability in the infant and, more important, will lessen the feeling of mutual alienation that is likely to pervade the relationship. Even very young infants express positive responses to short repetitive singing games that involve mother-child tactual contact, the manipulation of brightly colored objects, and balloon play, and older infants enjoy clapping activities, watching objects being removed from closed containers, and now-you-see-it, now-you-don't play.

The apparent helplessness of the neonate and infant suggest a unidirectional effect in the early mother-child relationship, but in fact it is bidirectional (Bell, 1968). Even in an uneventful mother-child relationship, the direction of effect from infant to mother is a strong one with the infant influencing the mother to adjust to him in a particular way as his characteristics evoke specific responses from her. When there is any prolonged difficulty, as in the case of the continually restless and irritable infant, the effect on the mother is intensified as she strives to adjust her behavior to cope with the demands of the infant. When she is unsuccessful, as she usually is, there is a deterioration in the mother-child relationship that reinforces the already existing difficulties and increases the negative influence of the infant's difficulties on the eventual outcome of the relationship. A preventive strategy should equip the mother to withstand the physical and psychological assault by the infant, an assault that is sometimes launched in the first day or two of extrauterine life.

The following is an extreme example of the influence of a particularly difficult neonate on the mother-child relationship when the mother, on leaving the hospital, was *not* equipped with a broad-based intervention strategy designed to cover as many facets of the infant's life as possible (Brazelton, 1961, pp. 509–511):

George was the first child of a 30-year-old research professor and his 28-year-old wife who also was a scientist. The baby arrived after 5 years of saving "to have a baby." The mother expressed delight in her pregnancy, voiced her determination to breast-feed her infant because it was a family tradition, and arranged for no medication to be given during labor. Her husband was at her side throughout labor, recording in detail every pain. After 12 hours of labor spinal anesthesia was administered and delivery followed immediately. The infant cried at once, his color was excellent, and he showed no signs of distress. The birth weight was 8-½ pounds. Findings of physical examination on the day of birth were normal.

On observation the baby characteristically exhibited two states and they were constant throughout his hospital stay. They were extreme states and the transition from one to the other was strikingly rapid, even though he showed a marked resistance to changing from one state to the other.

The first state was a deep sleep in which he was quite floppy, with poor muscle tone, and with little spontaneous movement or any startle reaction present. The baby was difficult to rouse; stimuli caused no change in alertness. When picked up he adjusted briefly with some muscle tone, eyes opened briefly, then he resumed his limp original state and one was struck by his refractoriness and his capacity to maintain this flaccid, relatively unresponsive state.

The second state consisted of screaming, hyperactivity, and hypersensitivity to stimuli. His activity consisted of constant thrusting, thrashing movements of the extremities intermingled with cyclic reflex startling to his own sudden movements. In this state, he seemed overreactive, and any mild stimulus seemed to perpetuate this activity. A major stimulus, such as a loud noise was able to briefly quiet him, following which his activity quickly reached a peak. This hyperactive state maintained itself for 15 to 20 minutes. The continuous hyperactivity interfered with any organized behavior such as sucking on a nipple, or any spontaneous quieting. Major restraints, such as swaddling were necessary to quiet him, and these restraints were finally instituted to facilitate nursing. As he became quiet, he very rapidly lapsed into the deep sleep state.

Since these two extreme states persisted after the first 5 days a neurological consultation was sought. The neurologist concluded that the infant was neurologically intact; however, he considered that the extremes of state, together with the refractoriness to stimuli and the capacity to maintain these two different states for such long periods, were definitely unusual.

The effect which this unreachable baby had on the new mother, with her determination to nurse, was dramatic. She became depressed over his "rejection of her," wept a great deal, ate poorly, and, as a result, was less and less effective in handling this maverick. With assistance from the nurses and the pediatrician, and by swaddling, after 7 days the baby began to nurse effectively and gained enough at the breast by the eighth day so that he could be discharged. At home, each breast feeding was a stormy 1½ to 2½ hour period, with the mother weeping and the baby screaming — "a nightmare of who would outlast the other." The mother remained determined to nurse. The baby had long periods of screaming each day, totaling 6 to 8 hours, and could not be quieted. The mother kept a detailed diary of each day and minute by minute recorded her unsuccessful, anxious attempts to reach her child. This screaming, thrashing pattern blended imperceptibly with another kind of unreachableness by 4 to 5 months in which he would lie staring at a bird mobile for long periods, and he seemed little gratified by being played with or held by his anxious, depressed mother. His father could get a better response but said "he is not as much fun as I expected him to be," and withdrew to his laboratory. The mother spent a part of every day in communication with her pediatrician and the baby was seen frequently to reassure her. No neurological or physical abnormality was ever found. The baby gained rapidly and seemed entirely healthy.

At the 5 months' examination the infant lay on the examining table and seemed unreachable. The examiner continued to talk to him in a soothing, quiet voice, and he began to look at the examiner. After some 20 minutes he even smiled briefly and allowed himself to be held, looking away from the examiner's face. (Earlier, he had screamed constantly until he was put down.) After 30 minutes, he responded by adapting his body to the examiner's arms, and with a look and a brief smile. The mother commented bitterly on how unusual this response was. As she took him from the pediatrician, he began to scream pitifully and her eagerness changed to rigid anger.

Motor development was slow but there was always evidence of a capacity to perform. The social responses were particularly uneven. He either cried when in new places or became silent and immobilized.

By 7 months his mother felt driven to seek psychotherapy and continued such treatment for 1½ years. After 2 months the mother observed, "at last I can see George as he really is. I always thought it was just my fault." The child began to make progress. He sat alone at 10 months, walked alone at 20, put words together by 28 months. At 6 or 7 months of age he could not be taken out of the house without screaming constantly. By 2½ he played on an equal level with 2-year-old children, and his mother and father had the courage to have another baby.

This second child, a boy also, was an easy, attractive, outgoing infant from the first. The mother nursed him for 9 months and had great delight in him. George regressed briefly after his mother's return from the hospital. Then he seemed to profit from the general happiness and relief in the family, and he has continued to progress more normally. His mother still says, "He knows how to win any struggle with me. He just screams or acts as if he cannot see or hear me, and I cannot fight back."[*]

This case provides a clear-cut example of the traumatic effects on the mother-child relationship of failure to discuss the infant's characteristics with the mother and to follow up with a strategy equipping her to handle her difficult infant. The pediatrician in this case recognized that "an early prediction of his difficult characteristics and some sort of elaboration of the limitations of his responses to *any* environment might have relieved some of the anxiety and guilt which furthered her incapacity as a mother to him" (Brazelton, 1961, p. 511), but cited two reasons for rejecting this course of action: one was the problem of reliable evaluation of the neonate and the other concerned the way in which the mother might use such predictions. The pediatrician appeared to view such predictions as possibly hazardous to the mother-child relationship. In our approach we would not consider that evaluation was uncertain given the description of the neonate's be-

Reprinted, by permission, from Brazelton, T. B.: Psychophysiologic reactions in the neonate. I. The value of observation of the neonate. *J. Pediatr. 58:* 509–512, 1961.

havior. Without making long-term predictions it was clear that an immediate problem existed. Furthermore, the way in which the mother might use the predictions would not be a decision that she would make. The pediatrician in our view should take an active part in developing strategies to help the mother handle the problem infant and would see that she had instruction in using the strategies correctly.

The management of this case is in marked contrast to the prevention strategies advocated here. It was clear in the first 5 days that the deviations were not chance fluctuations, so intervention was warranted. The child's characteristics would have been discussed with both parents and a specific strategy provided. The parents' tendencies to emphasize the negative aspects of the child's birth and behavior through detailed lists, and other secondary factors in the problem, would have been discouraged and the mother directed to focusing on positive aspects of the infant's behavior. With information gained from the nursing staff and the pediatrician's own observations, recommendations would have been made on how best to manage each of the basic care procedures. For example, the mother would have been strongly discouraged from breast feeding the infant in view of the trauma that this invoked. Emphasis would have been placed on the infant's contribution to the problem and the importance of working within and adapting to the confines of his temperament. The mother would have been enrolled immediately in a discussion group, instructed in behavior management techniques, and encouraged to engage in positive interactions such as play with the infant. The husband would have been urged to assume some regular responsibility for caretaking and to make provisions for some regular outside child care.

From the discussion of prevention in this chapter it is clear that the pediatrician has neither the time to carry out a preventive strategy nor the expertise to collect some of the data. His primary role is to decide whether an investigation should be undertaken and to set it in motion. He is in a strategic position to initiate such action because of his knowledge of the developmental process, his long association with the child and family and his observations of them, and his acceptance by the parents. However, effective prevention depends on a multidisciplinary or team approach. This topic has been described briefly in this chapter and will be developed further in the remaining two chapters.

# CHAPTER 8

# *Management*

The basic management procedure for the hyperactive child is a *comprehensive plan of action* designed to modify his behavior, with the immediate goal being more effective functioning in the home and school environments, and the long-term goal being optimal psychological development and educational progress. The assumption underlying this approach is that hyperactivity is a complex problem with potentially pervasive and long-lasting effects. The high activity level may decrease with age; however, the basic learning and emotional problems characteristic of hyperactivity tend to persist into adolescence and adulthood in the absence of an intensive treatment program (Stewart, Mendelson, & Johnson, 1973; Weiss, Minde, Werry, Douglas, & Nemeth, 1971). Treatment is the responsibility of a professional team rather than solely that of the pediatrician; it may be extensive and may involve any combination of three treatment modalities: psychotherapy, pharmacotherapy, and environmental manipulation.

The prerequisite to the design and implementation of a comprehensive management plan is a complete medical, psychoeducational, and behavioral evaluation of the child, including an assessment of his psychological environment, with particular attention to the pervasive effects of his problem behavior. The evaluation procedures serve the dual purpose of confirming the condition of hyperactivity and providing an objective and rational basis for the development of a management strategy. The competencies of individuals from several disciplines are required to conduct such an evaluation because of the expansion in the last 2 decades of assessment methodology coupled with the specialized nature of much of the knowledge in the area of behavior problems. Such an interdisciplinary group might function independently with each member contributing his skill as needed, as a team with one member making decisions on the procedures to be followed, or as a staffing conference with decisions being the consensus of the group. The goal of the evaluation is not just to arrive at a diagnosis, but rather to make a complete assessment of all potentially relevant aspects of the child and his family, with special attention to the identification of factors within the child or his environment that may be interacting to maintain his hyperactive behavior. All information that is acquired should be pooled and then used as a basis for devising a management program. Evaluation will be facilitated if each member of the group has a reasonable knowledge of the assessment and treatment procedures used by the other group members. Although the specific evaluative procedures used would depend on the training and experience of the participants, a comprehensive evaluation of the kind proposed here should include medical, psychoeducational, behavioral, and environmental assessments, and representative methods of assessment within each of these categories will be described.

At the present time and for most cases the comprehensive multidisciplinary evaluation recommended here would be done in a clinic setting or by the child's own pediatrician and other professionals that he recommends, rather than in the school setting. This locus may change since a new development has occurred in the school health program that may make evaluations within the child's own school setting the rule rather than the exception. During the last 5 years school health has come to be viewed as directly related to the learning process and advocates of this viewpoint (see, for example, Kappelman, Roberts, Rinaldi, & Cornblath, 1975) have urged the redefinition of school health to include the behavior and learning problems of childhood. Furthermore, Kappelman et al. and others (Menkes, 1972; Nader, Emmel, & Charney, 1972) have recommended that school health programs give these problems top priority. This approach requires a new pediatric specialist, the school health physician with specialized training and expertise about school facilities and educational methods, as well as a multidisciplinary team of educational, psychological, nursing, and other specialists. This team provides on-site diagnosis, makes recommendations for remedial action, conducts some of the remedial work, and follows up each case to evaluate the outcome. This type of program has been operating for several years with considerable success in the Baltimore area (Kappelman, Roberts, Rinaldi, & Cornblath, 1975). In describing its effectiveness Kappelman et al. note an increase in number of referrals over the previous year when no such program was available and attribute the increase to the presence of the team in the school. Concomitant with such a program should be in-service training for teachers in the school so that they maintain perspective on which problems lie appropriately within their own jurisdiction.

## MEDICAL EXAMINATION

The essential components of a complete medical examination are a basic clinical history, a complete physical examination, routine laboratory tests, and specialized physiological tests as required. In addition to routine information about the child and his family, the history and physical examination period should provide the pediatrician with three kinds of information relevant to the management of hyperactivity. One kind is provided by the opportunity for directly observing a sample of the mother-child relationship. The assumption is that the maternal behaviors observed, particularly the reinforcement style of the mother, are not idiosyncratic to the pediatrician's office situation but are characteristic of the mother-child interaction in many situations, and are therefore relevant to the behavior problem of the child. Another kind of information that the history provides concerns the mother's perception of the child and his problem and her evaluation of them. It is important to determine if the mother focuses on the difficulties that the child's behavior is creating for her and her husband or if she seems primarily concerned with the effects of the child's behavior on his own psychological development and well-being. The mother whose main concern is the inconvenience that the child is causing her is not likely to be an effective participant in any treatment strategy without increased understanding and new and more effective management skills. Ideally, the parents should be genuinely concerned about the child, and at the same time be apprehensive about the disruptive effects of his behavior on the rest of the family. A third kind of information concerns the type of family the child comes from. This information may pinpoint secondary etiological factors that interact with other facets of the case to exacerbate the hyperactivity. It also provides a basis for deciding what contribution the parents and siblings might be capable of making, and whether or not it is realistic to include them in the intervention program as active participants.

**History**

A basic clinical history should include detailed information on the pregnancy, birth process, and medical events of the neonatal and infancy periods similar to that described in the chapter on prevention. Compared to mothers of normal children, mothers of hyperactive children more often report a history of accidents and illnesses during pregnancy and delivery that could have caused brain damage although the pregnancy and delivery are often without difficulty (Werry, Weiss, & Douglas, 1964). A stormy neonatal and infant adjustment period characterized by marked restlessness, irritability, feeding difficulties, and sleep problems is also more prevalent (Barnard & Collar, 1973; Nichamin, 1972; Stewart, Pitts, Craig, & Dieruf, 1966).

In noting the medical events and pattern of development through infancy and childhood the pediatrician should be alert for evidence of accidents and accidental poisoning, which occur more often in the hyperactive child (Stewart, Thach, & Freidin, 1970), slow development especially in speech, and any conditions such as a history of allergy or failure of treatment with medication in which the use of medication for hyperactivity might be contraindicated. Information should also be obtained of evidence of the familial incidence of hyperactivity, severe behavior problems, and psychiatric disturbances, particularly in the first or second degree relatives of the child. Research by Cantwell (1972) and Stewart and Morrison (1973) has demonstrated an increased prevalence of alcoholism, sociopathy, hysteria, and a history of hyperactivity in the childhood of parents and relatives of hyperactive children. Knowing the incidence of such disorders may or may not be of help in making a diagnosis, but in any case knowledge of problems in the immediate family is essential in assessing the family's potential for participating in the treatment program.

The *age of onset* of the hyperactive behavior is important for diagnostic and treatment purposes. Hyperactive behavior that has its onset late in the preschool years and that appears suddenly is more likely to be etiologically related to noxious social or nonsocial environmental factors than is hyperactivity that appears in early infancy. Often hyperactivity is present in early infancy but is attributed to colic or is viewed only as evidence that the infant is a light sleeper and a restless child, so the mother may be unaware of any problem until the infant begins to move around. The pediatrician should elicit details of the characteristics of the hyperactive behavior, for example, whether it is constant, cyclic, or only occurs in highly stimulating situations. He should also use the dimensions of behavior identified by Chess, Thomas, and Birch (1968) to construct profiles of the present temperament of the child and his temperament in infancy.

## Physical Examination

The pediatrician may not see evidence of the child's hyperactive behavior in the examination situation. Most children are subdued in the doctor's office and the hyperactive child is no exception. In addition, he usually functions more effectively in a one-to-one situation.

The following components should be regarded as essential for a complete physical examination of the hyperactive child:

1. The child's physical condition should be evaluated to rule out the possibility of medical conditions such as hyperthyroidism that are characterized by extreme restlessness and emotional lability. During the physical examination the pediatrician should be alert to the presence of characteris-

tics such as head circumference out of the normal range, unusually fine hair that will not comb down, *epicanthus,* that is, a fold of skin covering the point at which the upper and lower eyelids join the nose, widely spaced eyes, malformed or asymmetrical ears, and a wide space between the first and second toes. Waldrop and her associates (Waldrop & Goering, 1971; Waldrop & Halverson, 1971; Waldrop, Pedersen, & Bell, 1968) have provided unequivocal evidence of a positive association between high anomaly scores and hyperactivity in young preschool and elementary school children. In general, a high incidence of minor physical anomalies was apt to be associated with hyperactive, aggressive, impatient, and intractable behavior in the preschool and elementary school settings although the behavior concomitants of the anomaly score tended to be less consistent for girls than for boys. Table 7 lists the anomalies used in their preschool study with brief definitions and scoring weights. Quinn and Rapoport (1974) believe that the presence of minor physical anomalies indicates that fetal insults have occurred and that hyperactivity is a result of the same insults affecting the central nervous system during early morphogenesis. Schain (1974) has pointed out that these anomalies may also be a sign of low intelligence and that the slow learner or child of borderline intelligence may react to the stress of academic demands that are beyond his ability with hyperactive or disruptive behavior. It follows that the pediatrician should be alert to the *possibility* that the presence of minor physical anomalies is associated with an intellectual deficit, which in turn is the primary etiological factor in the hyperactivity. If this is the case, the basic management strategy would be to initiate changes in the school situation rather than introduce intervention procedures such as pharmacotherapy that are aimed directly at the hyperactive behavior.

2. A neurological examination should be conducted to eliminate the possibility of a progressive disease of the central nervous system that may present as hyperactivity. If the child has major neurological handicaps an examination by a neurologist and the use of specialized tests may be required to rule out seizures, growths, or degenerative brain disease. A routine EEG is not justified in the absence of any suspected seizure activity. In discussing the value of the EEG in the workup of the hyperactive child, Cravens (Schmitt, Martin, Nellhaus, Cravens, Camp, & Jordan, 1973, p. 157) states:

First, in terms of diagnosis, the normal EEG does not mean that brain damage is absent; nor, reversely, does an abnormal EEG alone mean minimal cerebral dysfunction or minimal brain damage. Diagnosis must depend on the history and physical and neurologic findings — not on the EEG. The specific type of EEG abnormality might be of use to an investigator in neurophysiology but is not useful to the pediatrician dealing with a hyperactive child. Second, with respect to treatment, there is no EEG pattern which either compels or contraindicates a trial of medication.

With careful examination, soft neurologic signs can often be observed without special testing, the types of impaired neurological function often seen in hyperactivity being motor impersistence, incoordination, impaired alternating movements of the forearms, ataxia, inability to hop, Babinskis, synkinetic movements, involuntary movements, graphesthesia, and speech impairment (Millichap, 1968). Special techniques to detect soft signs have been described in detail by Aron (1972) and, as noted in the chapter on prevention, Goodman and Sours (1967) have described a "play" neurological examination. The significance of these signs is a matter of considerable controversy (Clements & Peters, 1962; Ingram, 1973; Wender, 1971; Werry & Sprague, 1970) but their presence is of some relevance to a management strategy.

3. An otological and ophthalmological examination should be conducted to rule out sensory defects that may be causing or contributing to the child's problem behavior. The child's level of speech development should be noted because speech abnormalities have been reported in a minority of hyperactive children (De Hirsch, 1973) and speech therapy may be required. Defects of vision and hearing are also present in a minority of hyperactive children (Stewart, Pitts, Craig, & Dieruf, 1966) and constitute a kind of sensory deprivation that may result in hyperactive behavior.

There is some controversy about the necessity for and value of a comprehensive medical examination (such as the one described above) in assessing hyperactivity in childhood. Kenny and his associates (Kenny, Clemmens, Hudson, Lentz, Cicci, & Nair, 1971) conducted evaluations on 100 children who were referred for hyperactivity to an interdisciplinary diagnostic and evaluation clinic. Each child received a thorough evaluation that included a complete medical and social history, a physical examination, and a neurological evaluation with emphasis on "soft signs." Electroencephalograms were obtained on 78 of the children. In the course of the evaluation each child was seen by three members of the evaluation staff who were instructed to make global judgments of the child's activity level. On the basis of the data, which showed no significant relationship among the neurological examination, EEG, and final diagnosis, these investigators concluded that requirements such as a medical diagnosis, neurological examination, and EEG prior to placement of hyperactive children in special education programs were inappropriate and that "the medical model has, at best, a minimal role to play in the evaluation of hyperactivity" (1971, p. 622).

We strongly disagree with this conclusion. Hyperactivity is a symptom, not a disease, so medical conditions such as metabolic problems, lead poisoning, and diseases of the central nervous system may present with hyperactivity as a primary symptom. In the absence of an adequate medical examination the child may be dismissed as hyperactive, given medication, and placed in a special class, when some other treatment may be indicated and urgently needed. Some good examples of the failure to initially pursue an intensive medical search for the etiology of hyperactivity in children are contained in an article by Walker (1974), in which he describes the case of a 5-year-old girl who was referred because she was hyperactive, had difficulties in school, and was prone to tantrums. A neurologist had diagnosed her as schizophrenic and prescribed loving care. The history revealed that the child had always tired easily and that both her fatigue and disruptive behavior were more evident at high altitudes than at sea level. Physical examination showed that certain veins at the back of the retina were congested with blood; such vein engorgement is sometimes a sign of cardiac problems and Walker did detect a moderate heart murmur. An EEG showed brain wave patterns indicative of an oxygenation problem. The child was referred to a cardiologist who found that she had an extra vessel between the heart and lung that was preventing a normal flow of oxygen to the brain. Following corrective surgery the child's hyperactivity, fatigue, rages, and tantrums disappeared and she progressed well in school without medication. Without a multidimensional approach to diagnosis, her hyperactivity would have continued and death would have occurred in a few years as a result of her cardiac problem. Walker reports several other cases in which hyperactivity was due to medical problems, including an 8-year-old boy with hypoglycemia whose inability to tolerate and assimilate glucose lead to hyperactivity which abated when he was put on a high protein, low carbohydrate diet; and a 9-year-old boy who had been on medication for over 2½ years whose hyperactivity abated as soon as he was treated for a calcium deficiency. Although we agree with Werry's (1968) statement that "the medical examination appears to have little role to play in the routine clinical assessment of the non-defective, physically healthy, hyperactive child," the cases reported by Walker (1974) and the discussion of etiology of hyperactivity in McMahon, Deem and Greenberg (1970) suggest that it is extremely important to establish first that the child *is* physically healthy and it is difficult to see how this can be achieved without a medical examination.

## PSYCHOEDUCATIONAL ASSESSMENT

The purpose of this assessment is to measure the basic intellectual capacity of the child and his academic performance. The intellectual assessment is essential to rule out the possibility that the child's behavior problem is a reaction to classroom demands far in excess of his capacity. For example, a retarded child or a child of borderline intelligence generally is unable to function effectively in a regular class without transitional help and may react to the frustrations in the situation with disruptive behavior. Assessment of school performance provides information on possible discrepancies between IQ test scores and actual achievement and is relevant to the subsequent management plan. The hyperactive child is often characterized by marked school dysfunction as a result of either his high level of activity, poor attention span, and generally disruptive behavior, or inadequate intelligence. Although most studies of hyperactive children have reported learning difficulties, the exact nature and reason for these difficulties is a matter of contention. The tests described below are among those frequently used to determine the functional intellectual ability and academic achievement of the hyperactive child. Many of these tests can be administered by personnel at the child's school.

## Intelligence Tests

A large number of individually administered intelligence tests are available. The two tests most often used are the Stanford-Binet Intelligence Test and the Wechsler Intelligence Scale for Children (WISC). Both tests have varied content: the Stanford-Binet is largely verbal and yields a single IQ, whereas the WISC includes performance as well as verbal tests and yields three scores, Verbal, Performance, and Full Scale. The Peabody Picture Vocabulary Test and the Goodenough Draw-A-Man Scale are also used extensively. Many clinicians consider the WISC to be superior to the other tests because it gives a performance score and the pattern of subtest scores yields more information than an overall IQ. Brief descriptions of these tests are given here, but for more detailed information the reader is referred to Anastasi (1968) and Buros (1972).

The *Stanford-Binet Intelligence Scale* has tests grouped into age levels ranging from II to Superior Adult. The test proceeds by half-year intervals for ages II to V and by yearly intervals for ages V to XIV. Each age level from II to XIV contains six tests with one alternative test; all seven are of approximately uniform difficulty. Each child is tested individually over a limited range of age levels suited to his own intellectual level. Testing usually takes 30 to 40 minutes for younger children and an hour or more for older children. There is a wide variety of item content including manipulation of objects and eye-hand coordination, observation and identification of common objects, similarities and differences between sets of objects, common-sense questions, tests of spatial orientation such as maze tracing and paper folding, numerical and memory tests, and many tests employing verbal content such as vocabulary, sentence completion, and proverb interpretation. The technical quality of the standardization procedures is high, with high scale reliability coefficients (.83 to .91 for ages 2½ to 5½, and .91 and above for ages 6 to 13) and criterion-related validity (correlates highly with performance in most academic courses, particularly the predominantly verbal ones).

The *Wechsler Intelligence Scale for Children* (WISC), for ages 5 to 15 years, provides a verbal score obtained from five subtests (general information, comprehension, arithmetic, similarities, vocabulary) and one alternate (digit span); and a performance score from five subtests (picture completion, picture arrangement, block design, object assembly, coding) and one alternate (mazes). Split-half reliabilities for the Full Scale, Verbal, and Performance Scales are satisfactory (for a 7½-year-old sample of 200 cases, .92, .88, and .86 respectively). However, subtest reliabilities are much lower, so judgments based on *differences between subtest scores,* including profile analysis, are on shaky ground. The WISC is well-standardized, stable over time (scores correlated .77 over a 4-year period), and correlates generally in the .80s with other tests of intelligence. However there are consistent discrepancies between the WISC and Stanford-Binet at different ages and intellectual levels. The main criticism of the test is the limited validity data.

The *Wechsler Preschool and Primary Scale of Intelligence* is a downward extension of the WISC for ages 4 to 6½ years. It follows the same format as the WISC, giving a Verbal, Performance, and Full Scale IQ. Three of the 11 subtests (Sentences, Animal House, and Geometric Design) are new. The remainder are adaptations or extensions of WISC subtests. Testing time is 50 to 75 minutes in one to two testing sessions. The standardization procedures were excellent, the reliabilities are satisfactorily high (.92 for the Full Scale after an 11-week interval), but validity data are minimal.

The *Peabody Picture Vocabulary Test* is a brief individual test of intelligence for ages 2½ to 18 years in which the test materials are cards, each with four pictures. The cards are arranged in ascending order of difficulty. The task on each item is to look at the four pictures on a card and point to the one that best illustrates the meaning of a test word spoken by the examiner. Testing proceeds from a basal age corresponding to eight consecutive correct responses to a ceiling corresponding to eight consecutive failures. No verbal response is required, so the test can also be administered to people with aphasia, speech impediments, and reading problems, as well as to the emotionally disturbed. Testing time is approximately 15 minutes. There are alternate forms, A and B, with reliability ranging from

.67 to .84. There are moderately high correlations with other intelligence tests (.60 with the WISC and .70 with the Stanford-Binet). There is some evidence of moderate predictive validity against academic achievement tests.

The *Goodenough Draw-A-Man Scale* is often used for a rapid assessment of intelligence. In this test the child is given a pencil and paper and instructed to "draw a whole man and the best man you can draw. Make *all* of him." The drawing is scored for detail and complexity. Although the test may appear to be a measure of visual motor coordination, it taps more complex functions. The test score correlates with the Stanford-Binet and the WISC, and correlates highly with social adjustment. It is attractive to children, can be easily administered and scored, and has good reliability. Research by Crowe (1972) has shown that hyperactive boys performed poorly on body image as measured by human figure drawings when compared to normal boys. The differences occurred independently of intelligence. When hyperactive boys were on psychoactive drugs they performed better than hyperactive boys on placebo.

## Achievement Tests

A number of tests have been developed for measuring the child's general educational achievement level in the basic academic subjects. When this type of test is used with children who are entering first grade it is usually called a *readiness test*. For the child who is already in school the test content becomes more advanced and the term *achievement test* is used. The following is a brief description of one of the most widely used readiness tests.

The *Metropolitan Readiness Tests* are group tests generally used to measure readiness to enter grade one. Each of the two forms consists of six subtests: word meaning (the child selects from a row of three pictures the one that the examiner names), listening (one or more sentences are used to identify the correct picture in a row), matching, alphabet (the child identifies on the page the letter named by the examiner), numbers (quantitative concepts and simple numerical operations), and copying (geometric forms, numbers, letters). Both the alternate-form and split-half reliabilities are over .90. There is evidence of predictive validity: correlations with end-of-year achievement test scores ranged from .57 to .67. The test appears to measure abilities believed to be associated with success in early school learning. Standardization procedures were satisfactory. Administration time is 60 minutes, in three sessions.

The *Wide Range Achievement Test Revised Edition* (WRAT) is a timed test with two levels, one for ages 5 to 11 years and the other for ages 12 years and over. It gives three scores, spelling, arithmetic, and reading. It is basically an individual test, but there is provision for group administration of some parts. It takes from 20 to 30 minutes to administer. It is mentioned here because it is used extensively in experiments evaluating the academic progress of hyperactive children under various treatment conditions, despite inadequate normative data, questionable test reliabilities, dubious content validity, and no supporting external criterion validity data. With these serious inadequacies, any conclusions that are based on experimental subjects' test performance are likely to be invalid, just as an elastic yardstick that may or may not be measuring linear distance is likely to give questionable measures of distance. Studies basing their conclusions concerning academic status solely on this one inadequate test do not advance the field because no confidence can be placed in the test results regardless of their direction in relation to the hypotheses being tested. For example, Wikler, Dixon, and Parker (1970) compared 24 children with scholastic-behavioral problems (forming two subgroups, hyperactive and nonhyperactive) and 24 matched controls on psychometric tests, neurological examination results, and EEG measures. On the psychometric scores Wikler et al. expressed surprise that the patients and controls did not differ on the WRAT as expected. Flynn and Rapoport (1975) reported no differences in the academic performance of hyperactive boys after a year in "open" as compared to "traditional" classrooms. Their finding was based on teachers' descriptions of the boys' academic functioning, and the reading and arithmetic scores of the WRAT. When the behavior being measured spans an extensive period of time, as in this study, it is particularly unproductive to use an inadequate measure of a major dependent variable. Denhoff, Hainsworth, and Hainsworth (1972) assessed the academic status (among other variables) of children aged seven who as infants had been part of a comprehensive investigation of events and complications of pregnancy, delivery, and the neonatal period thought to contribute to deficits in children. Of the 380 children, 184 scored less than 1.7 on the WRAT when a 2.0 grade level was the average expected. On the basis of these unreliable and sparse data the conclusion concerning academic performance was that major and minor neurological signs observable at birth were clearly associated with poor school performance at age seven. Conrad, Dworkin, Shai, and Tobiessen (1971) studied the effects of drug and/or tutoring conditions on the behavior, achievement, and perceptual-cognitive functioning of hyperactive children and reported that neither dextroamphetamine nor tutoring (for 20 weeks, twice a week) significantly influenced academic achievement as measured by the WRAT. In all of these studies the conclusions concerning academic status, which are unequivocally stated, have little or no basis and serve only to muddy the field further.

## ENVIRONMENTAL ASSESSMENT

The task here is to assess three major facets of the child's psychological ecosystem: pervasiveness of effect of the behavior problem, relevant etiological agents, and the presence of helpful resources. An adequate assessment of these facets requires information that must be obtained from relevant adults in the child's environment and from the child himself. The interview with the child may be conducted completely by the pediatrician if his interview skills and the nature of the problem are such that participation of a psychiatrist is not indicated. It is important that the interview be relaxed and nonthreatening; it should establish in the child's eyes that the pediatrician is aware of the difficulties the problem causes the child, is sympathetic about the problem, does not blame the child for it, and intends to take ameliorative action. The pediatrician should keep in mind that the information offered by the child is important for itself and for the extent to which it is consistent with his parents' and teacher's view of the problem. Areas in which discrepancies occur are of particular interest and effort should be directed at obtaining a clear picture of the child's view. Particular attention should be given to the child's account of his relationships with other children because peer relationships are generally considered to be the best single index of overall adjustment of the school-age child (Sundby & Kreyberg, 1969), and others may be unable to provide much information on this topic.

### Pervasiveness of Effect

In how many of the child's environments (e.g., home, school, organized groups, neighborhood) is his behavior problem causing trouble? To obtain information on this question each parent should be interviewed separately to determine how the child gets on at home and in the neighborhood and what the impact is of his behavior problem in these settings. If the child belongs to any formal neighborhood group, such as Cub Scouts, an interview with the adult in charge should be arranged. A report on the child's behavior should be obtained from his homeroom teacher and any other school personnel who have regular opportunities to observe him in different school settings and groups. Sociograms to evaluate his status in his homeroom would be helpful. The information obtained with a sociogram shows the child's place in the social structure of the group, whether he is very popular, disliked, anyone's best or second best friend, and whom he likes and dislikes. The administration of a sociogram to a class or a smaller subgroup need not in any way pinpoint a particular child as the object of an investigation. For the assessment of peer opinion of a child the Peer Nomination Inventory developed by Wiggins and Winder (1961) is particularly effective.

## Relevant Etiological Agents

Are there relevant etiological agents in the child's environment in the sense that social or nonsocial environmental factors, such as family tension or exposure to lead, might be causing, maintaining, or exacerbating the behavior problem? The identification of such agents would be based on the team's observations of the parents and other adults who regularly spend a substantial amount of time with the child. The team should decide to what extent, if any, one or both parents or the child's teacher might be contributing to his behavior either directly, through child rearing or classroom practices, or indirectly through mechanisms such as modeling. Different members of the team should be able to provide information on the presence of nonsocial etiological agents such as lead.

## Environmental Resources

What environmental resources are available? An assessment should be made of the psychological and financial potential of the family for embarking on a long-term plan of management. The *practicality* of requiring the family to participate should be established. If the family is to be of no help, this is the time to find out, *before* incorporating family help into the management program. Do the parents have the time, interest, stamina, and ability to put into action the kinds of intervention that would be recommended? It is important here to assess the school and community resources that would be available, since there is no point in making unrealistic recommendations, such as special class placement, if no special class is available.

## BEHAVIORAL ASSESSMENT

The assessment and interview procedures used here are concerned with the child's own behavior rather than with the effect he has on others or the quality of his interactions with them. The procedures have several purposes, one of which is to differentiate between hyperactivity and a level of activity that is at the extreme end of the normal range. In the case of the latter it would be important to determine if the high active child can inhibit his activity on command as well as the extent to which he exhibits overactivity in inappropriate settings. These qualitative aspects of the activity are the best indices of normality. Another purpose is to identify the primary targets for change in the child's behavior repertoire and, if there is a substantial number of these, assign priorities to them. A third purpose is to determine the child's areas of strength. In assessing a child with a behavior problem the usual procedure is to focus on his difficulties and develop a management program that attempts to remedy his weaknesses. It is our opinion that the assessment routine should also include the identification of the child's strong points, and the management program should then capitalize on these assets in effecting change in the deficit behaviors.

The questions here concern identifying the child's primary symptoms of hyperactivity and determining what secondary symptoms are present. These questions should be directed to his parents, teachers, a psychiatrist, and a psychologist. In addition, measures or estimates should be obtained of how the child sees himself and his world. To evaluate the symptoms of hyperactivity itself both parents should independently rate the child's behavior. We recommend the Werry-Weiss-Peters Activity Scale (see Table 8 and also page 311), although others are available, including the Conners' Parent's Questionnaire (Conners, 1970) and Behavior Problem Checklist (Quay & Peterson, 1967). It would be of value to have his teachers write a description of the child's problem as they see it, in addition to completing one of the several available teacher rating scales, such as Conners' Teacher Rating Scale or Conners' Abbreviated Teacher Rating Scale. Two others that are available are the Bell, Waldrop, and Weller Rating System and Davids' Rating Scales for Hyperkinesis. (See Appendix for copies of the Conners' Scales and the Bell et al. Scale.) These teacher rating scales, which are described briefly in the Appendix, have weaknesses that in our opinion reduce their value. The parents' and teachers' ratings and the teachers' description serve the dual purpose of providing immediate information that can serve as one basis for planning a management program, as well as baseline data for subsequent evaluation of the intervention strategies that are used. The purpose of the psychiatrist's interview is to determine how the child sees himself and his world. Information should be broken down into home, school, peers, formal activities such as Cub Scouts, and informal play outside. The psychologist should interview the parents and teacher using the Stewart, Pitts, Craig, and

## Table 8. Werry-Weiss-Peters Activity Scale

| | No | Yes–A Little Bit | Yes–Very Much |
|---|---|---|---|
| **During meals** | | | |
| Up and down at table | – | – | – |
| Interrupts without regard | – | – | – |
| Wriggling | – | – | – |
| Fiddles with things | – | – | – |
| Talks excessively | – | – | – |
| **Television** | | | |
| Gets up and down during program | – | – | – |
| Wriggles | – | – | – |
| Manipulates objects or body | – | – | – |
| Talks incessantly | – | – | – |
| Interrupts | – | – | – |
| **Doing home-work** | | | |
| Gets up and down | – | – | – |
| Wriggles | – | – | – |
| Manipulates objects or body | – | – | – |
| Talks incessantly | – | – | – |
| Requires adult supervision or attendance | – | – | – |
| **Play** | | | |
| Inability for quiet play | – | – | – |
| Constantly changing activity | – | – | – |
| Seeks parental attention | – | – | – |
| Talks excessively | – | – | – |
| Disrupts other's play | – | – | – |
| **Sleep** | | | |
| Difficulty settling down for sleep | – | – | – |
| Inadequate amount of sleep | – | – | – |
| Restless during sleep | – | – | – |
| **Behavior away from home (except school)** | | | |
| Restlessness during travel | – | – | – |
| Restlessness during shopping (includes touching everything) | – | – | – |
| Restlessness during church/movies | – | – | – |
| Restlessness during visiting friends, relatives, etc. | – | – | – |
| **School behavior** | | | |
| Up and down | – | – | – |
| Fidgets, wriggles, touches | – | – | – |
| Interrupts teacher or other children excessively | – | – | – |
| Constantly seeks teacher's attention | – | – | – |
| Total Score | _____ | _____ | _____ |

Reprinted, by permission, from Werry, J.S. Developmental hyperactivity. Pediatric Clinics of North America, 1968, 15, 581-599.

Dieruf (1966) list of behaviors characteristic of hyperactive children (see Table 2) and should rate the child's behavior in the classroom and in other natural environments, such as the recess period, because the child may be uncharacteristically well-behaved in one-to-one meetings.

Information on the child's hyperactivity typically is obtained from parents and teachers rather than from the child himself. In a recent paper Stone (1969) has described an objective nonverbal test of personality, the Missouri Children's Picture Series (Sines, Pauker, & Sines, 1973), which is administered to the child and includes an empirically-derived Hyperactivity Scale. The test procedure consists of having the child sort 200 pictures into two stacks, "looks like fun" and "does not look like fun." According to Stone (1969) the test has adequate test-retest reliability. However, the available data are as yet insufficient to warrant a recommendation that it be used in evaluating the hyperactive child. The test is mentioned here because the approach of allowing the child to provide information relevant to his own behavior is a potentially valuable one that has received little attention in the assessment of the behavior problems specific to the hyperactive child.

When the medical, psychoeducational, environmental, and behavioral assessments have been completed, the team of investigators must decide if the data support the diagnosis of hyperactivity. The criteria that have been used to arrive at this diagnosis by clinicians and researchers vary. Stewart, Thach, and Freidin (1970) assigned children to their hyperactive group if the child was hyperactive and/or distractible, exhibited any six of the 28 symptoms in Table 9, was attending school, and was free from chronic medical or neurological disease and orthopedic or special sensory handicaps. We recommend these criteria with one condition, that it be established that the child is not being subjected to academic or other pressures that might cause him to exhibit some of the behaviors characteristic of hyperactivity. Wikler, Dixon, and Parker (1970) classified a child as hyperactive if he was diagnosed as hyperactive in the psychiatrist's report and if, in addition, he exhibited at least 12 of the 18 characteristics in Table 10. David, Clark, and Voeller (1972) considered that the optimum basis for a diagnosis of hyperactivity required three sets of information: a doctor's diagnosis of hyperactivity, and teachers' and parents' ratings.

When the diagnosis of hyperactivity has been established the team must design a plan of management to present to the parents. Such a plan must be flexible enough to allow changes to keep abreast of current developments in the case, and would include some or all of the following components of treatment: psychotherapy which could include therapy, counselling, and/or participation in peer discussion groups for the child and his parents; environmental manipulation which could include special school arrange-

Table 9.  Symptoms on which the Diagnosis of Hyperactive Child Syndrome was Based

---

Overactivity (including unusual energy and restlessness) and Distractibility (including short attention span, never finishing work and projects) and any six of the following:

| | |
|---|---|
| Fidgets, rocks, etc. | Disobedient |
| Climbs on roof, etc. | Doesn't follow directions |
| Runs over furniture | Doesn't respond to discipline |
| Always into things | Defiant |
| Heedless of danger | Wakes early |
| Runs away | Hard to get to bed |
| Constant demands | Wets bed |
| Easily upset | Many accidents |
| Impatient | Lies often |
| Won't accept correction | Takes money, etc. |
| Tantrums | Neighborhood terror |
| Fights often | Sets fires |
| Teases | Reckless, daredevil |
| Destructive | Fears |

---

Reprinted, by permission, from Stewart, M.A., Thach, B.T., & Freidin, M.R.  Accidental poisoning and the hyperactive child syndrome.  Diseases of the Nervous System, 1970, 31, 403–407.

ments, tutoring, and special procedures for the parents to follow at home in handling the child and modifying his behavior; and medication. There is no clearcut answer to the question of when stimulant medication should be used. As Loney and Ordona (1975) have pointed out, the answers to this question range from advocating the use of medication with all children who are suspected of being hyperactive to recommendations that medication be used only when other forms of intervention have failed or when the child's hyperactivity is extreme. Our position on the question of medication is that stimulant drugs should be used only if three conditions are met: (1) The physician can confirm that all relevant aspects of the child's environment and development have been thoroughly assessed, (2) a remediation program is underway, and (3) the child's symptoms are so extremely debilitating that *temporary* medication is needed in order for him to benefit from the remediation program.

The research and treatment procedures within each of the major modes of intervention have already been discussed in detail. The purpose of the discussion here is to provide guidelines concerning what should be said to the parents and child concerning the management program.

Table 10.  Profile of the Hyperactive Child

---

I.   At home
  1. Cannot remain still
  2. Cannot conform to limits or prohibitions
  3. Makes excessive demands
  4. Has sleeping problems
  5. Shows unwarranted aggression
  6. Is general "pest"

II.  At school
  1. Is talkative
  2. Fidgets continuously
  3. Cannot concentrate
  4. Has short attention span
  5. Cannot conform to limits or prohibitions
  6. Shows poor school achievement

III. Relationships with other children
  1. Cannot make friends
  2. Fights without provocation
  3. Has poor manners
  4. Is extremely bossy
  5. Disregards rights of others
  6. Is constantly rejected

---

Courtesy, Parke, Davis & Company (C).

## What the Pediatrician Tells the Parents

It is usually the pediatrician's task to tell the parents that the investigation has confirmed the referral for hyperactivity. How the parents are told is of considerable importance. At this point they are anxious about their child and the school and home problems that have necessitated referral, but their anxiety is not formalized. The discussion with the pediatrician will shape their perception of the child's problem to a considerable degree; therefore, it is imperative that a careful explanation of the problem precede the use of labels or diagnosis that might arouse anxiety. In presenting the diagnosis it is essential to emphasize that the child is neither ill nor to blame for his hyperactivity. When parents treat hyperactivity as an illness and blame the child for it, the child receives many explicit messages that something is seriously wrong with him and it is his fault. The child's behavior may then conform to this parental input, with hyperactivity of longer duration and greater resistance to treatment accompanied by feelings of guilt. It is important to convey that the problem of hyperactivity creates difficulties in several areas of functioning. It is often helpful to provide the parents with a demonstration of the difficulties the child has in coping with school tasks. For example, the parents of one hyperactive child, who was so distractible that it was almost impossible for his teacher to keep his attention even in a one-to-one interaction, insisted that he could pay attention if he tried. These parents were each given rather detailed questionnaires and asked to complete them as quickly as possible. While they were completing them a series of highly distracting social and nonsocial events took place. Finally, the father complained rather angrily to the pediatrician, who then explained that this was how distracting even the quietest school environment was for their son. Similarly, Stover and Guerney (1967) have described a technique in which parents of a hyperactive child with perceptual-motor problems can experience the difficulty of having a deficit in this area. It is also important to stress that the hyperactivity is not insurmountable, is not likely to be permanent in the way mental retardation is, and will require hard work and active involvement on the part of the parents to deal with the problem. The parents should be reassured that expert help is available. It is essential that the pediatrician emphasize the child's strengths and the importance of helping the child acquire feelings of confidence about himself through successful experiences with some attribute or skill that is among or derived from those strengths. The pediatrician should briefly discuss other cases of hyperactivity and give information about other experts who can give the parents assistance.

The pediatrician should convey a feeling of optimism. Except in extreme cases of disability and IQ limitation, *no* prediction can be made with certainty about how a particular child will grow up, although Eisenberg (1966), presumably on the basis of his own clinical experience, has estimated that with an effective multimodality treatment strategy a successful outcome will be attained in only two-thirds of the hyperactive children. It is also essential that the parents not see the diagnosis of hyperactivity as indicative of permanent difficulties. Such a view would not only impose a heavy burden on the parent who is concerned about the child's future as well as the immediate problem, but it might also cause the child to acquire a pessimistic outlook about himself and jeopardize the progress that he might otherwise make. Since no predictions can be made with certainty, nothing is lost by taking a positive attitude about the child's potential progress and, in view of the extensive research on effects of expectation on subsequent performance, there is everything to gain from such an attitude. We have known some hyperactive children whose elementary school careers were chaotic and who were beset with difficulties in all major areas of their lives, but who became so capable and effective as adolescents that their high school teachers were incredulous about the consistently negative notations on their cumulative school records. Chess (1960) emphasizes the importance of conveying to the parents that they did not cause the hyperactivity by their handling of the child and the child is not deliberately creating havoc. At the same time the idea must be introduced here that the parents' behavioral responses to the child may be functioning as a powerful class of positive reinforcers for many of the child's irritating behaviors, thus serving to exacerbate the hyperactivity, and if these parental behaviors were systematically modified the result should be a marked improvement in the child's behavior. This idea should be introduced at this point to enhance the feeling of optimism about the child's prognosis and also to establish that the parents will play an important part in the intervention procedures.

## Medication — What to Tell the Parents

The pediatrician should explain why medication is needed if the team has decided that this form of treatment is needed. It is important to allay the parents' fears about the possibility of drug addiction as a result of the use of stimulant medication. There is no firm evidence either for or against the possibility that drug addiction occurs in these children. The only follow-up reported in the literature is the study by Laufer (1971) discussed in Chapter 4, which had several serious methodological weaknesses. Reports in the media, particularly those since the Omaha incident, appear to have conveyed the impression that stimulus medication is a form of mind control that turns children into zombies. Much of the parents' anxiety can be allayed by specifying what medication can and cannot do for the child. It is particularly important to explain that it will not make the child more intelligent; if he does better in school it is probably because he is better able to attend and the teacher feels more positively toward him (unfortunately often a factor in the child's grades regardless of his actual performance). The reason and procedure for medication trials should be explained and the importance of follow-up checks emphasized. It is essential to stress that the parents *must* consult the pediatrician before making any changes in the amount of medication (Solomons, 1973). Side effects should be discussed. With the most commonly used medications, the most frequent side effects are relatively mild, and include the *amphetamine look,* a pale, pinched, sad facial expression that is heightened by dark hollows under the eyes (this look alarms parents but there is no reason for alarm about the child's physical condition); *anorexia,* a marked loss of appetite that often can be controlled by the timing of medication and meals and that usually disappears after a few weeks; *insomnia,* which may result from the need for a bedtime dose of medication as a result of the daytime medication wearing off and leaving the child charged up with a rebound effect, it is often drug specific and may be eliminated by switching to another medication; and *headaches and abdominal pain,* which often occur simultaneously around the middle of the day, cause the child to feel quite uncomfortable, and can usually be relieved by the ingestion of a glucose-containing solid or liquid. There are several more serious short-term side effects such as psychotic episodes, delerium, hallucinations, bizarre body movements, petit mal seizures, and allergic reactions that occur much less frequently but cannot be discounted. It is essential that the parents report any side effects to the pediatrician immediately.

The following is a transcript of a doctor's inadequate discussion of the diagnosis and treatment of minimal brain dysfunction with a young mother. This interaction occurred in a university clinic where pediatricians from the community regularly gave volunteer hours; all interactions with the patients were routinely recorded for teaching purposes, and a red indicator light informed the doctor that his conversation was being taped.

Doctor:  It seems as though this young man (taps chart) has brain damage, well, uh, not brain *damage,* MBD, that is, minimal brain *dysfunction.*

Mother:  (clearly shocked) You mean it's his *brain?* All the school said was that he was hyperkinetic and very distractible.

Doctor:  Oh, sure, well, MBD and hyperkinetic are really the same thing. MBD just means that his brain isn't working properly right now so things get a bit out of control especially in school. But he'll probably grow out of it, a lot of these MBD kids are fine by the time they get to adolescence. It's not his intelligence, there isn't anything wrong with *that,* he's a bright boy.

Mother:  (sounds very troubled) I never thought of him having anything wrong with his *brain.* How does this brain dysfunction happen, like what caused it? Is it something we did?

Doctor:  Well, now, we don't really know what caused it. A lot of this kind of thing happens before birth or at birth. It's pretty difficult to pinpoint the cause. We aren't really sure most of the time how it happened.

Mother:  You mean he might have had it all his life?

Doctor:  That's right.

Mother:  How could he have had it all this time and never had any trouble until he's 7 years old and in the second grade?

Doctor:  Oh, well, that's when MBD shows up. In school. These MBD children often don't have any trouble until they get in school. But don't worry, we can fix him up with some medication. He'll be fine in school once he's on medication.

Mother: What will the medication do? It's not drugs, is it? What kind of medication is it?

Doctor: It'll quieten him down and he'll get on a lot better in school. . . the teacher'll love him now. The medication we're going to try first is a stimulant called

Mother: (interrupting) A *stimulant!* That's the last thing he needs. Is that some kind of drug?

Doctor: (coldly) Mrs. A., with these brain-damaged children stimulants have a quietening effect. You'll be *amazed* at the difference. We'll try one kind for a week or two and see how it goes; you just have to play it by ear at the beginning because we never know which kind will work best for a child, and if it doesn't do the trick we'll try another kind. Now you just take this prescription (hands it to the mother and starts to move toward the door) and be sure you don't forget to give them to him morning and afternoon. If these pills work and you forget to give him one you'll really know it, he'll go right back to being a nuisance in class. Now we'll check with you in a week, we have to watch out for side effects. . . they *can* be a problem. . . so we'll check with you in a week. O.K.?

Mother: (reluctantly) O.K., but you didn't tell me if this was drugs. I don't want him getting started on drugs.

Doctor: (showing patient out) Now, now, don't you worry about that, after all, you give him aspirin, don't you? Now you phone me. . . (Doctor terminates interview).

Note the defects in this interview. The doctor first suggested actual damage to the brain, then brushed aside the mother's concerned reaction, made no attempt to allay her concern about her role in the onset of the problem, did not answer her question about the medication being drugs, offered no other approach to the problem, lapsed back to using the term *brain damage* when she persisted in her questions about drugs, showed some annoyance at her persistence, and mentioned side effects without giving her sufficient information to use as a basis for detecting them.

## What the Pediatrician Tells the Child

It is our opinion that the pediatrician should discuss the child's problems with him without ever using the terms *brain damage, minimal brain dys-*

*function,* or other equivalents. The symptoms that were the reason for referral should be presented as temperamental or individual differences, and in concrete terms that even young children will readily understand (e.g., comparisons such as race horses versus farm horses, express trains versus freight trains, and teachers who are quick-tempered and excitable versus those who are slow to arouse and generally placid). Next, he should show clearly that he is aware of what a problem the child has and give reassurance that the situation can be improved with everyone working together. If the child is clearly distressed about his difficulties but unable to discuss his anxiety, the pediatrician could use the *third-person technique* of Rothenberg (1972) which often serves as an effective releaser. In this procedure, the adult talks about a hypothetical child of the same age and sex as the patient who experienced anxiety, dismay, despair, and other similar reactions to his school problems and then asks the patient if he ever felt that way. The pediatrician should then specify the changes that the team is recommending in the school and home settings. He must emphasize that he will meet regularly with the child and his parents to discuss progress and problems, and will keep in touch with his teacher.

## The Issue of Whether to Tell the Child that He is on Medication

A decision of major importance concerns whether the child should be told that he is on medication. The criterion for this decision should be the psychological wellbeing of the child and each case should be considered individually. Most clinicians (see, for example, Gardner, 1973; Millman, 1970; Stewart & Olds, 1973; Wender, 1971) believe that in most or all cases the child should be told and that a frank discussion about the child's condition and the purpose of medication is psychologically beneficial. Gardner (1973) has written a book for children with minimal brain dysfunction in which he discusses the medication aspect of treatment.

We strongly disagree with this decision. It is our opinion that while a small number of children *might* benefit from such candor, the large majority do not. In the small group who probably should be told are those who already have had considerable vicarious experience with stimulant medication, expect to be put on stimulants as a result of explicit and implicit information from their immediate family, teachers, and peers, and as a result have a number of misconceptions that should be cleared up with a frank discussion about the purpose of medication.

The arguments for telling the child are that he will feel more secure if he knows exactly where he stands, he can participate effectively in decisions about adjustment of dosage, the knowledge that he is on medication will make him more confident with a consequent improvement in performance, he should always be told the whole truth, and there will be an erosion of his trust in his parents and pediatrician if he is not told and subsequently finds out.

The arguments against telling the child are as follows. If the child is told that he is on medication he must be given some explanation for the reason and many children are distressed rather than relieved by the explanations that are given. It is difficult to explain to a child that there is some problem in his central nervous system without having him think that he is defective. Although the child may *say* that he understands, this reassurance should not be relied on because he is used to telling authority figures he understands, particularly when any sort of problem is involved; he has often been rewarded in the past for stating with assurance that he understands something when he does not, and he has learned that often the subject is dropped and he is left in peace as soon as he says he understands. The following excerpt is from a taped interview with a 10-year-old boy who clearly was disconcerted about the explanation that had been given:

He (the pediatrician) told me all about your brain sending messages and all that like in science only when it's *my* brain it gets mixed up, it sure is scary because I always thought I did those things myself but it wasn't me it was the messages go so fast that things go wrong and then I got in trouble. But now I have these pills and I won't get in no more trouble ever. It's really scary about my brain getting mixed up because I could have a bad accident or something.

No matter how carefully the child is told about the possible physiological reasons for his behavior difficulties, it usually is impossible for the parents and pediatrician to counteract other information from sources such as television and the peer group; when this other input is fear-arousing, the child may be uneasy, alarmed, or terrified. Consider the following statement from a 9-year-old boy:

The doctor says it's just some little thing wrong in my brain and it will go away after awhile and if I take these pills I'll do real good in school but I know there's really something terrible wrong. Like I'm probably soon going to die like in that program on TV they were all scared to tell this kid that he had a terrible thing growing in his brain and they all pretended everything was O.K. and they brought him lots of presents and he *knew* something funny was going on. And so do I because on the way home from the doctor my mom bought me a Ouija board and we had ice cream too and she never does that.

The child may become psychologically dependent on his pills, that is, he may view them as the real controllers of his behavior because he experiences success and reward when he takes them. Psychological dependence is dangerous because it robs the child of feelings of self-confidence and mastery of his already limited sphere of influence. It can be disastrous for him on occasions when he forgets to take his medication. Parents frequently express fears about addiction (Safer, 1971); if the child believes that pills can solve all his problems, parents may have some grounds for concern because the child's belief could contribute to the establishment of a predisposition for addiction. The following rather jubilant statement was made by a 7-year-old boy who clearly felt that all his school problems would be solved with medication:

See, I'm pretty jumpy and the teacher she gets mad and I break lots of things and I get a lot of wrong answers in number work. Well, the doctor said it's something wrong in my brain but when I'm big it'll be gone but right now all I have to do is take some pills and none of them things will happen any more. Boy, oh boy, I'm glad it's a school day tomorrow. Miss Matthews will sure be surprised when she sees me.

The belief that drugs are a complete and infallible solution is not uncommon, especially among younger children. Wender (1971, p. 91) reports one bright 8-year-old boy who referred to his dextroamphetamine as his "magic pills which make me into a good boy and makes everybody like me." His teacher confirmed that the boy felt that he could do no wrong when he was taking his pills. However, Kehne (1974) has suggested that a child's reaction to the drugs making him into a good boy might be one of guilt at a conscious level, that is, "if this drug makes me so *good,* I must otherwise be so *bad.*"

One argument for telling the child that he is on medication concerns the issue of erosion of trust in his parents if he is not told and then finds out from outside sources. To reduce the chances of this situation occurring, the pediatrician should strongly recommend that the parents not tell anyone that the child is on medication. If others comment on his appearance (should he have the "amphetamine look") the parents should state firmly that he has been to the doctor and is fine. However, should the child find out or at any point ask if the pills he is taking are stimulants, we strongly advocate an immediate and unequivocal affirmative response backed up by a discussion of the function of the pills. There is no reason for an erosion of trust if the parents have in the past shown clearly by their behavior that they act in the child's best interests, and if they answer him truthfully on this question. We are not advocating lying to the child at any time in this management program. The pediatrician should discuss with both parents the possibility that the child may raise this question, outline the principles that they should adhere to in their discussion with the child (for example, avoiding the use of terms such as *brain damage*), and have them rehearse answers with the pediatrician. In view of the pseudo-sophistication of the present elementary school group about such matters it is essential that both parents have an answer ready so that when confronted with the question they can respond truthfully, calmly, and objectively, making no excuses for the fact that the child was not previously informed about the stimulant medication but instead referring to it as "just one part of the whole treatment plan."

In not telling the child that he is on medication (unless he asks) what we are advocating is the withholding of information that may have an immediate and long-term negative effect on the child. We have seen several children who have been psychologically devastated by hearing the "whole truth," and adults who were diagnosed as minimal brain dysfunction as children have told us that it was a long time before they were able to think of themselves as "normal." In two cases adults who were apparently well-adjusted in other respects reported that they never were able to forget that they had some brain damage or dysfunction.

### Summary of Pediatrician's Discussion with Child

1. Discuss the actual problems the child is having.
2. Describe the problems in terms of individual differences.
3. Do not use terms such as *brain damage*; do not describe the problem as something wrong with the child's brain; make *no* attempt to give a factual account of hyperactivity.
4. Convey your understanding that it is a real problem to the child *now*.
5. Describe the changes in school and home that you are recommending.
6. Emphasize that you will meet regularly with the child (and his parents) to discuss his progress and problems.
7. If a prescription for medication has been given to the mother say something like, "I'd like you to take some pills, I've talked to your mother and she knows when to give them to you," and do not discuss the reasons.
8. If the child asks point blank if he is now on stimulants say "yes" and discuss the reason for them, but make sure the discussion conforms to the points listed in #3.

### Psychotherapy

The parents and child may all benefit from such therapeutic procedures as counselling and group discussion. The most helpful groups for parents are those in which free discussion is combined with training in procedures to modify some of the child's behaviors. Such groups can be useful in instructing the parents in what they should and should not expect from the child, and in helping them to distinguish behaviors that can be attributed to hyperactivity from those which should not be attributed to it. Schaefer, Palkes, and Stewart (1974) have described in detail a group counselling procedure in which the parents of hyperactive children learned how to make and enforce rules, and modify their children's problem behavior. In this procedure the parents met once a week for 10 weeks, discussed specific behavior problems and their solutions, made and enforced rules, and were instructed in the use of behavior shaping procedures. Group or individual counselling for the parents may also demonstrate that it is the parents' behavior and attitudes that are of etiological importance in the child's hyperactivity. It is well-documented in the clinical literature that treatment of the parent is often of crucial importance for the successful modification of the child's hyperactivity. Ricks (1974) reports the case of a boy who was considered to be hyperactive but did not benefit from drug intervention. As more facts were accumulated about the boy's case it became apparent that his hyperactivity stemmed from environmental restriction of the type reported by McNamara (1972) and Thomas, Chess, Sillen, and Mendez (1974). The restriction was imposed by his mother so it was decided to direct therapeutic intervention towards helping her to become more active, assertive, and able to enjoy her highly active son. After two years of therapy the mother was happier, socially more active, and had a markedly improved relationship with her son, who was functioning effectively in school and was no longer considered hyperactive. Note that with the management procedures that we are advocating, the environmental restrictions imposed on the boy would have been identified prior to the onset of *any* treatment program, including drug intervention.

It is important that the pediatrician and other members of the team work actively with the child and his family to effect a harmonious household. The inclusion of both parents in the treatment process allows the pediatrician to deal simultaneously with the child's problem and with family difficulties related to the hyperactivity. The child's father should be involved in the treatment procedure and should assume some responsibility on a regular basis for the child. While the demands of the father's occupation almost invariably will limit his available time, they should not excuse him from all responsibility. Too often in these cases the father escapes thankfully to work, abdicates all responsibility, and consequently has very little understanding of the child's day-to-day problems. We have frequently noticed that mothers are much more tolerant than fathers of the hyperactive child's behavior in the home possibly because they have learned methods of response that minimize psychological wear and tear, and Nelson (1973) reported that mothers were more effective in communicating with their hyperactive children. These apparent differences in parental reactions may be a function of time spent with the child: the mother spends more time with him and consequently has more practice in handling his outbursts and other upsets. One approach to minimizing distress in interactions with the hyperactive child is to have *planned responses* for handling events that are likely to occur, for example, the parent decides in advance what he will say or do if the child has a tantrum, breaks something, or starts throwing things. One goal for the pediatrician and other members of the team is to see that the child is not allowed either to become a scapegoat or to get away with misbehavior that ordinarily would be unacceptable to his parents. They should learn to differentiate behaviors that are truly beyond the child's control and should be ignored and those that are of a deliberate nature and should be dealt with firmly and decisively, and adopt a socialization procedure for the hyperactive child that is consonant with his needs, problems, and abilities. Any parent of a hyperactive child (and most parents of normal children) would benefit greatly from reading *Raising a hyperactive child* (Stewart & Olds, 1973). It is essential that the parents not feel guilty or responsible for the child's hyperactive behavior, or be exploited or tyrannized by the child. If the child is allowed to exploit any feelings of guilt that his parents have he will rapidly get out of hand, a state of affairs that will be detrimental to his interactions with both peers and adults. The guilt problem should be discussed, with the pediatrician using concrete examples of what the child might say in specific situations (e.g., when reprimanded, the child says, "You don't love me the way you love [sibling]"). Techniques based on family therapy, such as the brief therapy of Weakland, Fisch, Watzlawick, and Bodin (1974) can be extremely helpful to the parents in coping with and modifying the child's behavior.

### Environmental Manipulation

Procedures here are related to the school and home. The management plan may include changes in school arrangements ranging from special class placement to private tutoring. It is important to inform the school concerning changes that are being recommended (having first determined that the school-related changes are feasible) and to maintain contact with the school as a valuable source of subsequent information about the child's progress. If the intervention strategies that are being initiated for a child constitute the first systematic help that has been given him for his hyperactivity, it would be wise to postpone special class placement for several weeks in order to determine if the intervention strategies result in sufficient behavioral improvement to allow the child to remain in the regular class.

Special class placement is a serious decision with effects that often are of a magnitude and duration that impose serious limitations on the child's intellectual and social development. Although special class placement may alleviate the stress, failure, and negative effects on the child's self-esteem of the regular classroom, it is important to recognize that it may also produce a whole new set of enduring stresses. For some hyperactive children it is a psychological haven that is essential for a short and temporary period or a long-term period, but for others it is not essential at all *if* the school will show some tolerance and modify some of the regular class demands, *and* special training is provided to help the child cope with the demands of the regular class environment. In a discussion of intervention in hyperactivity Chess (1972, pp. 34–35) states:

> As far as possible one would wish to avoid undue reduction of environmental expectations, particularly if the social and educational situation is in fact not a deviant one. Reduction of expectations may actually be limiting a child's opportunities for full choice of social and economic activity in adult life. Of course, if his capacities are genuinely limited then nothing is to be gained by making him face repeated failure and a sense of unworthiness. But if his capacities are adequate, and only his prior experience and training inadequate, then intervention should be designed to remediate the experiential deficit at a pace and in a manner optimum for the child.

An important supplement to such a school program would be extracurricular activities that provide the child with opportunities to capitalize on his assets; such activities might consist of special coaching in some athletic activity, special family interactions or responsibilities, or hobbies.

Most hyperactive children will benefit from a well-ordered and structured home environment. By structure we mean rules, routines, and predictability, rather than rigidity. Limits should be set that are reasonable, consistent, and firmly but not punitively enforced. Disciplinary measures should be appropriate and consistent. For most hyperactive children symbolic punishment such as withdrawal of privilege or response cost measures are more effective than physical punishment. Reasonable efforts should be made to keep the child's environment structured, simple, and consistent with his developmental age. Large birthday parties and other exciting events should be avoided until it is established that the child can cope satisfactorily with lesser events. Peer group play should be supervised and kept at a simple level while the child is learning to function well in small group situations. With sensible management the home environment can become a powerful positive adjunct to the school program and can do much to determine the eventual prognosis for the child.

# CHAPTER 9

# *Conclusion*

Hyperactivity is one of the most common symptoms of disordered behavior in childhood. In this text hyperactivity has been defined as a consistently high level of activity that is manifested in situations where it is clearly inappropriate, and is coupled with an inability to inhibit activity on command. Hyperactivity can exist as a single functional disturbance. However, it more often occurs as a primary symptom in a variety of medical and psychological disorders, one of the latter disorders being a cluster of symptoms characterized by a variety of behavioral problems including distractibility, poor attention span, perceptual problems, emotional lability, impulsivity, learning problems, and low frustration tolerance. In the United States, conservative estimates (Huessy, 1967; Stewart & Olds, 1973) indicate that this cluster of symptoms is present in from 4 to 10 percent, or 1.4 to 3.5 million children (National Center for Education Statistics, 1975), whereas educators (Yanow, 1973) believe that 15 to 20 percent represents a more realistic estimate. The fact that hyperactivity has been reported in other major Western countries suggests that this problem is not unique to one culture or school system. However, the sweeping statement (Office of Child Development, 1971) that "hyperkinetic disorders are found in children of all socio-economic groups and in countries throughout the world" receives little support from the literature on Chinese-American children in New York (Sollenberger, 1968), mainland Chinese children (Greene, 1961; Wray, 1975), school children from urban and rural areas of England (Bax, 1972), and primitive Pacific cultures (Prescott, 1968, 1970), to cite just a few instances of groups in which hyperactivity is reported to be virtually nonexistent.

Although the first systematic description of hyperactivity was published early in this century (Still, 1902), most of our knowledge about this behavior has accumulated in the last 25 years. Research and related attempts to delineate the causes and treatment of hyperactivity have burgeoned in the last decade with a marked increase in the number of conferences, special education courses, and official expressions of interest and concern by major professional groups. It can be seen from Table 11 that this trend has been accompanied by an exponential increase in the number of articles,

288

Table 11.   A Comparison of the Number of Articles, Theses, and Books on Hyperactivity Published in Three Different Four-Year Periods

| Publications | 1950–1953 | 1960–1963 | 1970–1973 |
|---|---|---|---|
| Articles | 13 | 82 | 315 |
| Theses | 1 | 4 | 31 |
| Books | 1 | 12 | 33 |

Source: Winchell, C.A. *The hyperkinetic child*. (A bibliography.) Westport, Conn.: Greenwood Press, 1975.

dissertations, and text books published on this topic. The period since 1970 has been notable for research that is broader in scope and far more varied than that of the two previous decades. Accompanying these trends and reflecting an increased awareness of the complexities of the hyperactivity problem has been the use of highly sophisticated empirical analysis techniques. The result has been the accumulation of some important new facts and the discarding of some previously accepted findings. In part the advances reflect diverse contributions from a number of different disciplines, but in the main they can be attributed to the intensive and specialized research of several small groups of investigators, particularly those in some of the major university settings.

One important advance pertains to the increased awareness of the *duration of effect of hyperactivity*. Although for a number of years it has been recognized at a theoretical level (Anderson & Plymate, 1962; Laufer & Denhoff, 1957) that the point of onset of hyperactivity could be early in the preschool years and that different manifestations of the behavior sometimes persisted into adulthood (Menkes, Rowe, & Menkes, 1967), for all practical purposes hyperactivity has been viewed as a problem of middle childhood and early adolescence, the hyperactive behavior itself has been seen as the major symptom, and the whole problem has been considered to be over when the high levels of activity diminished. There is now evidence that hyperactivity may span the major developmental stages, often being apparent in the last trimester of pregnancy and continuing well into adulthood (Arnold, 1972; Gross & Wilson, 1974; Huessy, 1974; Oettinger, 1971). In addition to the evidence for a sustained and long-term duration of effect, a number of recent studies (Mendelson, Johnson, & Stewart, 1971) have placed the hyperactive behavior of the middle childhood period in a new and sobering perspective. It is now conceptualized as the tip of the iceberg, a catalytic agent which, in the absence of effective intervention, can trigger off a chain reaction of secondary problems in childhood. These problems, in turn, interact with the stresses of adolescence to significantly decrease the probability of effective adjustment in adulthood. This conceptualization of the scope, impact, and aftermath of hyperactivity is one that changes a relatively transitory disturbance of childhood into a chronic disorder of potentially major importance throughout much of the life span.

Another major advance has been *the more precise specification of the nature of the learning and performance problems that typify the hyperactive child.* At one time the cause of the child's problems was attributed to a vague and poorly defined general intellectual deficit supposedly the result of demonstrable or assumed brain damage. More recently, the problems were attributed to an incompatibility between hyperactive behavior and well-organized, integrated performance. The fact that drug-induced cessation of the hyperactive behavior was accompanied by marked improvement in performance was viewed as supportive of this explanation. Now it is generally accepted that central to the hyperactive child's learning and performance difficulties is his inability to focus and sustain attention. Although some investigations of the nature of this attentional problem unequivocally accept the global assumption that the problem represents a generalized and pervasive attention deficit, the work of Douglas and her associates at McGill University (Douglas, 1972, 1974) clearly suggests that the problem is far more subtle and complex than this description would indicate. Specifically, these investigators have demonstrated that the hyperactive child is indistinguishable from the normal child in some aspects of attention and characterized by major deficits in others; starting from this empirical base they have examined in detail the role of attentional problems in performance on a wide range of cognitive tasks, specified a variety of procedural interventions that can facilitate the acquisition of such tasks, and currently are engaged in testing the validity of their approach within the experimental framework of a special classroom program for the hyperactive child. The more refined approach to this problem is evident also in the investigation of such indices of attention as heart rate deceleration in the foreperiod of task presentation (Lacey, 1967; Porges, Walter, Korb, & Sprague, 1975; Sroufe, Sonies, West, & Wright, 1973) and in the increased awareness of the importance of separating attention effects from motivation effects (Sroufe, 1975). The sophistication of the approach to the problem of attention that is inherent in the work of investigators such as Douglas and Sroufe represents a major contribution to the embryo theory of hyperactivity in that it establishes a sound empirical base for the precise specification of the nature of the hyperactive child's learning problems, and consequently lays the groundwork for the development of effective remediation programs.

A third significant development concerns the *etiology of hyperactivity.* For most of this century it has been assumed that in the majority of cases the locus of the problem of hyperactivity resides within the child in the form of brain damage or minimal brain dsyfunction with a biochemical, genetic, or perinatal trauma base. The apparent increase in prevalence of hyperactivity over the past quarter of a century has been difficult to reconcile with these explanations and they are further discredited by the growing body of evidence that discounts the presence of brain damage in most hyperactive children. Now recent research has suggested that many hyperactive children may be the products, and victims, of technological advances and that the locus of the problem is not almost invariably within the child but, instead, may originate in the environment in the form of *pollutants* such as lead and radiation, *environmental nonsocial factors* such as the constraints of inner city living, or *social factors* such as socialization practices. These findings must at present be viewed as tentative but if they are confirmed they will set a definite and predictable course for preventive strategies as well as for treatment intervention, in the same way that the identification of environmental carcinogenic agents has determined the course of action for the control of some kinds of cancer.

The period since 1970 has also been notable for a clear trend toward *a more sophisticated approach to the experimental assessment of drugs*. We are not referring here to the increasing number of methodologically adequate studies in the literature. The trend that we have noted is represented by isolated but major sets of events such as the first report (Safer, Allen, & Barr, 1972) of a possible growth suppression effect of the amphetamines being followed immediately by a strong editorial commentary (Eisenberg, 1972) on the need for further definitive study of the problem and very shortly afterward by a flurry of statements all supported by empirical data relevant to the growth issue (Beck, Langford, MacKay, & Sum, 1975; Gross & Wilson, 1974; Levitis, 1974), and finally by a second, more extensive, study by Safer, Allen, and Barr (1975) as well as a long-term ongoing investigation by Sachar, Greenhill, and Sassin (Smithsonian Science Information Exchange, 1975) of the effect of the amphetamines on *growth hormone response* as well as growth pattern. The important point here is not the issue of growth suppression, rather it is the quality and degree of response elicited by the suggestion of a potentially serious long-term drug effect.

The extremes of optimism and negativism that characterized the reactions to psychoactive drugs in the 1950s and early 1960s are in marked contrast to the more restrained approach of the 1970s, as reflected in the calm and judicial assimilation of reports of possible serious long-term side effects of these drugs and in the cautious optimism concerning reports of the efficacy of new drugs. Unfortunately, the line between calm assimilation of negative reports and research inactivity concerning the verification of these reports is a fine one that is further obscured by the tendency to continue using the questionable drug in the absence of definitive research data. The change that has occurred in attitudes to stimulant medications is surprisingly similar to a graphical illustration used by Williams (1954) to depict the usual course of events in the introduction of a drug into clinical use (see Figure 10). According to Williams' formulation, after a period of initial skepticism uncontrolled trials lead to uncritical acceptance and widespread use until the first reports of side effects cause a disproportionate decrease in its use. Finally, an equilibrium position is reached in which the drug is deemed acceptable in proportion to the associated benefits and risks. A similar course of events, depicted graphically in Figure 11, has characterized attitudes about the clinical usage of the amphetamines. The early reports (Bradley, 1937; Molitch & Eccles, 1937; Lindsley & Henry, 1942) of their efficacy met with skepticism and indifference. It was not until the early 1950s that the amphetamines were accepted and it was only in the mid-1950s that they became widely used. A decade of enthusiastic and largely uncritical acceptance of the amphetamines ended in the mid-1960s with the publication of several very negative critical reviews of the field of psychopharmacology. The stimulant medications continued to be widely used but the dissenting voices were powerful and competent and this opposing force received strong support from the Omaha incident. The

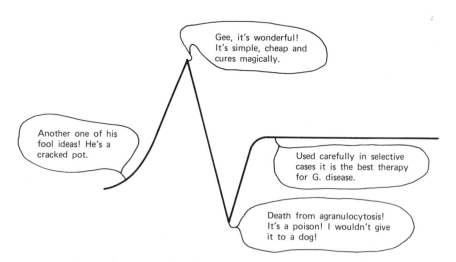

**Figure 10.** Oscillations in the development of a drug. (Reprinted from Williams, R. H. The clinical investigator and his role in teaching, administration, and the care of the patient, *Journal of the American Medical Association,* 156, 127–136. Copyright 1954, American Medical Association.)

present decade has been marked by a far more cautious attitude to these drugs.

Finally, as an offshoot of the research of the last decade, *a new concept in school health care* has emerged in the United States in a scattering of school districts whose administration has a sophisticated view of the importance of behavior problems in the school setting. In this concept school health is viewed as directly related to the learning process, so that high priority is assigned to the on-site management of behavior and learning problems. This redefinition of school health care represents a major shift that is almost a reversal of the traditional school health program with its focus on physical examinations, sensory deficit screening, immunization procedures, and customary referral to outside agencies of children with behavior and learning problems. Having always *professed* concern about the whole child, the school system is for the first time now assuming its rightful responsibility in this area, a change that represents a breakthrough in the care of the hyperactive child and those with other behavior problems or learning disabilities. The concept of treating behavior problems within the school setting has placed disorders such as hyperactivity squarely

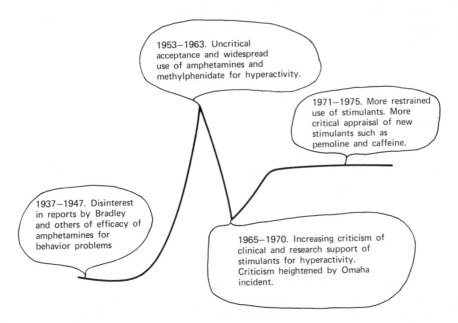

**Figure 11.** Changes in attitude to central nervous system stimulants. (After Williams, R. H. The clinical investigator and his role in teaching, administration, and the care of the patient. *Journal of the American Medical Association,* 1954, **156,** 127–136.)

within an educational context. The potential contribution of this shift in school health care to the effective *management* of the hyperactive child is considerable, but of even greater importance may be its impact on *prevention:* a well-established management program is a sound basis for the logical next step of developing a prevention program within the same framework. If the criterion of value for a major innovation in the area of behavior and learning problems is the number of children who benefit from it, this new concept of school health care has the potential to be the most important of all the major advances of the 1970s.

Despite the foregoing major advances, there is an urgent need for more rapid progress in the development of preventive and management strategies. One reason for the urgency is the sheer number of children involved, with 1.4 to 3.5 million being a conservative estimate of the hyperactive children in the United States who are presumed to be in need of some kind of intervention (Huessy, 1967; National Center for Education Statistics, 1975; Sroufe, 1975). If these numbers represented the estimated incidence of a disease, the public outcry would make wide-scale federal and state level intervention mandatory, but because hyperactivity is a behavior disorder, and particularly a nonviolent behavior disorder, there is no widespread reaction of alarm despite the fact that some of the sequelae of hyperactivity are more serious in duration and effect than those of many childhood diseases. An analogous situation exists in attitudes to acute versus chronic diseases. For example, in 1900 diphtheria was widespread but by 1960 this disease had been virtually eliminated as a result of active immunization programs by public health authorities. In sharp contrast is the marked indifference to the incidence of secondary anemia, that is, iron deficiency. In one major urban area the incidence in 1937 was 25 to 30 percent for all 2-year-old children and these figures remained unchanged in 1957. Although secondary anemia has potentially serious long-term effects it is still the most common nutritional deficiency of infants and young preschool children and has elicited little or no public health action on a national scale.

Related to the high incidence of hyperactivity is the sobering fact that we are not at the present time coping effectively with the problem. Many hyperactive children are not receiving treatment of any kind (Gorin & Kramer, 1973), and many of the 150,000 to 200,000 children who currently are receiving treatment in the form of stimulant medication are being treated for long periods despite inadequate knowledge about the effects of this intervention (Sroufe & Stewart, 1973). Furthermore, drug intervention is often the only treatment given these children and there is substantial evidence of the inadequacy of drugs as the sole treatment process. In a recent commentary on the frequency and potential results of such drug usage, Rie (1975, p. 788–789) stated:

> It is my personal conviction that the stimulant drugs are being used excessively. I believe that in many instances when medication is the sole mode of intervention, when there is limited communication among relevant professionals, when monitoring of drug response is minimal, or when effectiveness is judged by a child's response in a single area of functioning, the result may well be to obscure the remaining problems . . . while satisfying the needs of the child's caretakers and teachers . . .

Despite the inadequacies inherent in the present use of drug intervention, the age-range and number of children so treated can be expected to increase sharply in the next few years. There is increasing evidence and endorsement in the literature of the use of stimulants with infants and preschool children (McMahon, Deem, & Greenberg, 1970; Nichamin, 1972) despite research (Conners, 1973; Schleifer, Weiss, Cohen, Elman, Cvejic, & Kruger, 1975) that contraindicates their use at these age levels, and a lack of knowledge about their effects on the developing nervous system. In addition, there are two school-related procedures which, if put into effect, would cause a sharp increase in the use of stimulant medication: one is *mainstreaming*, which refers to the reassignment of children with special learning needs or handicaps to the regular classroom, and the other is the *mass routine screening* of school children to identify those who might benefit from the stimulants. Many hyperactive children function successfully in special classes and without medication because these classes offer features such as modified demands and low pupil-teacher ratios. Without some special help it is highly unlikely that these children could continue to function effectively without medication if they were returned to regular classrooms. The mass screening proposal advanced by Steinberg, Troshinsky, and Steinberg (1971) advocates teacher nomination of elementary school children who might benefit from a trial of stimulant medication. If this disastrous proposal were put into effect it would result in a massive increase in the number of children on medication. Unfortunately there are a number of factors that favor its implementation: Educators are showing increasing concern about the problem of hyperactivity and other behavior problems in the schools and their estimates of the prevalence of these problems (15 to 20 percent of the children) far exceed those of other professionals. Teachers know relatively little about the short- and long-term negative effects of the stimulants and therefore would be expected to have few misgivings about making such recommendations (Robin & Bosco, 1973). Many parents freely use a variety of drugs themselves and would be likely to agree to a medication trial for their children, particularly if such a proposal were presented as a means to increase achievement. Also, many nominations would come from inner-city schools where the parents may be ill-equipped to judge the merits of stimulants, evaluate potential outcomes for their children, or influence the quality of their education. The drugs themselves are firmly entrenched and have many advantages such as ease and economy of time for all concerned, and often they relieve the parents and teachers of feelings of responsibility for further action. Perhaps the most important of all the factors that might facilitate such an increase in the use of stimulant medications is the present lack of an effective, multimodality procedure for the treatment and management of the hyperactive child that is readily available to parents, teachers, and pediatricians and that is practical for wide-scale usage. In short, the crux of the problem is that drugs are the treatment of choice and often are the only treatment given to the child because *in the main* pediatricians, teachers, and parents do not know of any other way to handle the problem or are unwilling to expend the necessary time and effort to incorporate other modes of treatment. This situation is almost certain to be maintained unless a concerted effort directed toward change is launched by the medical profession, educational establishment, and federal government.

To begin to cope effectively with the problem of hyperactivity, changes will have to be made in the two major areas of the field, that is, basic and applied research, and clinical and educational applications of knowledge related to the field. Such a strategy would first require a consensus of experts to develop a master plan incorporating what is known and what needs to be investigated in relation to what is known.

## RESEARCH CHANGES

A coordinated research strategy should be developed with substantial federal funding allocated to those few groups of researchers who have already contributed substantially to the field, whose areas of investigation are potentially valuable in terms of the master plan, and whose methodology is above reproach. The current state of research on hyperactivity is characterized by overlap, methodological weaknesses that render findings useless, a narrowness of focus that makes inter-study comparisons impossible, and general confusion and disorganization. One area of research that should be developed is the early identification of children at risk for hyperactivity. Although there has been a steady body of work on the development of screening procedures for the problem of learning disabilities (Denhoff, 1973; Denhoff, Hainsworth, & Hainsworth, 1972;

Eaves, Kendall, & Crichton, 1972) the early identification of hyperactive children has been virtually ignored, with the exception of peripheral research with serious methodological weaknesses by Broussard and Hartner (1970, 1971) and an intensive long-term study in progress at the University of Washington (Barnard & Collar, 1973). More research attention should be given to some of the less obvious effects of treatment on the child and to etiological factors such as child rearing that have been extensively investigated in other groups of children but not in hyperactive children.

One topic of research that should be investigated is the *psychological cost* to the hyperactive child of being on stimulant medication. A survey of the research literature would lead one to conclude that the psychological effects of the stimulants are largely positive because there are only occasional accounts of negative effects (Kehne, 1974) other than mild transitory ones. An adequate model of a treatment procedure should predict both positive and negative effects and in this respect our current state of knowledge about the psychological cost of drug treatment is almost zero. The advocates of stimulant medications typically present them as the means of terminating a downward spiral of misery for the child. In fact, some of the children's comments in this text suggest that the mere act of taking drugs with other children's knowledge can have a detrimental effect on both peer relations and self-esteem. Further, a recent report by Rie (1975) has identified a change in *affect* that occurs as a function of stimulant medication. Rie described this phenomenon as an ''affectless, humorless, and apathetic demeanor'' and noted that in a double-blind study of primary grade children, those on methylphenidate could be distinguished without error from the controls solely on the basis of this diminished affect. In a discussion of this drug effect Rie (1975, p. 788) stated:

The implications of children developing for any period of time with substantially diminished affective arousal may be considerable. At the least, those whose emotional status is a major determinant of their hyperactivity and related problems are inaccessible, under this condition, to any mode of intervention that seeks to alter their characteristic affective responses, simply because the responses fail to occur. It remains to be determined whether children treated continuously for prolonged periods of time are able to develop age-adequate patterns of emotional adaptation.

These kinds of general psychological cost of being on medication should be carefully investigated as should the possibility that stimulant medication treatment might be an antecedent of various kinds of drug abuse.

The foregoing are *general* effects of the stimulant medication regimen. Research attention should also be focused on the specific behavioral effects of drugs. One topic that has greatly interested us is the potential effect of the stimulants on incidental learning, particularly in the middle childhood years. According to Erikson's (1937) concept of the eight stages of man, the middle childhood years are a period of industry in which the central task is learning. Learning can be categorized on various parameters, but two that are frequently used in socialization theories are *intentional* and *incidental learning*. Intentional learning refers to the learning that occurs as a result of formal training as, for example, when a mother teaches her child to drink from a cup or cross a street safely, or when a teacher instructs a child in multiplication or reading. Incidental learning refers to learning that occurs in the absence of an induced set or motivation to learn. The label "incidental" in no way implies that the learning is unimportant, nonessential, or of little permanent value to the child. Much of what a child learns is acquired under incidental learning conditions, with some estimates putting the amount as high as 80 percent of the child's total learning (Postman, 1964). When a child acquires mannerisms from his parents through casual observation, or gleans information or misinformation from conversations that he overhears, this is incidental learning. Incidental learning is of considerable importance in the middle childhood years when the child is striving for entry into the peer group. It follows that any procedure that serves to inhibit or interfere with the acquisition of incidental learning during this period may seriously disrupt the socialization process.

In clinical descriptions of the behavior of children on stimulant drugs and in some research reports there are enthusiastic accounts of the way in which the stimulants cause the child to focus closely on the task at hand: Fowlie (1973) described how her son concentrated on a puzzle with a single-mindedness that was unique for him, Wender (1971) reported the astonishment and delight of the parents whose daughter had to be literally pried loose from her homework, and teachers and parents have often commented that there could be an earthquake and the child on drugs would not notice. In these accounts the implication is that the narrowness of the focus is beneficial to the child and as such is a state that should be fostered. The point that disturbs us is this: If the child focuses on the intentional training task in school to the almost total exclusion of other visual and auditory input he almost certainly would be being deprived of incidental learning opportunities that in the long run may be as valuable or more valuable to him than the school learning task, and if he is consistently deprived through drug intervention of incidental learning opportunities the long-range cost of such deprivation may be quite severe. This question is of considerable importance to the socialization of the hyperactive child and should be intensively investigated particularly since the hyperactive child is usually deficient in social behavior skills. One piece of research evidence is available in support of the above speculation that there may be a drug-induced incidental learning deficit. Several years ago we conducted an experiment to investigate the effect of type of reward (tangible reward, praise, and neutral comment) for intentional learning on the incidental learning of young mentally retarded children in social game situations (Ross, 1970). Briefly, the experimental task was a two-person discrimination box game in which the players (an adult and a mentally retarded child) took turns trying to catch fish. Prior to the game the adult who was running the experimental sessions taught the two players the *rules of the game* (the intentional learning) using discussion, demonstration, and where appropriate, promises of reward. When the game started the adult player exhibited a variety of *verbal and nonverbal mannerisms* (incidental learning) when she took her turn. The mannerisms were game-related in the same way that certain verbal and nonverbal mannerisms are related to games such as baseball. On the basis of previous research (Bahrick, 1954) an inverse relationship between motivational level and incidental learning was hypothesized and this hypothesis was supported by the data. Subjects who were rewarded either tangibly or with praise learned and retained more of the rules (intentional learning) and less of the mannerisms (incidental learning), whereas subjects who were exposed to neutral comments learned more of the mannerisms and fewer of the rules. In the school where the research was conducted there was a group of eight hyperactive boys of borderline intelligence who could not formally participate in the experiment because they were not mentally retarded and they were on stimulant medication. Each of these boys was given a turn in this game and three other games similar in format but differing markedly in appearance. The results were consistent across games and reward conditions. The boys made almost perfect scores on the intentional learning tasks and near-zero scores on the incidental learning, regardless of type of reward. One of our research assistants described their concentration on the game as "ferocious." In this experiment the incidental learning was a set of mannerisms of little value so in this instance the hyperactive boys were not missing anything by focusing almost exclusively on the intentional learning. However, this is seldom the case in everyday activities, where instead, the content of the incidental learning opportunities is of considerable value to the child who is able to take advantage of the situation. Consequently, this finding raises serious questions about the effects of stimulant drugs on incidental learning in real-life situations, particularly in the classroom, and underlines the need for investigation of this and other psychological effects of medication.

A research topic that has considerable relevance to the *management* of the hyperactive child concerns the fact that some hyperactive children cope effectively despite their high level of activity, whereas others flounder. Are there environmental influences or other factors common to hyperactive children who function effectively in adolescence and adulthood? The longitudinal studies needed to investigate this question have not yet been done, however, some empirical data of relevance are available. In the Shelley and Riester (1972) study the young adults who were diagnosed retrospectively as minimal brain dysfunction had progressed through school, and in some cases, through college, without any major difficulty although they had clearly exhibited many of the behaviors characteristic of hyperactivity. Several factors emerged from the retrospective data that may have facilitated their successful adjustment in school and college: the group had experienced firm parental handling, been exposed to consistent demands for achievement, and at the same time had been encouraged to develop compensatory skills. In the Battle and Lacey (1972) study the finding that high active girls appeared to encounter little social difficulty with adults or peers in childhood and adolescence, were physically competent, and placed positive valuation on their intellectual ability and were confident about it, also appeared to be related to parental factors, specifically to mothers who were well-educated themselves and encouraged their daughters to strive for achievement in academic areas. In contrast, high active boys experienced considerable social difficulty with adults from infancy on, with their peer group in the school years, and exhibited evidence of poor self-esteem particularly in respect to estimates of their own intellectual ability. These boys experienced a very different kind of mother-child interaction, one that was cold, rejecting, critical, and derogatory. Halverson and Victor (1975) also report sex differences in the social adjustment of hyperactive children, with boys who were hyperactive in school being judged negatively by the peer group while hyperactive girls were not. The foregoing results suggest that parental handling and particularly the early mother-child interaction may be an important determinant of the ability of the hyperactive child to cope adequately with the demands of school and home in the middle childhood period. The fact that the subjects of both sexes in the Shelley and Riester (1972) and Battle and Lacey (1972) studies experienced difficulty in young adulthood also suggests that for the girls as well as the boys the earlier adequate functioning rested on a psychologically fragile structure. Of considerable relevance to an examination of the effect of maternal handling on outcome are the reports of differential early handling of infant boys and girls by their mothers, with boys being given more physical stimulation and girls being exposed to more verbal input (Kagan, 1971); the extent to which early maternal behavior seems to be an important determinant of subsequent intellectual development in children (Willerman, 1973); the lack of hyperactive behaviors in Chinese-American children in New York, which appears to be related to socialization procedures that are markedly different from those most

American children experience (Sollenberger, 1968); and marked differences in the early handling of American and Japanese infants, with American infants being subjected to considerable active verbal and nonverbal stimulation and Japanese infants being treated more passively and soothingly with a concomitant difference in activity levels (Caudill & Weinstein, 1969). Taken together, this rather diverse set of findings suggests that both the onset and the cause of some instances of hyperactivity may be determined by maternal handling. If confirmed, this finding would have major implications for both the prevention and management of hyperactivity.

## CLINICAL AND EDUCATIONAL CHANGES

The concept of school health care that assigns priority to the management of behavior and learning problems has already been discussed and programs have been reported that hold great promise for improved care of children with behavior and learning problems. It is our opinion that a major goal of such programs should be prevention; and this goal could best be accomplished by establishing new training requirements for professional personnel involved with children with school behavior problems, and conducting parent education programs (geared to all parents within a school) on instruction and practical training relevant to the prevention and management of problems. Within a 5-year period a parent program of this type could have a marked positive effect on the behavior of children in a school. The training program we envisage would enable those concerned with the child to modify his immediate problems through effective management and prevent future problems by understanding the application of general principles of behavior control. The program proposed here differs in several respects from the few programs already in existence: It assigns a coordinating role to the psychologist rather than to the pediatrician on the team; it focuses on prevention at both the professional *and* parent level; and it assigns much of the responsibility for teaching behavioral control principles to the school nurse.

We recommend the establishment of a pediatric subspecialty in hyperactivity, learning disabilities, and other problems that commonly occur in the school setting. Such an area of specialization would require a knowledge and understanding of the nonmedical diagnostic procedures used with the hyperactive child; drug, psychotherapeutic, and educational remediation techniques; a solid grounding in developmental psychology; some knowledge of clinical psychology; and some skill in communicating with other disciplines. With this training the pediatrician would be far more cognizant about the problems of hyperactivity than most pediatricians are. At the present time the parents of a child who elicits formal complaints about hyperactivity from the school usually turn first to the pediatrician, who typically is neither adequately trained for assuming full responsibility for the management of the problem nor enthusiastic about it (Solomons, 1973). In view of the current statistics on the impending acute shortage of pediatricians in this country, it is neither practical nor logical to expect the pediatrician to manage the problem. Instead, within our proposal the pediatrician would be one of a team jointly responsible for the child. The coordinator of the team should be a psychologist, preferably a pediatric psychologist, whose tasks would include consulting initially with the parents, assessing the child and delegating some aspects of the assessment to other team members, instructing the parents and teachers in the principles of behavior modification and other management procedures, determining whether psychiatric referral is advisable for the parents or child, and evaluating the success of the nonmedical procedures. A social worker would be needed to assess the home environment and could assist with training the parents in child management. However, the major part of the training of parents and teachers in such procedures as recording the child's behaviors, monitoring his progress on stimulant medication, administering medication, helping the parents and teachers on class management techniques, such as behavior modification procedures (the psychologist having been responsible for the initial discussion of these procedures), and supervising the completion of checklist records by parents, would be the responsibility of the school nurse. Unequivocal support for the feasibility of this role for the school nurse can be found in the approach of Barnard and Collar (1973). The nurse and social worker would both have to be conversant with the general psychological testing procedures, related norms, and other aspects of the problem of hyperactivity so that all members of the team could communicate knowledgeably with each other and the parents about most aspects of the child's hyperactivity.

## Training

The pediatrician's subspecialty training, and the psychologist's and social worker's graduate school training should adequately equip these members of the team for their responsibilities. However, a 6-month post-graduate federally funded course should be available to them and should be required for the school nurse. Teachers constitute a special case because their university training generally is inadequate to meet the requirements of a contributing team member as envisaged here. Their participation in the 6-month course would be essential since there is little point in developing a management team if the agents closest to the problem at school, that is, the teachers, continue to function in ways that are likely to provoke some cases of hyperactivity and exacerbate others. However, the crux of the teacher's problem lies in the inadequacy of the university teacher-training programs, and we would recommend exposure to course content and a general philosophy of teaching that differs in several important respects from current practices.

On the basis of extensive contact with the teaching and administrative personnel in special education departments, we have noted the following deficits and weaknesses inherent in teacher-training programs that contribute markedly to difficulties in the classroom and that could be eliminated. There is a *research-application gap* that is particularly costly to classroom functioning. A very small percentage of the empirical findings relevant to specific problems in special education are directly taught in teacher-training programs and when these findings are taught they are not presented within a format that allows the beginning teacher to see how they can be used effectively in an actual classroom situation. These programs spend an exorbitant amount of time on transmitting established knowledge of a course-content nature and omit or neglect to instill in the teacher a strong determination to find out how her pupils can best learn and to select from her repertoire of general learning principles those procedures most appropriate to the individual problem. Too little time is allocated to the problem of *classroom control,* yet this problem probably causes the most difficulties for the beginning teacher. It should be presented as a skill that can be analyzed in terms of the principles of modern behavior theories. For example, the student teacher would need only a few empirical examples *and* practical demonstrations of the duration of effect of aperiodic positive reinforcement of a misbehavior to appreciate the folly of such a response in the classroom setting. It is also essential that teachers understand the behavior modification process for what it is, that is, behavior maintained by its consequences, and that they not confuse it with bribery, mind control, or other nefarious developments. With any child, but particularly a child with special learning needs, teachers should learn to *teach to the child's strengths* rather than to focus on his weaknesses, a procedure guaranteed to have a devastating effect on a child's self-esteem. Teachers seldom seem to recognize that capitalization on strengths can compensate for weaknesses. In the case of the hyperactive child it is essential that the teacher be aware that the child can be trained to respond in the ways that drugs enable him to respond, and that the training she provides can do much to eliminate the need for drugs. The acceptance of such an approach would return the education of the hyperactive child to a more holistic approach in which the child and the teacher are required to take more responsibility for his behavior and in the process both acquire an increased sense of mastery. Although federal funding might be obtained for some aspects of the teacher-training for the kind of team effort we have described here, the impetus for these changes would have to come from the faculty and administration of schools of education. If such changes were put into action, even a beginning teacher would require only a minimum of help to become a smoothly functioning member of the interdisciplinary team that we have described.

## Location

Although space is at a premium in many schools, the optimal center for the team operation is the school. Regular school space should be available for the school nurse to carry out her activities, and space should also be available for large-group meetings. In addition, a mobile trailer unit would allow one set of expensive equipment to be readily available to several schools. Centering the whole project at the local school has many advantages: having the program there places hyperactivity within the context of a behavior problem, the school is within easy reach for most mothers, a child would be out of class the minimum amount of time necessary for testing and training activities and there are unlimited opportunities for recording the child's behavior in naturalistic but controlled settings.

## Development of New Programs

Establishing a cooperative team effort with specialized training for team members is an essential facet of the proposed attack on the problem of hyperactivity. But in order to make maximum use of the team, training programs must be available to them either for their own use with the child or for parents' or outside help such as college students' use in working with the child at home. Major large-scale attempts to change the existing social-educational system have generally been far less successful than the expenditures of time, money, and ideas would indicate; one reason for the minimal success has been that no attempts were made to replace the old inadequate programs with new content and procedures based on current psychological and educational research data. The Headstart and Early Childhood Education programs have been far less successful than they should have been because no programs strong enough and detailed enough to accommodate a wide range of teacher expertise were available when the organizational framework was set up for these projects.

For the hyperactive child, a major research and development drive should be launched to develop programs to modify the child's experiential deficits. For example, we have described successful single-case efforts to modify the impulsive behavior and speed and range of response of hyperactive children. Programs such as these, and a large number of other programs geared to modify the wide range of inappropriate behaviors and deficits of the hyperactive child and capitalize on his strengths, should be written out in detail so that they can first be subjected to experimental evaluation and then made available on a national basis and in a form that reasonably competent adults could follow with help from the team. The ultimate goal would be to have a complete school program with accompanying home programs to accommodate the special needs of the hyperactive child at all age levels.

It can be seen from these proposals for change in the management of the hyperactive child that the federal and state costs would be high for the interdisciplinary team approach, together with the concomitant program development. In a recent report on the problems of adequate drug therapy in private practice, Solomons (1973, p. 342) recommended regional centers for a more adequate monitoring of children on stimulant medications:

. . . a regional facility is needed, where these children can have a multidisciplinary assessment, a diagnosis can be made, the decision to initiate drug therapy can be made and the appropriate medication determined, and periodic contacts and long-term follow-up can be maintained by telephone and visitation. Such centers should also be able to initiate and provide the necessary care to parents and other family members relevant to the child's problems. Liaison could be maintained between the center and school personnel (e.g., nurse, psychologist, educators) involved with specific patients. Group sessions with parents and other involved family members could be carried out.

Solomons prefaced his recommendation with an apologetic recognition of the enormity of his suggestion. We strongly disagree. Hyperactivity is a major problem in the United States and it will not be solved with small-scale solutions. The kind of systematic interdisciplinary team approach that we are advocating, backed up by the research and educational changes in training and program development, and the local school centers that we are proposing would involve large expenditures. But it is time to think about the potential costs of the present ineffective approach to the whole problem, and to ponder the immediate and long-term costs of hyperactivity to the 1.4 to 3.5 million children who are estimated to be hyperactive, their parents and siblings, their school districts, and society in general.

# APPENDIX

# *Assessment of Activity Level and Hyperactivity*

## MECHANICAL MEASURES OF ACTIVITY

A number of mechanical devices for measuring activity have been described in the literature (see, for example, Cromwell, Baumeister, & Hawkins, 1963) along with discussions of their limits in measuring children (Johnson, 1972). For example, it is the qualitative aspects of the activity level that distinguish the hyperactive child from his normal counterpart, but the mechanical measures are limited to a quantitative assessment of the behavior; it is difficult to relate the data collected to the actual activity of the subject; there is no way of knowing whether or not the level of activity is appropriate for the situation; and inappropriate behavior that is significant cannot be distinguished from inappropriate behavior that is not significant. The devices can be grouped into the following categories.

In the *kinetometer approach* a device is attached to the subject's body. The most commonly used device in this category is the *pedometer*. It is attached to the subject's leg and measures his activity in terms of the number of leg movements needed to make a unit change in the pedometer. The *actometer* is a modified self-winding calendar watch (developed by Schulman & Reisman, 1959) whose dial hands are activated by movement of the arm or leg to which the watch is strapped. Depending on the numbers of watches used, the axes that can be obtained are a vertical recording axis, a horizontal left to right axis, and a horizontal front to back axis. Although the actometer has the advantage of being small, inexpensive, usable in naturalistic settings and for long periods of time, it has a number of disadvantages: Reliability within and between watches is questionable (Johnson, 1971; Schulman, Kaspar, & Throne, 1965); the range of measurement is limited to the body parts to which the actometer is attached; the way in which a body part is moved greatly influences the reading; slight variations in placement position provide different readings; and, as Johnson (1971) says, the actometer and other similar devices do not identify the hyperactive child if the criteria for hyperactivity are "repetitive, unsocial, annoying, or inappropriate activities."

The *fidgetometer approach* measures the amount of vibration when the subject moves on a surface. Devices here are the stabilimeter, ballistographic chair, and the stabilimetric chair. The *stabilimeter* has been used to study activity in infants by using a special crib (Irwin, 1932) which Lipsitt and DeLucia (1960) have further modified to obtain measures of generalized activity and of specific movements in infants. The *ballistographic chair* developed by Foshee (1958) measures movement as the subject sits in it. Reported test-retest reliability on successive days is high ($r = .95$) and correlations between observer measures and chair measures were .89. The *stabilimetric chair* developed by Sprague and Toppe (1966) is a small cushion for use on any chair. It is similar in principle to the ballistographic chair. A movement of about 1/16 inch or more in a backward-forward or left-right direction is recorded. High reliability ($r = .97$) is reported for alternating 12-second intervals. The fidgetometer approach provides data that can be analyzed for both temporal pattern and amplitude of single bursts of activity. A reliable measure of total activity can be obtained in a given time period when the amplitude and frequency of the waveform are combined by using an electronic interpreter. However, gross versus fine movements cannot be studied and the weight of the subject influences the amount of activity recorded, with small subjects likely to show less recorded activity than large ones.

*Traversal activity measures* include overhead filming, pneumatic pads, photoelectric equipment, ultrasonic generators, and grid rooms. *Film measurement* provides a precise and permanent measure of variations in laterality in potentially naturalistic settings but has the disadvantage of being expensive and the limitation of restricting the area of activity. Hutt and Hutt (1970) describe a wide angle lens camera for filming children's movements during play in a room with a checkerboard pattern of squares marked on the floor. Kessen, Hendry, and Leutzendorff (1961) used an overhead camera to photograph infants for five 30-second periods for several days. For each period six frames at equal distances along the film were selected for analysis of frame-to-frame displacement of seven body points. They reported stable individual differences, even within one 30-second period, with systematic increases occuring in the first 5 days of life. Sainesbury (1954) introduced a light flash at equal intervals during filming of activity to eliminate any ambiguity about interval boundaries for later evaluation by judges. Using this system, inter-judge reliability was .86, odd-even reliability for 100 feet of film was .93, correlation between the film scores and scores from an electromyograph during a 20-minute period was .83, and between film scores and observer scores was .87 for the same period of time. Montagu and Swarbrick (1974) used a matrix of electric pressure mats under the carpet. Each mat had its own switch so that a counter kept a cumulative record of the subject's movement around the room. Ellis and Pryer (1959) have used *photoelectric equipment* in developing an eight-foot square activity room. The apparatus uses lamps and photoelectric cells embedded in opposite walls and 18 inches from the floor so that the room is criss-crossed by a light grid. When movement by the subject interferes with a light beam making contact with a photoelectric cell, the interruption is recorded on a counter. Reliability of .92 was obtained for two neuropathologic children measured for one 20-minute period a day for eight days; for 10-minute periods it was .87. The equipment for this method is relatively inexpensive and no observer is needed. One disadvantage is that upper torso movements are not recorded because the lamps are 18 inches from the floor. The *ultrasonic generator* developed by Peacock and Williams (1962) also measures activity within a special room. As the subject moves, standing waves set up by signals radiated into the room by the ultrasonic generator are disturbed and a receiver detects the signal. One difficulty is that the size of the signal detected by the receiver has some relationship to the distance between the moving subject and the transmitter, so that a small movement near the transmitter and a large movement far from it may produce similar output. The electrical output of the device is adaptable to counting, ink-writing, and storage on magnetic tape. The equipment is expensive but it can be adjusted to measure small or large movements. Newbury (1956) has developed a simple *magnetic relay system* that can be used with any type of cage, bed, or situation in which electrical contact can be produced by the subject's activity and is particularly useful in time-sampling studies. The system records and counts the number of time units in which activity occurs. It describes equal time-intervals, permanently records which intervals contain activity, and gives a cumulative interval total. *Grid rooms* are rooms in which the floor is divided into equal squares forming a grid pattern. The subject's activity score is in terms of how many squares he traverses during the period of observation. By laying down strips of removable tape, any floor area can become a grid room.

The traversal methods described above have the advantage of allowing unrestricted movement within the room and of providing a reliable measure of activity without the subject being aware that his activity is being recorded. With the exception of the grid room, observer time is at a minimum (although most young children would dislike being left in a room by themselves so some familiarization sessions would be essential). Scores can be distorted depending on the position of the subject and the kind of recording device. For example, vigorous activity such as hammering would produce no score because the subject is not traversing a grid or interrupting a light beam. In setting up a room it should be established *first* that the stimuli used are homogeneous in appeal in order to avoid variations in activity level as a function of variations in the attention value of the stimulus objects. Similarly, if subjects at different age levels are being compared, great care should be taken to select sets of objects that are appropriate for each age level and at the same time do not differ in attention value across age levels. For example, Routh, Schroeder, and O'Tuama (1974) reported a cross-sectional developmental study on open-field locomotor activity of 140 children from 3 to 9 years of age. Each quadrant in the experimental room contained an identical set of 5 different toys. The same toys were used for all age levels. It is difficult to see how toys that might appeal to a 3-year-old would be equally appealing to a 9-year-old. One measure concerned the number of quadrants entered. It would be far more difficult for the younger children to perceive that the sets of toys in each quadrant were identical since this judgment requires an understanding of the concepts "same" and "different," so one would expect that on this basis alone, the younger children would enter more quadrants than the older children. This result was reported as a function of age, when in fact other variables were contributing to it.

In *radio telemetry* radio waves convey information picked up by transducers. A device is taped to the body and is connected to a small transmitter in the subject's pocket. Information on movement changes is transmitted to a distant receiver where it is recorded. These devices require subject cooperation in placing them, but this need not be a drawback if the child is properly prepared. Rubenstein (1962) collected characteristic wave forms over a pre-arranged course for common movements such as walking. Following the administration of sodium amytal, distinct changes occurred in the wave forms. Herron and Ramsden (1967a) have developed a radio telemetry-transducer system for measuring children's activity patterns under "natural" environmental conditions. A miniature transmitter-transducer is installed in the heel of the child's shoe and is not noticeable to the wearer. The range for this device is about 100 feet, it identifies walking and running, and is very inexpensive (in 1967 the parts cost less than $10). Its disadvantage is that of all the radio telemetry systems: the F.C.C. restricts the strength of transmitted signals, so the monitoring range is limited.

## OBSERVATIONS OF BEHAVIOR

As a part of the diagnostic work-up, direct observation of the child in the school environment provides an important source of data concerning the child's behavior as well as of the classroom environment, particularly the teacher's behavior. Whatever the focus of interest, the categories of behavior that are of interest are precisely defined and a selected time period for the observation is broken down into equal sub-units, usually ranging from five or more seconds to a minute or two (depending on the behaviors being observed). Observations are usually made at different times during the day and over several days. During each sub-unit of time the observer puts a check mark in any categories of behavior that the child (or whoever is being observed) exhibits in that sub-unit. When the categories are well-defined it is possible to obtain high inter-rater agreement with a minimum of rater training. Agreement is usually calculated by the percent-agreement method, with blank categories not included in the computation because their effect is to spuriously inflate the inter-rater agreement figure. Accuracy of observation is facilitated by having a timer tick the interval boundaries so that the observer need not watch the clock in addition to watching the child. When the timer ticks the observer automatically moves to the next column unit of time. Even in a classroom setting observations can be made quite unobtrusively. It is best if the teacher is given only a general description of the purpose of the observation, without singling out any particular child or any specific behavior, because it is impossible for a teacher to remain unaffected by prior knowledge of the purpose of the observation. It is much better to provide the teacher with all relevant information after the assessment has been completed and the management plan prepared. In addition to having satisfactory reliability, the direct observation approach is simple and requires a minimum of equipment. Although it does require one full-time observer, an astute observer can provide additional information concerning general aspects of the classroom scene, and this information can be of substantial help in planning a management strategy.

For direct observation in the laboratory and some naturalistic settings Lovaas, Freitag, Gold, and Kassorla (1965) developed an apparatus that provides a precise record of the duration and time of onset of each category of behavior and reduces the time spent by the observer on recording. The apparatus consists of a panel of up to 12 buttons, each representing a specific behavior category and each attached to its own pen recorder. When the subject starts a categorized behavior the observer presses the appropriate button, which activates the corresponding pen on an automatic cumulative recorder, and then releases the button when the behavior ends.

## RATING SCALES

Data from rating scales are useful in making a decision as to whether a problem does exist, in helping to determine what aspects of the problem should have priority as targets for change, and in evaluating the effectiveness of the management and change program. The scales are inexpensive and simple to use and so are particularly appropriate for parents and teachers as well as for others having long-term contact with the child. When selecting a scale first consider the adequacy of the rater reliability, test reliability, and validity data, then scan the response categories for ambiguity usually due to a failure to define the terms operationally. For example, Simpson (1944) reported great differences among raters in applying the category "frequently": 25 percent used this term to describe events occurring at least 80 percent of the time, whereas another 25 percent used it for events occurring less than 40 percent of the time. Next, determine if the items are operationally defined and are descriptive rather than interpretive. On descriptive items the observer rates the presence, absence, or frequency of certain behaviors, whereas on interpretive items he must extrapolate well beyond direct observation so that his own background and experience become his standards for judgment (Mischel, 1968). If no clear operational definition is provided for the behavior the rater must rely on his personal definition of such descriptions as "easily frustrated." Consider the following rating scales in the light of the above discussion.

### Werry-Weiss-Peters Activity Scale

This scale (see Table 8) consists of seven categories, five for specific contexts of activity engaged in by the child and two for more general areas of activity. The item categories are clearly delineated and differentiated (e.g., during meals, television). The behaviors within a category are all directly observable so that the rater is rating specific behaviors in specific contexts. The response choices could be improved. For example, "No" in a 3-response choice is too restrictive since if the person exhibits the behavior only once he must be scored in the middle category. It is preferable to have a "never or seldom" choice with each response choice accompanied by a frequency description. The school behavior item would have been better omitted. It is too short an assessment of so large and complex a sample of behavior and its rating would be based on second-hand information from the teacher. It would be better to have the teacher do a parallel rating of the child's school behavior in specific situations representative of the school in the way that the Werry-Weiss-Peters items are representative of the home.

### Conners' Teacher Rating Scale

This 39-item rating scale (see Table 12) consists of three clusters of items: classroom behavior, group participation, and attitude toward authority.

## Table 12. Conners' Teacher Rating Scale

IV.  Listed below are descriptive terms of behavior. Place a check mark in the column which best describes this child. ANSWER ALL ITEMS.

| Observation | Degree of Activity | | | |
|---|---|---|---|---|
| | Not at all | Just a little | Pretty much | Very much |
| **CLASSROOM BEHAVIOR** | | | | |
| 1. Constantly fidgeting | | | | |
| 2. Hums and makes other odd noises | | | | |
| 3. Demands must be met immediately—easily frustrated | | | | |
| 4. Coordination poor | | | | |
| 5. Restless or overactive | | | | |
| 6. Excitable, impulsive | | | | |
| 7. Inattentive, easily distracted | | | | |
| 8. Fails to finish things he starts—short attention span | | | | |
| 9. Overly sensitive | | | | |
| 10. Overly serious or sad | | | | |
| 11. Daydreams | | | | |
| 12. Sullen or sulky | | | | |
| 13. Cries often and easily | | | | |
| 14. Disturbs other children | | | | |
| 15. Quarrelsome | | | | |
| 16. Mood changes quickly and drastically | | | | |
| 17. Acts "smart" | | | | |
| 18. Destructive | | | | |
| 19. Steals | | | | |
| 20. Lies | | | | |
| 21. Temper outbursts, explosive and unpredictable behavior | | | | |
| | | | | |
| **GROUP PARTICIPATION** | | | | |
| 22. Isolates himself from other children | | | | |
| 23. Appears to be unaccepted by group | | | | |
| 24. Appears to be easily led | | | | |
| 25. No sense of fair play | | | | |
| 26. Appears to lack leadership | | | | |
| 27. Does not get along with opposite sex | | | | |
| 28. Does not get along with same sex | | | | |
| 29. Teases other children or interferes with their activities | | | | |
| | | | | |
| **ATTITUDE TOWARD AUTHORITY** | | | | |
| 30. Submissive | | | | |
| 31. Defiant | | | | |
| 32. Impudent | | | | |
| 33. Shy | | | | |
| 34. Fearful | | | | |
| 35. Excessive demands for teacher's attention | | | | |
| 36. Stubborn | | | | |
| 37. Overly anxious to please | | | | |
| 38. Uncooperative | | | | |
| 39. Attendance problem | | | | |

Reproduced, by permission, from C. Keith Conners.

The items are rated on a four-point scale in which "Not at all" is scored 0, "Just a little" is 1, "Pretty much" is 2, and "Very much" is 3. Factor analysis (Sprague, Cohen, & Werry, 1974) has identified four factors that were labeled Conduct Problem, Inattentive-Passive, Tension-Anxiety, and Hyperactivity. Research by Kupietz, Bialer, and Winsberg (1972) and Sprague, Christensen, and Werry (1974) has confirmed the efficacy of the scale for assessing and diagnosing hyperactive children in the classroom setting, and a study by Sprague, Cohen, and Werry (1974) has provided normative data.

Both the items and the response choices are open to criticism. In the items the behaviors are labeled but no behavioral description is provided, so the respondent must generalize rather than rate specific behaviors in specific contexts, for example, Item 4 — Coordination poor, or Item 30 — Submissive; there is overlap, for example, Item 14 — Disturbs other children and Item 29 — Teases other children or interferes with their activities; the wording is ambiguous and confusing particularly when a negatively worded item is considered in relation to the scale point Not at all, for example, Item 28 — Does not get along with same sex; both descriptive and interpretive items are included, for example, Item 20 — Lies and Item 34 — Fearful; more than one behavior is included in one item, for example, Item 29 — Teases other children or interferes with their activities. The *response choices* are ambiguous, for example, *Pretty much* is scale point 3 and *Very much* is scale point 4. The first scale point *Not at all* is a weak one if it is taken literally, as it should be. (Scale point 3 in Conners' Preliminary School Report and in a shortened version of the scale [Conners, 1972] was different from the one originally used [Scale point 3, Pretty much, replaced Quite a bit], but unfortunately has the same problems.)

## Conners' Abbreviated Teacher Rating Scale

This 10-item rating scale (see Table 13) consists of items from the 39-item rating scale. The 10 items were selected from those most often checked by teachers and have proven to be reliable in identifying hyperactive children and in assessing drug changes. The items are rated on the same four-point scale used in the full scale. A child would be classified as hyperactive on this scale with a total score of 15 points or more. Sprague, Cohen, and Werry (1974) reported satisfactory correlations between the abbreviated and complete scales.

**Table 13. Conners' Abbreviated Teacher Rating Scale**

CONNERS' ABBREVIATED TEACHER RATING SCALE

Child's Name _____

TEACHER'S OBSERVATIONS

Information obtained _____ By _____
                     Month    Day    Year

| Observation | Degree of Activity | | | |
| --- | --- | --- | --- | --- |
| | Not at all 0 | Just a little 1 | Pretty much 2 | Very much 3 |
| 1. Restless or overactive | | | | |
| 2. Excitable, impulsive | | | | |
| 3. Disturbs other children | | | | |
| 4. Fails to finish things he starts, short attention span | | | | |
| 5. Constantly fidgeting | | | | |
| 6. Inattentive, easily distracted | | | | |
| 7. Demands must be met immediately—easily frustrated | | | | |
| 8. Cries often and easily | | | | |
| 9. Mood changes quickly and drastically | | | | |
| 10. Temper outbursts, explosive and unpredictable behavior | | | | |

OTHER OBSERVATIONS OF TEACHER (Use reverse side if more space is required.)

_____

_____

_____

_____

## Conners' Parents Questionnaire

Conners (1970) has also developed a 93-item parent symptom checklist that assesses many other problems besides those that are often seen in the hyperactive child. These include fears and worries, bowel problems, sex problems, and perfectionism. Factor analysis identified six factors that were labeled aggressive conduct disorder, anxious-inhibited, antisocial, enuresis-encopresis, psychosomatic, and anxious-immature. The items are rated on the same four-point scale as that in the Conners' Teacher Rating Scale. Children previously diagnosed as hyperactive were correctly identified as hyperactive in 74 percent of the cases ($n = 133$) rated by parents. As previously noted, we prefer the Werry-Weiss-Peters Scale for use with parents.

One question with the Conners rating scales is what numerical value the respondent attaches to the categories Not at all, Just a little, Pretty much, and Very much. If one parent regards 10 instances of bullying (Item 39) over the previous month as sufficient for a rating of Very much (Scale Point 3) and another parent categorizes the same number of bullying incidents as Just a little (Scale Point 1), the diagnostic value of the information supplied by the rating scale is limited, as is the value of the scale for research in which the dependent variable is between-child comparisons based on parental ratings. To obtain some information on the numerical values that parents assign to the four categories, we conducted individual interviews with white, middle-class mothers of elementary school children. All of the mothers had attended college for two or more years. Following a brief explanatory statement and opportunity for questions, each mother was given a total of three items, one at a time. She was handed a card with a single item and the four categories on it and was asked how often in the past month her child would have had to exhibit the behavior described in the item for her to use each of the categories. For each of the three items the mother gave four numerical values that would result in her rating her child in the different categories. The three items given to each mother were Item 32 — Wants help doing things he should do alone, Item 39 — Bullying, and Item 57 — Throws and breaks things.

As can be seen from Table 14 the results from this rather homogeneous group of respondents showed a wide range of numerical values for each category except Not at all (Scale Point 0), to which the majority responded with a zero. We recognize that these mothers were stating how they thought a child would have to behave to be rated in each of the four categories and, as such, are clearly somewhat different from mothers who are completing the rating scale because their children do have problems serious enough to warrant a consultation. Nonetheless, the results suggest that the Conners scales and, indeed, most scales with this type of undefined

**Table 14　Numerical Values Assigned by Mothers (n = 40) to Categories on Conners' Parents Questionnaire**

| Item | | Not at all | Just a little | Pretty much | Very much |
|---|---|---|---|---|---|
| 32. Wants help doing things he should do alone | Mean | 1.58 | 14.73 | 33.30 | 51.60 |
| | Range | 0–15 | 2–120 | 3–200 | 7–300 |
| 39. Bullying | Mean | 0.75 | 7.60 | 15.45 | 29.17 |
| | Range | 0–10 | 1–80 | 2–100 | 5–200 |
| 57. Throws and breaks things | Mean | 0.50 | 3.65 | 6.70 | 12.02 |
| | Range | 0–10 | 1–30 | 4–60 | 5–90 |

descriptive categories might be of more value to the professional if the respondent was simply asked, ''Approximately how many times in the past month has your child exhibited this behavior?''

### The Bell, Waldrop, and Weller Rating System

Bell, Waldrop, and Weller (1972, p. 24) say that this is ''a rating system for the various facets of hyperactivity and withdrawal'' (see Table 15). It consists of six hyperactivity rating scales and three withdrawal rating scales. Each is an 11-point scale with descriptive statements provided for from three to five of the 11 scale points. The scales all involve direct behavior observation so that the rater does not have to go beyond this level, a plus feature; however, the descriptive statements for points within a scale are ambiguous. For example, the Frenetic Play scale includes frequency, intensity, and location unsystematically placed along the scale. As the scale points are described, the selection of a point along the scale is arbitrary. The sixth point on the Induction of Intervention scale is defined as ''three to four interventions per day required'' and the first point as ''never plays in such a way that requires intervention.'' If one or two interventions a day are required the rater has four scale points (2, 3, 4, 5) to choose from and still remain within the defined points. Having 11 points in each scale would appear to contribute to rater error. Behaviors within a scale do not all relate to the topic of the category so that two different continua are treated as one. For example, in the Nomadic Play scale, three scale points (11, 6, 3) concern amount of shifting from one activity to the next, but the first scale point (1) is a withdrawal-from-activity behavior, ''Very hesitant to engage in play. Stands and watches or leans on mother or teacher." There is overlap between scales. Although the distinction between Frenetic Play and Nomadic Play is clear in the Bell, Waldrop, and Weller (1970) article (*frenetic* has an intensity and disorganization quality, whereas *nomadic* concerns rapid movement from activity to activity), this distinction is unclear in the descriptions given the rater: the descriptions for the eleventh point on both scales are difficult to differentiate. The scales vary greatly in breadth. Frenetic Play is a characteristic applying to a wide range of activities while Spilling and Throwing is a very specific behavior. It is dificult to see how satisfactory full-scale reliability could be obtained by two raters independently rating one child on the entire scale, with the limited number of *defined* scale points and without excessive training for the observers. Full-scale inter-observer reliability for behavior ratings should be in the high .90's, and this level is not difficult to achieve with operationally defined response categories and descriptive items. Some validity support is provided by the finding that most (no data given) but not all of the children identified by the staff as having definite adjustment problems had scores above the cutting point delineating the presence of adjustment problems.

## Davids' Rating Scale for Hyperkinesis

This scale (Davids, 1971) is intended to provide an assessment of the hyperkinetic syndrome. Seven traits or behaviors are rated on a 6-point scale ranging from "much less than most children" to "much more than most children." The first six traits used to assess the hyperkinetic syndrome are hyperactivity, short attention span, variability, impulsiveness and inability to delay gratification, irritability, and explosiveness. The possible score ranges from 6 to 36; scores of 24 or more suggest hyperkinesis, scores of 19 to 23 are in the suspicious range, and those of 18 or less indicate no significant hyperkinesis. No reliability and no validity data are reported. The author says only that the rating scales have "adequate reliability" (but gives no breakdown into test and observer reliability) and "considerable clinical utility." It is presented as a less than fully developed tool, lacking reliability, validity, and normative data. Davids hopes that these data will be forthcoming from scale users. Specific weaknesses of the scale include categories that overlap, for example, Category 1. Hyperactivity, includes the description "always on the move, rarely sits still" and Category 2. Short attention span, includes "frequent shifting from one activity to another." The categories require the respondent to extrapolate well beyond direct observation, the behaviors are described in general contexts rather than in specific situations, the categories lack clear opera-

| SCALE POINTS | DEFINITIONS |
|---|---|
| | HYPERACTIVITY |

**FRENETIC PLAY**

11. Much more than others, shows impulsive, fast moving, ineffective, incomplete play.
9. During play and transitions shows behavior with only two or three of the components listed in 11, or play showing all components but with less intensity.
6. Only during transitions or in vehicle shows frenetic behavior.
4. During transitions shows mild frenetic behavior.
1. Never shows any frenetic behavior.

| Scale | 11 | 10 | 9 | 8 | 7 | 6 | 5 | 4 | 3 | 2 | 1 |
|---|---|---|---|---|---|---|---|---|---|---|---|
| Percentage distribution ª | 0 | .2 | .2 | 1 | 1 | 2 | 2 | 4 | 8 | 16 | 64 |

**INDUCTION OF INTERVENTION**

11. Very frequently plays in such a way as to make it highly likely teacher in area would feel compelled to intervene either to prevent injury to the child or others, or to prevent damage to physical objects.
6. Three to four interventions per day required.
1. Never plays in such a way that requires intervention.

| Scale | 11 | 10 | 9 | 8 | 7 | 6 | 5 | 4 | 3 | 2 | 1 |
|---|---|---|---|---|---|---|---|---|---|---|---|
| Percentage distribution | 0 | 0 | .1 | 1 | 1 | 2 | 2 | 4 | 8 | 16 | 66 |

**INABILITY TO DELAY**

11. When waiting turn for food, toy or any other object which is of interest, or when waiting to take part in some activity, seems unusually unable to wait for gratification.
9. Same as 11, except behavior is shown only during certain situations, such as transitions, or in the car.
6. In only a few instances seemed unable to wait for gratification.
1. Under above circumstances seems definitely able to contain self and wait for gratification.

| Scale | 11 | 10 | 9 | 8 | 7 | 6 | 5 | 4 | 3 | 2 | 1 |
|---|---|---|---|---|---|---|---|---|---|---|---|
| Percentage distribution | 0 | .2 | 1 | 1 | 2 | 7 | 10 | 13 | 17 | 20 | 30 |

**EMOTIONAL AGGRESSION**

11. Frequently throws toys, tears things down, breaks toys, pushes objects over, attacks, pushes or hits, takes things from others even though not needed to achieve an objective and even though may or may not be upset.
6. Usually interested in other activities but will occasionally throw toys, tear things down, break toys, etc., as a reaction to frustration, when just wandering, or during transitions.
1. Never takes from others.

| Scale | 11 | 10 | 9 | 8 | 7 | 6 | 5 | 4 | 3 | 2 | 1 |
|---|---|---|---|---|---|---|---|---|---|---|---|
| Percentage distribution | 0 | 0 | .1 | .1 | .1 | 2 | 1 | 2 | 6 | 10 | 80 |

**NOMADIC PLAY**

11. Shifts rapidly from one setting or toy to another, typically trying out an item for only an instant and then moving on, showing no sustained play or engagement of interest unless assisted.
6. Shifts between toys or settings but finds two or three activities during the session which engage interest for approximately five minutes.
3. Goes straight to a single setting or toy on arrival and remains engaged for most of session.
1. Very hesitant to engage in any play. Stands and watches or leans on mother or teacher.

| Scale | 11 | 10 | 9 | 8 | 7 | 6 | 5 | 4 | 3 | 2 | 1 |
|---|---|---|---|---|---|---|---|---|---|---|---|
| Percentage distribution | .1 | .2 | 2 | 6 | 13 | 28 | 22 | 18 | 10 | 2 | .2 |

318

DEFINITIONS

## HYPERACTIVITY—(Continued)

### SPILLING, THROWING
11. Spills water, containers, salt or other substances and/or throws food or other objects much more often than others (playful throwing of a ball should not be considered under this heading).
9. In certain situations, such as in the car or in transitions, shows frequent spilling and throwing.
6. Usually interested in other activities, but will occasionally spill and/or throw either as a reaction to frustration or when just wandering.
1. Never spills water or throws objects.

| Scale | 11 | 10 | 9 | 8 | 7 | 6 | 5 | 4 | 3 | 2 | 1 |
|---|---|---|---|---|---|---|---|---|---|---|---|
| Percentage distribution | 0 | 1 | 2 | 3 | 6 | 14 | 18 | 21 | 18 | 12 | 5 |

## WITHDRAWAL

### VACANT STARING
11. Is immobile and staring without apparent focus much more than others.
9. Spends a large amount of time staring in a single direction, at a single object, setting or area, or occasionally shows staring without focus. (This can accompany relatively disorganized or aimless play.)
3. Seldom shows fixed or vacant staring and then as a reaction to some specific strange or fearful incident.
1. Never shows fixed or vacant staring.

| Scale | 11 | 10 | 9 | 8 | 7 | 6 | 5 | 4 | 3 | 2 | 1 |
|---|---|---|---|---|---|---|---|---|---|---|---|
| Percentage distribution | 0 | .1 | 1 | 1 | 2 | 6 | 10 | 14 | 20 | 24 | 24 |

### CLOSENESS TO ADULT BASE
11. Spends an unusually large amount of time clinging tightly to mother or teacher, hiding eyes, not exploring the situation either visually or otherwise.
9. Almost continuously follows or remains close to mother or teacher.
6. Alternates staying close to mother or teacher with occasional efforts to play separately.
4. Plays separately, except during transitions.
2. Only comes to mother or teacher and stays close when there is something strange or novel in situation.
1. Never spends time in activities listed.

| Scale | 11 | 10 | 9 | 8 | 7 | 6 | 5 | 4 | 3 | 2 | 1 |
|---|---|---|---|---|---|---|---|---|---|---|---|
| Percentage distribution | 0 | 0 | 1 | 1 | 2 | 3 | 6 | 15 | 19 | 28 | 28 |

### CHRONIC FEARFULNESS
11. Characteristically appears to be guarded, wary, defensive, apprehensive, frightened, or panicky.
6. Neither characteristically bold or guarded; shows some of each.
1. Seems to be bold rather than fearful; seldom, if ever, shows fearfulness, even in situations which might ordinarily be expected to produce this effect.

| Scale | 11 | 10 | 9 | 8 | 7 | 6 | 5 | 4 | 3 | 2 | 1 |
|---|---|---|---|---|---|---|---|---|---|---|---|
| Percentage distribution | 0 | .2 | 1 | 1 | 2 | 8 | 12 | 18 | 23 | 20 | 14 |

a Smoothed percentages for scale points 11 through 1, based on combined data for 43 males and 31 females (test samples).

tional definitions, and there is some question that they adequately describe the hyperkinetic child. The response choices are ambiguous. The standard is "behavior displayed by other 'normal' children." The respondents' definitions of 'normal' and their experience with children would lead to fluctuating standards across raters. No attempt is made to define the scale points and an important scale point, "same as," is omitted so that the respondent is forced to use either "slightly less" or "slightly more" when in fact he may regard the child as "the same as other children." The "slightly less" point is scored as 3 and the "slightly more" as 4. A respondent who tends to mark the latter category in lieu of a "same as" category would end up with a rating in the "suspicious range" as opposed to one in the "absence of significant hyperkinesis" range. The instructions reduce accuracy: the author says the instructions can be modified somewhat for more specific purposes but does not clarify why or how. The respondent is in effect instructed to guess if he is unable to place the child's behavior: "Even though it may sometimes be difficult to make a judgment, please make a rating on one or the other side of the scale."

# REFERENCES

Abrams, A. L. Delayed and irregular maturation versus minimal brain injury. *Clinical Pediatrics*, 1968, **7**, 344–349.

Alabiso, F. Inhibitory functions of attention in reducing hyperactive behavior. *American Journal of Mental Deficiency*, 1972, **77**, 259–282.

Alderton, H. R. Imipramine in childhood enuresis: Further studies on the relationship of time and administration to effect. *Canadian Medical Association Journal*, 1970, **102**, 1179–1180.

Allen, K. E., Henke, L. B., Harris, F. R., Baer, D. M., and Reynolds, N. J. Control of hyperactivity by social reinforcement of attending behavior. *Journal of Educational Psychology*, 1967, **58**, 231–237.

Allen, R. P., Safer, D., and Covi, L. Effects of psychostimulants on aggression. *Journal of Nervous and Mental Diseases*, 1975, **160**, 138–145.

Aman, M. G. and Sprague, R. L. The state-dependent effects of methylphenidate and dextroamphetamine. *Journal of Nervous and Mental Diseases*, 1974, **158**, 268–279.

Aman, M. G., & Werry, J. S. Methylphenidate in children: Effects upon cardiorespiratory. *International Journal of Mental Health*, 1975, **4**, No. 1–2, 119–131.

Ament, A. Treatment of hyperactive children (letter). *Journal of the American Medical Association*, 1974, **230**, No. 3, 372.

Ambrose, A. (Ed.), *Stimulation in early infancy*. New York: Academic Press, 1969.

American Academy of Pediatrics, Committee on Drugs. Statement issued June, 1970.

American Psychiatric Association. *Diagnostic and statistical manual of mental disorders*. Washington, D.C., 1968.

Anastasi, A. *Psychological testing*, 3rd ed. New York: Macmillan, 1968.

Anderson, C. M. and Plymate, H. B. Management of the brain-damaged adolescent. *American Journal of Orthopsychiatry*, 1962, **32**, 492–500.

Anderson, D. Application of a behavior modification technique to the control of a hyperactive child. Unpublished M.A. Thesis, University of Oregon, 1964.

Anderson, W. W. The hyperkinetic child: A neurological appraisal. *Neurology*, 1963, **13**, 968–973.

Ariès, P. *Centuries of childhood: A social history of family life*. New York: Knopf, 1962.

Arnold, L. E. Hyperkinetic adult. Study of the "paradoxical" amphetamine response. *Journal of the American Medical Association*, 1972, **222**, 693–694.

Arnold, L. E., Kirilcuk, V., Corson, S., and Corson, E. O. Levoamphetamine and dextroamphetamine: Differential effect on aggression and hyperkinesis in children and dogs. *American Journal of Psychiatry*, 1973, **130**, 165–170.

Arnold, L. E. and Knopf, W. The making of a myth. *Journal of the American Medical Association*, 1973, **223**, 1273–1274.

Arnold, L. E. and Smeltzer, D. J. Behavior checklist factor analysis for children and adolescents. *Archives of General Psychiatry*, 1974, **30**, 799–804.

Arnold, L. E., Strobl, D., and Weisenberg, A. Hyperkinetic adult. *Journal of the American Medical Association*, 1972, **222**, 693–694.

Arnold, L. E., Wender, P. H., McCloskey, K., and Snyder, S. H. Levoamphetamine and dextroamphetamine: Comparative efficacy in the hyperkinetic syndrome. *Archives of General Psychiatry*, 1972, **27**, 816–822.

Aron, A. M. Minimal cerebral dysfunction in childhood. *Journal of Communication Disorders*, 1972, **5**, 142–153.

Atkinson, B. R. The effect of activity and social stimulation on attention. Unpublished doctoral dissertation, University of Western Ontario, 1970.

Aub, J. C., Fairhall, L. T., Minot, A. S., and Resnikoff, P. *Lead poisoning*. Baltimore: Williams & Wilkins, 1926.

Ayllon, T., Layman, D., and Kandel, H. J. A behavioral-educational alternative to drug control of hyperactive children. *Journal of Applied Behavior Analysis*, 1975, **8**, 137–146.

Bahrick, H. P. Incidental learning under two incentive conditions. *Journal of Experimental Psychology*, 1954, **47**, 170–172.

Baker, R. R. The effects of psychotropic drugs on psychological testing. *Psychological Bulletin*, 1968, **69**, 377–387.

Bakwin, H. and Bakwin, R. M. *Clinical management of behavior disorders in children*. Philadelphia: Saunders, 1966.

Baldwin, D. G., Kittler, F. J., and Ramsay, R. G. The relationship of allergy to cerebral dysfunction. *Southern Medical Journal*, 1968, **61**, 1039.

Bandura, A. Modeling approaches to the modification of phobic disorders. In *CIBA Foundation Symposium: The role of learning in psychotherapy*. London: Churchill, 1968.

Bandura, A. *Principles of behavior modification*. New York: Holt, Rinehart, & Winston, 1969.

Bandura, A. Psychotherapy based upon modeling principles. In A. E. Bergin and S. L. Garfield (Eds.), *Handbook of psychotherapy and behavior change*. New York: Wiley, 1971, Chapter 17.

Bandura, A. Behavior theory and the models of man. *American Psychologist*, 1974, **29**, 859–869.

Bandura, A., Blanchard, E. B., and Ritter, B. J. The relative efficacy of desensitization and modeling treatment approaches for inducing affective, behavioral, and attitudinal changes. *Journal of Personality and Social Psychology*, 1969, **13**, 173–199.

Bandura, A., Ross, D., and Ross, S. A. Transmission of aggression through imitation of aggressive models. *Journal of Abnormal and Social Psychology,* 1961, **63,** 575–582.

Bandura, A., Ross, D., and Ross, S. A. Imitation of film-mediated aggressive models. *Journal of Abnormal and Social Psychology,* 1963, **66,** 3–11.

Bandura, A. and Walters, R. H. *Adolescent aggression.* New York: Ronald, 1959.

Bandura, A. and Walters, R. H. *Social learning and personality development.* New York: Holt, Rinehart, & Winston, 1963.

Barcai, A. The emergence of neurotic conflict in some children after successful administration of dextroamphetamine. *Journal of Child Psychology and Psychiatry,* 1969, **10,** 269–276.

Barcai, A. Predicting the response of children with learning disabilities and behavior problems to dextroamphetamine sulphate. *Pediatrics,* 1971, **47,** 73–80.

Barkley, R. A. and Routh, D. K. Reduction of children's locomotor activity by modeling and the promise of contingent reward. *Journal of Abnormal Child Psychology,* 1974, **2,** 117–131.

Barnard, K. and Collar, B. S. Early diagnosis, interpretation, and intervention: A commentary on the nurse's role. *Annals of the New York Academy of Sciences,* 1973, **205,** 373–382.

Barrett, B. Reduction in rate of multiple tics by free operant conditioning methods. *Journal of Nervous and Mental Diseases,* 1962, **135,** 187–195.

Barrett, R. J., Leith, N. J. and Ray, O. S. Permanent facilitation of avoidance behavior by d-amphetamine and scopolamine. *Psychopharmacologia,* 1972, **25,** 321–331.

Barten, H. (Ed.), *Brief therapies.* New York: Behavioral Publications, 1971.

Bass, H. N. and Schulman, J. L. Quantitative assessment of children's activity in and out of bed. *American Journal of Diseases of Children,* 1967, **113,** 242–244.

Battle, E. S. and Lacey, B. A context for hyperactivity in children, over time. *Child Development,* 1972, **43,** 757–773.

Bauer, R. and Kenny, T. An ego disturbance model of MBD. *Child Psychiatry and Human Development,* 1974, **4,** 238–245.

Bauman, S. S. and Greene, S. K. Brain dysfunction in adolescence: II. Life styles. *American Journal of Orthopsychiatry,* 1970, **40,** 334–335.

Bax, M. The active and the overactive school child. *Developmental Medicine and Child Neurology,* 1972, **14,** 83–86.

Bax, M. and MacKeith, R. (Eds.), Minimal cerebral dysfunction. *Little Club Clinics in Developmental Medicine,* 1963, **10,** London: Heineman.

Bazell, R. J. Panel sanctions amphetamines for hyperkinetic children. *Science,* 1971, **171,** 1223.

Beck, L., Langford, W. S., MacKay, M., and Sum, G. Childhood chemotherapy and later drug abuse and growth curve: A follow-up study of 30 adolescents. *American Journal of Psychiatry,* 1975, **132,** 436–438.

Becker, W. C., Madsen, C. H., Jr., Arnold, C. R., and Thomas, D. R. The contingent use of teacher attention and praise in reducing classroom behavior problems. *Journal of Special Education,* 1967, **1,** 287–307.

Beecher, H. K. The powerful placebo. *Journal of the American Medical Association,* 1955, **159,** 1602–1606.

Begelman, D. A. Ethical issues in behavior control. *Journal of Nervous and Mental Diseases,* 1973, **156,** 412–419.

Bell, R. Q. A reinterpretation of the direction of effects in studies of socialization. *Psychological Review,* 1968, **75,** 81–95.

Bell, R. Q. Stimulus control of parent or caretaker behavior by offspring. *Developmental Psychology,* 1971, **4,** 63–72.

Bell, R. Q., Waldrop, M. F., and Weller, G. M. A rating system for the assessment of hyperactive and withdrawn children in preschool samples. *American Journal of Orthopsychiatry,* 1972, **42,** 23–34.

Bellak, L. and Chassan, J. B. An approach to the evaluation of drug effect during psychotherapy: A double-blind study of a single case. *Journal of Nervous and Mental Diseases,* 1964, **139,** 20–30.

Bender, L. *Aggression, hostility, and anxiety in children.* Springfield, Illinois: Thomas, 1953.

Bensberg, G. J. (Ed.), *Teaching the mentally retarded: A handbook for ward personnel.* Atlanta: Southern Regional Education Board, 1965.

Benton, A. L. Review of *Brain damage and behavior: A clinical-experimental study. Neurology,* 1966, **16,** 1228.

Bergin, A. E. The effects of psychotherapy: Negative results revisited. *Journal of Counseling Psychology,* 1963, **10,** 244–250.

Bergin, A. E. The evaluation of therapeutic outcomes. In A. E. Bergin and S. L. Garfield (Eds.), *Handbook of psychotherapy and behavior change: An empirical analysis.* New York: Wiley, 1971, pp. 217–270.

Bergin, A. E. and Garfield, S. L. (Eds.), *Handbook of psychotherapy and behavior change.* New York: Wiley, 1971.

Berkowitz, B. T. and Graziano, A. M. Training parents as behavior therapists: A review. *Behavior Research and Therapy,* 1972, **10,** 297–317.

Berlin, I. Minimal brain dysfunction. Management of family distress. *Journal of the American Medical Association,* 1974, **229,** No. 11, 1454–1456.

Berlyne, D. E. *Conflict, arousal, and curiosity.* New York: McGraw-Hill, 1960.

Bernal, G., Jacobson, L. I., and Lopez, G. N. Do the effects of behavior modification programs endure? *Behavior Research and Therapy,* 1975, **13,** 61–64.

Bernal, M. E. Behavioral feedback and the modification of "brat" behaviors. *Journal of Nervous and Mental Diseases,* 1969, **148,** 375–385.

Bernal, M. E., Duryee, J. S., Pruett, H. L., and Burns, B. J. Behavior modification and the brat syndrome. *Journal of Consulting and Clinical Psychology,* 1968, **32,** 447–455.

Berne, E. *Transactional analysis in psychotherapy.* New York: Grove, 1961.

Berne, E. *Games people play.* New York: Grove, 1964.

Berne, E. *What do you say after you say Hello?* New York: Grove, 1972.

Berwick, D. M. Prevalence and management of hyperactive children (letter). *New England Journal of Medicine,* 1975, **292,** 536.

Bettelheim, B. Bringing up children. *Ladies Home Journal,* 1973, **90,** 28.

Bijou, S. W. Experimental studies of child behavior, normal and deviant. In L. Krasner and L. P. Ullman (Eds.), *Research in behavior modification.* New York: Holt, Rinehart, & Winston, 1965, pp. 56–81.

Bijou, S. W. and Baer, D. M. Operant methods in child behavior and development. In W. K. Honig (Ed.), *Operant behavior: Areas of research and application.* Springfield, Ill.: Appleton-Century-Crofts, 1966.

Bijou, S. W., Peterson, R. F., Harris, F. R., Allen, K. E., and Johnston, M. S. Methodology for experimental studies of young children in natural settings. In E. J. Thomas (Ed.), *Behavior modification procedure: A sourcebook.* Chicago: Aldine, 1974, pp. 61–95.

Blackwood, R. O. *Mediated self-control: An operant model of rational behavior.* Akron, Ohio: Exordium Press, 1972.

Block, J., Block, J. H., and Harrington, D. M. Some misgivings about the Matching Familiar Figures Test as a measure of reflection-impulsivity. *Developmental Psychology,* 1974, **10,** 611–632.

Block, J., Block, J. H., and Harrington, D. M. Comment on the Kagan-Messer reply. *Developmental Psychology,* 1975, **11,** 249–252.

Bolstad, O. D. and Johnson, S. M. Self-regulation in the modification of disruptive classroom behavior. *Journal of Applied Behavior Analysis,* 1972, **5,** 443–454.

Bond, E. D. and Appel, K. E. *The treatment of behavior disorders following encephalitis.* New York: Commonwealth Fund, Division of Publications, 1931.

Bond, E. D. and Smith, L. H. Post-encephalitic behavior disorders. *American Journal of Psychiatry,* 1935, **92,** 17–33.

Borgstedt, A. D. and Rosen, M. G. Fetal electroencephalography: Relationship to neonatal and one-year developmental neurological examinations in high-risk infants. *American Journal of Diseases of Children,* 1975, **129,** 35–38.

Boszormenyi-Nagy, I. and Framo, J. (Eds.), *Intensive family therapy.* New York: Harper & Row, 1965.

Bower, T. G. R. Development of infant behavior. *British Medical Bulletin,* 1974, **30,** 175–178.

Bradley, C. The behavior of children receiving benzedrine. *American Journal of Psychiatry,* 1937, **94,** 577–585.

Bradley, C. Benzedrine and dexedrine in the treatment of children's behavior disorders. *Pediatrics,* 1950, **5,** 24–37.

Bradley, C. Characteristics and management of children with behavior problems associated with organic brain damage. *Pediatric Clinics of North America,* 1957, **4,** 1049–1060.

Bradley, C. and Bowen, M. Amphetamine (Benzedrine) therapy of children's behavior disorders. *American Journal of Orthopsychiatry,* 1941, **11**, 92–103.

Bradley, J. E. and Baumgartner, R. J. Subsequent mental development of children with lead encephalopathy, as related to type of treatment. *Journal of Pediatrics,* 1958, **53**, 311–315.

Braud, L. W., Lupin, M. N., & Braud, W. G. The use of electromyographic biofeedback in the control of hyperactivity. *Journal of Learning Disabilities,* 1975, **8**, 420–425.

Brazelton, T. B. Psychophysiologic reactions of the neonate: I. The value of observation of the neonate. *Journal of Pediatrics,* 1961, **58**, 508–512.

Bremer, D. A. Attention during reading in hyperactive boys: Reactions to distracting stimuli and to rewards. *Dissertation Abstracts International,* 1974, **34B**, 6206–6207.

Broadbent, D. E. *Perception and communication.* London: Pergamon Press, 1958.

Broden, M., Bruce, M., Mitchell, M., Carter, V., and Hall, R. V. Effects of teacher attention on attending behavior of two boys at adjacent desks. *Journal of Applied Behavior Analysis,* 1970, **3**, 199–203.

Broussard, E. R., and Hartner, M. S. S. Maternal perception of the neonate as related to development. *Child Psychiatry and Human Development,* 1970, **1**, 16–25.

Broussard, E. R., and Hartner, M. S. S. Further considerations regarding maternal perception of the first born. In J. Hellmuth (Ed.), *Exceptional infant, Vol 2. Studies in abnormalities,* New York: Brunner/Mazel, 1971.

Browder, J. A. Appropriate use of psychic drugs in school children. *American Journal of Diseases of Children,* 1972, **124**, 606–607.

Brown, A. J. A longitudinal study of hyperkinetic syndrome in children: Kindergarten through grade three. *Dissertation Abstracts International,* 1969, **30A**, 1857–1858.

Brown, D., Winsberg, B. G., Bialer, I., and Press, M. Imipramine therapy and seizures. Three children treated for hyperactive behavior disorders. *American Journal of Psychiatry,* 1973, **130**, 210–212.

Browning, R. Effect of irrelevant peripheral visual stimuli on discrimination learning in minimally brain-damaged children. *Journal of Consulting Psychology,* 1967, **31**, 371–376.

Buchsbaum, M. and Wender, P. Average evoked responses in normal and minimally brain dysfunctioned children treated with amphetamine: A preliminary report. *Archives of General Psychiatry,* 1973, **29**, 764–770.

Buckley, N. K. and Walker, H. M. *Modifying classroom behavior.* Champaign, Ill.: Research Press, 1970.

Buckley, R. E. Neurophysiologic proposal for the amphetamine response in hyperkinetic children. *Psychosomatics,* 1972, **13**, 93–99.

Buddenhagen, R. G. and Sickler, P. Hyperactivity: A forty-eight hour sample plus a note on etiology. *American Journal of Mental Deficiency,* 1969, **73**, 580–589.

Bullen, B. A., Reed, R. B., and Mayer, J. Physical activity of obese and nonobese adolescent girls appraised by motion picture sampling. *American Journal of Clinical Nutrition,* 1964, **14**, 211–223.

Burns, B. J. The effect of self-directed verbal commands on arithmetic performance and activity level of urban hyperactive children. Boston College, Ph.D. Dissertation, 1972.

Buros, O. K. (Ed.), *The seventh mental measurements yearbook.* Highland Park, N.J.: Gryphon Press, 1972.

Bustamante, J. A., Jordan, A., Vila, M., Gonzalez, A., and Insua, A. State dependent learning in humans. *Physiology and Behavior,* 1969, **5**, 793–796.

Bustamante, J. A., Rossello, A., Jordan, A., Pradera, E., and Insua, A. Learning and drugs. *Physiology and Behavior,* 1967, **3**, 553–555.

Butter, H. J., and Lapierre, Y. D. The effect of methylphenidate on sensory perception and integration in hyperactive children. *International Pharmacopsychiatry,* 1974, **9**, 235–244.

Byers, R. K. and Lord, E. E. Late effects of lead poisoning on mental development. *American Journal of Diseases of Children,* 1943, **66**, 471–494.

Campbell, S. B. Cognitive styles in reflective, impulsive and hyperactive boys and their mothers. *Perceptual and Motor Skills,* 1973, **36**, 747–752.

Campbell, S. B., Douglas, V. I., and Morgenstern, G. Cognitive styles in hyperactive children and the effect of methylphenidate. *Journal of Child Psychology and Psychiatry,* 1971, **12**, 55–67.

Campbell, W. A., Cheeseman, E. A., and Kilpatrick, A. W. The effects of neonatal asphyxia on physical and mental development. *Archives of Diseases of Childhood,* 1950, **25**, 351–359.

Cantrell, R. P., Cantrell, M. L., Huddleston, C. M., and Wooldridge, R. L. Contingency contracting with school problems. *Journal of Applied Behavior Analysis,* 1969, **2**, 215–220.

Cantwell, D. P. Psychiatric illness in the families of hyperactive children. *Archives of General Psychiatry,* 1972, **27**, 414–417.

Cantwell, D. P. Epidemiology, clinical picture and classification of the hyperactive child syndrome. In D. P. Cantwell (Ed.), *The hyperactive child.* New York: Spectrum, 1975, pp. 3–15.

Cantwell, D. P. Natural history and prognosis in the hyperactive child syndrome. In D. P. Cantwell (Ed.), *The hyperactive child.* New York: Spectrum, 1975a, pp. 51–64.

Cantwell, D. P. Genetic studies of hyperactive children. In R. R. Fieve, D. Rosenthal, and H. Brill (Eds.), *Genetic research in psychiatry.* Baltimore, Md.: Johns Hopkins University Press, 1975b, pp. 273–280.

Carter, C. O. *An ABC of medical genetics.* Boston: Little, Brown, 1969.

Carter, C. O. Multifactorial genetic disease. *Hospital Practice,* 1970, **5**, 45–49, 55–59.

Casey, G. A. Behavior rehearsal: Principles and procedures. *Psychotherapy: Theory, Research, and Practice,* 1973, **10**, 331–333.

Cash, W. M. and Evans, I. M. Training pre-school children to modify their retarded siblings' behavior. *Journal of Behavior Therapy and Experimental Psychiatry,* 1975, **6,** 13–16.

Caudill, W. and Weinstein, H. Maternal care and infant behavior in Japan and America. *Psychiatry,* 1969, **32,** 12–43.

Cautela, J. R. and Kastenbaum, R. A reinforcement survey schedule for use in therapy, training, and research. *Psychological Reports,* 1967, **20,** 1115–1130.

Chamberlain, R. W. Convulsions and Ritalin? (letter). *Pediatrics,* 1974, **54,** 658–659.

Chess, S. Diagnosis and treatment of the hyperactive child. *New York State Journal of Medicine,* 1960, **60,** 2379–2385.

Chess, S. Hyperactive children: A rational approach to medication. *Urban Review,* 1972, **5,** 33–35.

Chess, S., Thomas, A., and Birch, H. G. Behavior problems revisited. In S. Chess and T. Birch (Eds.), *Annual progress in child psychiatry and child development.* New York: Brunner/Mazel, 1968, pp. 335–344.

Chess, S., Thomas, A., Rutter, M., and Birch, H. G. Interaction of temperament and environment in the production of behavioral disturbances in children. *American Journal of Psychiatry,* 1963, **120,** 142–148.

Childers, A. T. Hyperactivity in children having behavior disorders. *American Journal of Orthopsychiatry,* 1935, **5,** 227–243.

Chisolm, J. J., Jr. Lead poisoning. *Scientific American,* 1971, **224,** 15–23.

Christensen, D. E. and Sprague, R. L. Reduction of hyperactive behavior by conditioning procedures alone and combined with methylphenidate (Ritalin). *Behavior Research and Therapy,* 1973, **11,** 331–334.

Cleland, C. C. Severe retardation: Program suggestions. Paper read at Regional Council on Exceptional Children, Austin, Texas, 1961.

Clements, S. D. *Task Force One: Minimal brain dysfunction in children.* National Institute of Neurological Diseases and Blindness, Monograph No. 3, U.S. Department of Health, Education and Welfare, 1966.

Clements, S. D. and Peters, J. Minimal brain dysfunctions in the school-age child. *Archives of General Psychiatry,* 1962, **6,** 185–197.

Close, J. Scored neurological examination. *Psychopharmacology Bulletin,* National Institute of Mental Health, Washington, D.C., 1973, pp. 142–150.

Cohen, A. R. Tricyclic antidepressants and brain dysfunction (Letter). *Journal of the American Medical Association,* 1973, **225,** 177–179.

Cohen, N. J. and Douglas, V. I. Characteristics of the orienting response in hyperactive and normal children. *Psychophysiology,* 1972, **9,** 238–245.

Cohen, N. J., Douglas, V. I., and Morgenstern, G. Psychophysiological concomitants of hyperactivity in children. *Canadian Psychology,* 1969, **10,** 199 (Abstract).

Cohen, N. J., Douglas, V. I., and Morgenstern, G. The effect of methylphenidate on attentive behavior and automatic activity in hyperactive children. *Psychopharmacologia,* 1971, **22,** 282–294.

Cohen, N. J., Weiss, G., and Minde, K. Cognitive styles in adolescents previously diagnosed as hyperactive. *Journal of Child Psychology and Psychiatry*, 1972, **13**, 203–209.

Collard, R. R. Review of Bayley Scales of Infant Development (1969). In O. K. Buros (Ed.), *The seventh mental measurements yearbook, Vol. 1*. Highland Park, N.J.: Gryphon Press, 1972, pp. 727–729.

Conners, C. K. The effect of dexedrine on rapid discrimination and motor control of hyperkinetic children under mild stress. *Journal of Nervous and Mental Diseases*, 1966, **142**, 429–433.

Conners, C. K. A teacher rating scale for use in drug studies with children. *American Journal of Psychiatry*, 1969, **126**, 884–888.

Conners, C. K. Symptom patterns in hyperkinetic, neurotic, and normal children. *Child Development*, 1970, **41**, 667–682.

Conners, C. K. Recent drug studies with hyperkinetic children. *Journal of Learning Disabilities*, 1971, **4**, 476–483.

Conners, C. K. The effect of stimulant drugs on human figure drawings in children with minimal brain dysfunction. *Psychopharmacologia*, 1971a, **19**, 329–333.

Conners, C. K. Pharmacotherapy of psychopathology in children. In H. C. Quay and J. S. Werry (Eds.), *Psychopathological disorders of childhood*. New York: Wiley, 1972, pp. 316–347.

Conners, C. K. Symposium: Behavior modification by drugs. II. Psychological effects of stimulant drugs in children with minimal brain dysfunction. *Pediatrics*, 1972a, **49**, 702–708.

Conners, C. K. A clinical comparison of methylphenidate and placebo in the treatment of children with minimal brain dysfunction. Paper presented at the Meetings of the American Psychological Association, Montreal, August, 1973.

Conners, C. K. What parents need to know about stimulant drugs and special education. *Journal of Learning Disabilities*, 1973a, **6**, 349–351.

Conners, C. K. A placebo-crossover study of caffeine treatment of hyperkinetic children. *International Journal of Mental Health*, 1975, **4**, No. 1–2, 132–143.

Conners, C. K. and Eisenberg, L. The effects of methylphenidate on symptomatology and learning in disturbed children. *American Journal of Psychiatry*, 1963, **120**, 458–464.

Conners, C. K., Eisenberg, L., and Barcai, A. Effect of dextroamphetamine in children. *Archives of General Psychiatry*, 1967, **17**, 478–485.

Conners, C. K., Eisenberg, L., and Sharpe, L. Effects of methylphenidate (Ritalin) on paired-associate learning and Porteus Maze performance in emotionally disturbed children. *Journal of Consulting Psychology*, 1964, **28**, 14–22.

Conners, C. K. and Rothschild, G. H. Drugs and learning in children. In J. Hellmuth (Ed.), *Learning disorders, Vol. 3*. Seattle, Wash.: Special Child Publications, 1968, pp. 191–223.

Conners, C. K., Rothschild, G. H., Eisenberg, L., Stone, L., and Robinson, E. Dextroamphetamine in children with learning disorders. *Archives of General Psychiatry*, 1969, **21**, 182–190.

Conners, C. K., Taylor, E., Meo, G., Kurtz, M. A., and Fournier, M. Magnesium pemoline and dextroamphetamine: A controlled study in children with minimal brain dysfunction. *Psychopharmacologia,* 1972, **26,** 321–336.

Conrad, W. G., Dworkin, E. S., Shai, A., and Tobiessen, J. E. Effects of amphetamine therapy and prescriptive tutoring on the behavior and achievement of lower class hyperactive children. *Journal of Learning Disabilities,* 1971, **4,** 509–517.

Conrad, W. G. and Insel, J. Anticipating the response to amphetamine therapy in the treatment of hyperkinetic children. *Pediatrics,* 1967, **40,** 96–98.

Council for Exceptional Children. Impressions of special education Soviet style. *Exceptional Children,* 1973, **40,** 111–117.

Creager, R. O. and Van Riper, C. The effect of methylphenidate on the verbal productivity of children with cerebral dysfunction. *Journal of Speech and Hearing Research,* 1967, **10,** 623–628.

Cromwell, R. L., Baumeister, A., and Hawkins, W. F. Research in activity level. In N. R. Ellis (Ed.), *Handbook of mental deficiency.* New York: McGraw-Hill, 1963, pp. 632–663.

Crook, W. G. An alternate method of managing the hyperactive child (letter). *Pediatrics,* 1974, **54,** 656.

Crowe, P. B. *Aspects of body image in children with the symptoms of hyperkinesis.* Unpublished doctoral dissertation, George Washington University, 1972.

Cruickshank, W. M., Bentzen, F. A., Ratzeburg, F. H., and Tannhauser, M. T. *A teaching method for brain injured and hyperactive children.* Syracuse, N.Y.: Syracuse University Press, 1961.

Cunningham, C. P. An exploratory study of the long term effects of drug use in hyperkinesis. *Dissertation Abstracts International,* 1974, **A34,** 5752.

Dahlin, I., Engelsing, E. L., and Henderson, A. T. Directive family therapy for hyperkinetic children. Paper presented at the CIBA Medical Horizons Symposium on Minimal Brain Dysfunction, Ohio State University, 1975.

Daniels, L. K. Parental treatment of hyperactivity in a child with ulcerative colitis. *Journal of Behavior Therapy and Experimental Psychiatry,* 1973, **4,** 183–185.

David, O. J. Association between lower level lead concentrations and hyperactivity in children. *Environmental Health Perspectives,* 1974, No. 7, 17–25.

David, O., Clark, J., and Voeller, K. Lead and hyperactivity. *Lancet,* 1972, **2,** 900–903.

Davids, A. An objective instrument for assessing hyperkinesis in children. *Journal of Learning Disabilities,* 1971, **4,** 499–501.

Davis, G. D. Effects of central excitant and depressant drugs on locomotor activity in the monkey. *American Journal of Physiology,* 1957, **188,** 619–623.

Davison, G. C. and Stuart, R. B. Behavior therapy and civil liberties. *American Psychologist,* 1975, **30,** 755–763.

De Hirsch, K. Early language development and minimal brain dysfunction. *Annals of the New York Academy of Sciences,* 1973, **205,** 158–163.

de la Cruz, F. F., Fox, B. H., and Roberts, R. H. (Eds.), Minimal brain dysfunction. *Annals of the New York Academy of Sciences*, 1973, **205.**

DeLong, A. R. What have we learned from psychoactive drug research on hyperactives? *American Journal of Diseases of Children*, 1972, **123,** 177–180.

Denenberg, V. H. Discussant in A. Ambrose (Ed.), *Stimulation in early infancy.* New York: Academic Press, 1969, pp. 99–100.

Denhoff, E. To medicate — to debate — or to validate. *Journal of Learning Disabilities*, 1971, **4,** 467–469.

Denhoff, E. The natural life history of children with minimal brain dysfunction. *Annals of the New York Academy of Sciences*, 1973, **205,** 188–205.

Denhoff, E., Davids, A., and Hawkins, R. Effects of dextroamphetamine on hyperkinetic children: A controlled double blind study. *Journal of Learning Disabilities*, 1971, **4,** 27–34.

Denhoff, E., Hainsworth, P. K., and Hainsworth, M. S. The child at-risk for learning disorder. *Clinical Pediatrics*, 1972, **11,** 164–170.

Denson, R., Nanson, J. L., and McWatters, M. A. Hyperkinesis and maternal smoking. *Canadian Psychiatric Association Journal*, 1975, **20,** 183–187.

Department of Health, Education, and Welfare. Testimony before the House Privacy Subcommittee Hearings. September 29, 1970.

Dielman, T. E., Cattell, R. B., and Lepper, C. Dimensions of problem behavior in the early grades. *Journal of Consulting and Clinical Psychology*, 1971, **37,** 243–249.

Digman, J. M. A test of a multiple-factor model of child personality. *Progress Report NIMH MH 08659-01,* Washington, D.C.: United States Public Health Service. March, 1965.

Divoky, D. Toward a nation of sedated children. *Learning*, 1973, **1,** 7–13.

Doll, E. A., Phelps, W. M., and Melcher, R. T. *Mental deficiency due to birth injuries.* New York: Macmillan, 1932.

Doubros, S. G. and Daniels, G. J. An experimental approach to the reduction of overactive behavior. *Behavior Research and Therapy*, 1966, **4,** 251–258.

Douglas, V. I. Stop, look and listen: The problem of sustained attention and impulse control in hyperactive and normal children. *Canadian Journal of Behavioral Science*, 1972, **4,** 259–282.

Douglas, V. I. Sustained attention and impulse control: Implications for the handicapped child. In J. A. Swets and L. L. Elliott (Eds.), *Psychology and the handicapped child.* Washington, D.C.: U.S. Department of Health, Education, and Welfare, DHEW Pub. No. (OE) 73-05000, 1974.

Douglas, V. I. Are drugs enough? — To treat or train the hyperactive child. *International Journal of Mental Health*, 1975, **4,** No. 1–2, 199–212.

Douglas, V. I., Weiss, G., and Minde, K. Learning disabilities in hyperactive children and the effect of methylphenidate. *Canadian Psychology*, 1969, **10,** 201 (Abstract).

Drabman, R. S. Child-versus teacher-administered token programs in a psychiatric hospital school. *Journal of Abnormal Child Psychology*, 1973, **1**, 68–87.

Drash, P. W. Treatment of hyperactivity in the two-year-old. *Pediatric Psychology*, 1975, **3**, 17–20.

Durfee, K. Crooked ears and the bad boy syndrome: Asymmetry as an indicator of minimal brain dysfunction. *Bulletin of the Menninger Clinic*, 1974, **38**, 305–316.

Dykman, R., Ackerman, P. T., Clements, S. D., and Peters, J. E. Specific learning disabilities: An attentional deficit syndrome. In H. Mykelbust (Ed.), *Progress in learning disabilities*, Vol. II. New York: Grune & Stratton, 1971.

Eaves, L. C., Kendall, D. C., and Crichton, J. U. The early detection of minimal brain dysfunction. *Journal of Learning Disabilities*, 1972, **5**, 454–462.

Ebaugh, F. G. Neuropsychiatric sequelae of acute epidemic encephalitis in children. *American Journal of Diseases of Children*, 1923, **25**, 89–97.

Edelson, R. I. and Sprague, R. L. Conditioning of activity level in a classroom with institutionalized retarded boys. *American Journal of Mental Deficiency*, 1974, **78**, 384–388.

Edson, T. Physical education: A substitute for hyperactivity and violence. *Journal of Health, Physical Education, and Recreation*, 1969, **40**, 79–81.

Egeland, B. Training impulsive children in the use of more efficient scanning techniques. *Child Development*, 1974, **45**, 165–171.

Ehrenfest, H. Birth injuries of the child. *Gynecological and Obstetrical Monographs*. New York: Appleton, 1926.

Eisenberg, L. Psychiatric implications of brain damage in children. *Psychiatric Quarterly*, 1957, **31**, 72–92.

Eisenberg, L. Basic issues in drug research with children: Opportunities and limitations of a pediatric age group. In S. Fisher (Ed.), *Child research in psychopharmacology*. Springfield, Ill.: Thomas, 1959, pp. 21–47.

Eisenberg, L. The management of the hyperkinetic child. *Developmental Medicine and Child Neurology*, 1966, **8**, 593–632.

Eisenberg, L. Psychopharmacology in childhood: A critique. In E. Miller (Ed.), *Foundations of child psychiatry*. Oxford: Pergamon Press, 1968.

Eisenberg, L. The hyperkinetic child and stimulant drugs. *New England Journal of Medicine*, 1972, **287**, 249–250.

Eisenberg, L. Symposium: Behavior modification by drugs. III. The clinical use of stimulant drugs in children. *Pediatrics*, 1972a, **49**, 709–715.

Eisenberg, L. and Conners, C. K. Psychopharmacology in childhood. In N. B. Talbot, J. Kagan, and L. Eisenberg (Eds.), *Behavioral science in pediatric medicine*. Philadelphia: Saunders, 1971.

Eisenberg, L., Gilbert, A., Cytryn, L., and Molling, P. A. The effectiveness of psychotherapy alone and in conjunction with perphenazine or placebo in the treatment of neurotic and hyperkinetic children. *American Journal of Psychiatry*, 1961, **117**, 1088–1093.

Erikson, E. H. *Childhood and society.* New York: Norton, 1937.

Ellinwood, E. H. and Cohen, S. (Eds.), *Current concepts on amphetamine abuse.* Proceedings of a workshop at Duke University Medical Center, June, 1970. Washington, D.C.: U.S. Government Printing Office DHEW No. (HSM) 72-9085, 1972.

Ellis, M. J., Witt, P. A., Reynolds, R., and Sprague, R. L. Methylphenidate and the activity of hyperactives in the informal setting. *Child Development,* 1974, **45,** 217–220.

Ellis, N. R. and Pryer, R. S. Quantification of gross bodily activity in children with severe neuropathology. *American Journal of Mental Deficiency,* 1959, **63,** 1034–1037.

English, H. B. and English, A. C. *A comprehensive dictionary of psychological and psychoanalytical terms.* New York: Longmans, Green, 1958.

Environmental Protection Agency Report. *Health hazards of lead* (mimeo), 1972.

Epstein, L. C., Lasagna, L., Conners, C. K., and Rodriguez, A. Correlation of dextroamphetamine excretion and drug response in hyperkinetic children. *Journal of Nervous and Mental Diseases,* 1968, **146,** 136–146.

Epstein, Y. M. and Karlin, R. A. Effects of acute experimental crowding. *Journal of Applied Social Psychology,* 1975, **5,** 34–53.

Erenberg, G. Drug therapy in minimal brain dysfunction: A commentary. *Pediatric Pharmacology and Therapeutics,* 1972, **81,** 359–365.

Ernst, J. L. Using Transactional Analysis in a high school learning disability grouping. *Transactional Analysis Journal,* 1971, **1,** 209–213.

Eysenck, H. J. (Ed.), *Behavior therapy and the neuroses.* New York: Pergamon, 1960.

Fagot, B. I. and Patterson, G. R. An in vivo analysis of reinforcing contingencies for sex-role behaviors in the preschool child. *Developmental Psychology,* 1969, **1,** 563–568.

Feighner, A. C. and Feighner, J. P. Multimodality treatment of the hyperkinetic child. *American Journal of Psychiatry,* 1974, **131,** 459–463.

Feinberg, I., Hibi, S., Braun, M., Cavness, C., Westerman, G., and Small, A. Sleep amphetamine effects on MBDS and normal subjects. *Archives of General Psychiatry,* 1974, **31,** 723–731.

Feingold, B. F. *Introduction to clinical allergy.* Springfield, Ill.: Thomas, 1973.

Feingold, B. F. Hyperkinesis and learning disabilities linked to artificial food flavors and colors. *American Journal of Nursing,* 1975, **75,** 797–803.

Feldstone, C. S. Developmental studies of negatively correlated reinforcement in children. *Developmental Psychology,* 1969, **1,** 528–542.

Ferber, A., Mendellsohn, M., and Napier, A. *The book of family therapy.* New York: Science House, 1972.

Finnerty, R. J., Soltys, J. J., and Cole, J. O. The use of d-amphetamine with hyperkinetic children. *Psychopharmacologia,* 1971, **21,** 302–308.

Firestone, P. The effects of reinforcement contingencies and caffeine on hyperactive children. Unpublished doctoral dissertation, McGill University, Montreal, Quebec, 1974.

Fischer, K. C. and Wilson, W. P. Methylphenidate and the hyperkinetic state. *Diseases of the Nervous System,* 1971, **32,** 695–698.

Fish, B. Limitations of the new nomenclature for children's disorders. *International Journal of Psychiatry,* 1969, **7,** 393–398.

Fish, B. The "one child, one drug" myth of stimulants in hyperkinesis. *Archives of General Psychiatry,* 1971, **25,** 193–203.

Fish, B. The importance of diagnostic syndromes in the drug treatment of hyperkinesis. *Psychopharmacology Bulletin,* 1971a, **7,** 40–41.

Fish, B. Stimulant drug treatment of hyperactive children. In D. P. Cantwell (Ed.), *The hyperactive child.* Holliswood, New York: Spectrum Publications, 1975, pp. 109–127.

Flynn, N. M. and Rapoport, J. L. Hyperactivity in open and traditional classroom environments. (Submitted for publication, 1975.)

Flynn, R. and Hopson, B. Inhibitory training: An alternative approach to development of controls in hyperactive children. Paper presented at the National Association of School Psychologists Meetings, Chicago, Illinois, March, 1972.

Forehand, R. and Baumeister, A. A. Effects of variations in auditory-visual stimulation on activity levels of severe mental retardates. *American Journal of Mental Deficiency,* 1970, **74,** 470–474.

Forness, S. Educational approaches with hyperactive children. In D. P. Cantwell (Ed.), *The hyperactive child.* Holliswood, New York: Spectrum Publications, 1975, pp. 159–172.

Foshee, J. G. Studies in activity level. I. Simple and complex task performance in defectives. *American Journal of Mental Deficiency,* 1958, **62,** 882–886.

Fowlie, B. A parent's guide to amphetamine treatment of hyperkinesis. *Journal of Learning Disabilities,* 1973, **6,** 352–355.

Fras, I. Alternating caffeine and stimulants (letter). *American Journal of Psychiatry,* 1974, **131,** 228–229.

Freedman, D. G. Discussant in A. Ambrose (Ed.), *Stimulation in early infancy.* New York: Academic Press, 1969, pp. 102–103.

Freeman, R. D. Drug effects on learning in children. A selective review of the past thirty years. *Journal of Special Education,* 1966, **1,** 17–44.

Freibergs, V. and Douglas, V. I. Concept learning in hyperactive and normal children. *Journal of Abnormal Psychology,* 1969, **74,** 388–395.

French, G. M. and Harlow, H. F. Locomotor reaction decrement in normal and brain damaged Rhesus monkeys. *Journal of Comparative and Physiological Psychology,* 1955, **48,** 496–501.

Frey, A. H. Behavioral biophysics. *Psychological Bulletin,* 1965, **63,** 322–337.

Friedman, R., Dale, E. P., and Wagner, J. H. A long-term comparison of two treatment regimens for minimal brain dysfunction. Drug therapy versus combined therapy. *Clinical Pediatrics,* 1973, **12,** 666–671.

Fromm, G. H., Amores, C. Y., and Thies, W. Imipramine in epilepsy. *Archives of Neurology,* 1972, **27,** 198–204.

Furman, S. and Feighner, A. Video feedback in treating hyperkinetic children: A preliminary report. *American Journal of Psychiatry,* 1973, **130,** 792–795.

Gallagher, C. C. Federal involvement in the use of behavior modification drugs on grammar school children. Hearing before a subcommittee of the Committee of Government Operations, House of Representatives, September 29, 1970.

Gallagher, J. J. Children with developmental imbalances: A psycho-educational definition. In W. M. Cruickshank (Ed.), *The teacher of brain-injured children.* Syracuse, N.Y.: Syracuse University Press, 1966.

Gallagher, J. J. (Ed.), *Windows on Russia.* Washington, D.C.: U.S. Department of Health, Education, and Welfare, DHEW Publication No. (OE) 74-05001, 1974.

Gardner, R. A. *MBD: The family book about minimal brain dysfunction.* New York: Aronson, 1973.

Gardner, W. I., Cromwell, R. L., and Foshee, J. G. Studies in activity level: II. Effects of distal visual stimulation in organics, familials, hyperactives, and hypoactives. *American Journal of Mental Deficiency,* 1959, **63,** 1028–1033.

Garfinkel, B. D., Webster, C. D., and Sloman, L. Methylphenidate and caffeine in the treatment of children with minimal brain dysfunction. *American Journal of Psychiatry,* 1975, **132,** 723–728.

Gastaut, H. Combined photic and Metrazol activation of the brain. *Electroencephalography and Clinical Neurophysiology,* 1950, **2,** 249–261.

Gelfand, C. C. The effects of an altered interpersonal environment on minimally brain-damaged children. *Dissertation Abstracts International,* 1973, **34B,** 1274–1275.

Gellhorn, E. *Autonomic imbalance and the hypothalamus.* Minneapolis: University of Minnesota Press, 1957.

Gellner, L. *A neurophysiological concept of mental retardation and its educational implications.* Chicago: J. Levinson Research Foundation, 1959.

Gersten, J. W., Foppe, K. B., Gersten, R., Maxwell, S., Mirrett, P., Gipson, M., Houston, H., and Grueter, B. Effectiveness of aides in a perceptual motor training program for children with learning disabilities. *Archives of Physical Medicine and Rehabilitation,* 1975, **56,** 104–110.

Gesell, A. L. and Ilg, F. L. *Infant and child in the culture of today: The guidance of development in home and nursery school.* New York: Harper, 1943.

Gilfillan, S. C. Lead poisoning and the fall of Rome. *Journal of Occupational Medicine,* 1965, **7,** 53–60.

Glasser, W. *Schools without failure.* New York: Harper & Row, 1968.

Glennon, C. A. and Nason, D. E. Managing the behavior of the hyperkinetic child: What research says. *The Reading Teacher,* 1974, **27,** 815–824.

Goertzel, V. and Goertzel, M. G. *Cradles of eminence.* Boston: Little Brown, 1962.

Gofman, H. F. and Allmond, B. W. Learning and language disorders in children. Part II: The school-age child. *Current Problems in Pediatrics,* 1971, **1,** No. 11.

Golden, G. S. Gilles de la Tourette's syndrome following methylphenidate administration. *Developmental Medicine and Child Neurology,* 1974, **16,** 76–78.

Goodman, E. O., Jr. Modeling: A method of parent education. *The Family Coordinator,* 1975, **24,** No. 1, 7–12.

Goodman, J. and Sours, J. *The child mental status examination.* New York: Basic Books, 1967.

Goodman, L. S. and Gilman, A. *The pharmacological basis of therapeutics.* New York: Macmillan, 1970.

Gorin, T. and Kramer, R. A. The hyperkinetic behavior syndrome. *Connecticut Medicine,* 1973, **37,** 559–563.

Goyette, C. H. Personal communication, May, 1975.

Graham, F. K., Caldwell, B. M., Ernhart, C. B., Pennoyer, M. M., and Hartmann, A. F., Sr. Anoxia as a significant perinatal experience: A critique. *Journal of Pediatrics,* 1957, **50,** 556–569.

Graham, F. K., Ernhart, C., Thurston, D., and Craft, M. Development three years after perinatal anoxia and other potentially damaging newborn experiences. *Psychological Monographs,* 1962, **76,** 1–53.

Graham, P., Rutter, M., and George, S. Temperamental characteristics as predictors of behavior disorders in children. *American Journal of Orthopsychiatry,* 1973, **43,** 328–339.

Grant, Q. R. Psychopharmacology in childhood emotional and mental disorders. *Journal of Pediatrics,* 1962, **61,** 626–637.

Greenberg, L. M., Deem, M. A., and McMahon, S. Effects of dextroamphetamine, chlorpromazine, and hydroxyzine on behavior and performance in hyperactive children. *American Journal of Psychiatry,* 1972, **129,** 532–539.

Greenberg, L. M., McMahon, S. A., and Deem, M. A. Side effects of dextroamphetamine therapy of hyperactive children. *Western Journal of Medicine,* 1974, **120,** 105–109.

Greene, F. *Awakened China.* New York: Doubleday, 1961.

Greenspan, S. I. The clinical use of operant learning approaches: Some complex issues. *American Journal of Psychiatry,* 1974, **131,** No. 8, 852–857.

Grinspoon, L. and Singer, S. Amphetamine in the treatment of hyperkinetic children. *Harvard Educational Review,* 1973, **43,** 515–555.

Groover, R. V. The hyperkinetic child. *Psychiatric Annals,* 1972, **2,** 36–44.

Gross, M. B. and Wilson, W. C. *Minimal brain dysfunction.* New York: Brunner/Mazel, 1974.

Grossman, M. Late results in epidemic encephalitis. *Archives of Neurology and Psychiatry,* 1921, **5,** 580–584.

Guerney, B. G., Jr. Filial therapy: Description and rationale. *Journal of Consulting Psychology,* 1964, **28,** 304–310.

Guerney, B. G., Jr. and Guerney, L. F. Choices in initiating family therapy, *Psychotherapy: Theory, Research, and Practice,* 1964, **1,** 119–123.

Guerney, B. G., Jr. Guerney, L., and Andronico, M. Filial therapy. *Yale Scientific Magazine*, 1966, **40**, 6–14.

Haig, J. R., Schroeder, C. S., and Schroeder, S. R. Effects of methylphenidate on hyperactive children's sleep. *Psychopharmacologia*, 1974, **37**, 185–188.

Hall, P. H. The effect of a stimulant drug (methamphetamine) on cognitive impulsivity, planning, new learning, and social behavior in hyperactive children. *Dissertation Abstracts International*, 1973, **33**, 5584.

Hall, R. V., Axelrod, S., Tyler, L., Grief, E., Jones, F. C., and Robertson, R. Modification of behavior problems in the home with a parent as observer and experimenter. *Journal of Applied Behavior Analysis*, 1972, **5**, 53–66.

Hall, R. V. and Broden, M. Behavior changes in brain-injured children through social reinforcement. *Journal of Experimental Child Psychology*, 1967, **5**, 463–479.

Halverson, C. F. and Victor, J. B. Minor physical anomalies and problem behavior in elementary school children. In press, 1975.

Halverson, C. F. and Waldrop, M. F. The relations of mechanically recorded activity level to varieties of preschool play behavior. *Child Development*, 1973, **44**, 678–681.

Handford, H. A. Brain hypoxia, minimal brain dysfunction, and schizophrenia. *American Journal of Psychiatry*, 1975, **132**, 192–194.

Hanley, E. M. Review of research involving applied behavior analysis in the classroom. *Review of Educational Research*, 1970, **40**, 597–625.

Haring, N. G. and Phillips, E. L. *Educating emotionally disturbed children*. New York: McGraw-Hill, 1962.

Harris, T. *I'm OK – you're OK: A practical guide to transactional Analysis*. New York: Harper & Row, 1969.

Hartley, E. R. Radiation that's good for you. *Science Digest*, 1974, **76**, 39–45.

Hartocollis, P. The syndrome of minimal brain dysfunction in young adult patients. *Bulletin of the Menninger Clinic*, 1968, **32**, 102–114.

Havard, J. School problems and allergies. *Journal of Learning Disabilities*, 1973, **6**, 492–494.

Havighurst, R. J. *Developmental tasks and education*. (3rd ed.) New York: McKay, 1972.

Hawkins, R. P., Peterson, R. F., Schweid, E., and Bijou, S. W. Behavior therapy in the home: Amelioration of problem parent-child relations with the parent in a therapeutic role. *Journal of Experimental Child Psychology*, 1966, **4**, 99–107.

Hawley, C. and Buckley, R. Food dyes and hyperkinetic children. *Academic Therapy*, 1974, **10**, 27–32.

Hayes, T. A., Panitch, M. L., and Barker, E. Imipramine dosage in children: A comment on "Imipramine and electrocardiographic abnormalities in hyperactive children." *American Journal of Psychiatry*, 1975, **132**, 546–547.

Henderson, A. T., Dahlin, I., Partridge, C. R., and Engelsing, E. L. A hypothesis on the etiology of hyperactivity, with a pilot-study report of related non-drug therapy. *Pediatrics,* 1973, **52,** 625.

Henderson, A. T., Dahlin, I., Partridge, C. R., and Engelsing, E. L. Hyperactivity: The Henderson-Dahlin-Partridge-Engelsing hypothesis (letter). *Pediatrics,* 1974, **54,** 514.

Hentoff, N. Dealing with drugs and children. *Current,* 1971, **126,** 40–45.

Hentoff, N. Drug-pushing in the schools: The professionals (1). *The Village Voice,* May 25, 1972, pp. 20–22.

Herron, R. E. and Ramsden, R. W. A telepedometer for remote measurement of human locomotor activity. *Psychophysiology,* 1967a, **4,** 112–115.

Herron, R. E. and Ramsden, R. W. Continuous monitoring of overt human body movement by radio telemetry: A brief review. *Perceptual and Motor Skills,* 1967, **24,** 1303–1308.

Hewett, F. M., Taylor, F. D., and Artuso, A. A. The Santa Monica Project: Evaluation of an engineered classroom design with emotionally disturbed children. *Exceptional Children,* 1969, **35,** 523–529.

Hoffman, H. *Der Struwwelpeter: Oder lustige geschichten und drollige bilder.* Leipzig: Insel-Verlag, 1845.

Hoffman, S. P., Engelhardt, D. M., Margolis, R. A., Polizos, P., Waizer, J., and Rosenfeld, R. Response to methylphenidate in low socioeconomic hyperactive children. *Archives of General Psychiatry,* 1974, **30,** 354–359.

Hohman, L. B. Post-encephalitic behavior disorders in children. *Johns Hopkins Hospital Bulletin,* 1922, **33,** 372–375.

Holt, J. *How children fail.* New York: Pitman, 1964.

Homme, L. E. *How to use contingency contracting in the classroom.* Champaign, Illinois: Research Press, 1971.

Howell, M. C., Rever, G. W., Scholl, M. L., Trowbridge, F., and Rutledge, A. Hyperactivity in children. Types, diagnosis, drug therapy, approaches to management. *Clinical Pediatrics,* 1972, **11,** 30–39.

Hoy, E., Weiss, G., Minde, K., and Cohen, N. J. Characteristics of cognitive and emotional functioning in adolescents previously diagnosed as hyperactive. Unpublished manuscript, McGill University, 1972.

Huessy, H. R. Study of the prevalence and therapy of the choreatiform syndrome or hyperkinesis in rural Vermont. *Acta Paedopsychiatrica,* 1967, **34,** 130–135.

Huessy, H. R. The adult hyperkinetic (letter). *American Journal of Psychiatry,* 1974, **131,** 724–725.

Huessy, H. R. Effect on growth of long-term administration of antidepressant drugs. Research in progress, University of Vermont, 1975.

Huessy, H. R., Metoyer, M., and Townsend, M. 8-10 year follow-up of 84 children treated for behavioral disorder in rural Vermont. *Acta Paedopsychiatrica,* 1974, **40,** 230–235.

Huessy, H. R. and Wright, A. L. The use of imipramine in children's behavior disorders. *Acta Paedopsychiatrica,* 1970, **37,** 194–199.

Huestis, R. D. and Arnold, L. E. Possible antagonism of amphetamine by decongestant-antihistamine compounds. *Journal of Pediatrics*, 1974, **85**, 579–580.

Huestis, R. D., Arnold, L. E., & Smeltzer, M. A. Caffeine versus methylphenidate and d-amphetamine in minimal brain dysfunction: A double-blind comparison. *American Journal of Psychiatry*, 1975, **132**, 868–870.

Hunsinger, S. School storm: Drugs for children. *Christian Science Monitor*, October 31, 1970, pp. 1, 6.

Hurst, M., Radlow, R., Chubb, N. C., and Bagley, S. K. Effect of d-amphetamine on acquisition, persistence, and recall. *American Journal of Psychology*, 1969, **82**, 307–319.

Hutchinson, R. R. and Azrin, N. H. Conditioning of mental-hospital patients to fixed-ratio schedules of reinforcement. *Journal of the Experimental Analysis of Behavior*, 1961, **4**, 87–95.

Hutt, S. J. and Hutt, C. *Direct observation and measurement of behavior.* Springfield, Ill.: Thomas, 1970.

Ingram, T. T. Soft signs. *Developmental Medicine and Child Neurology*, 1973, **15**, 527–530.

Irwin, O. C. The amount of motility of seventy-three newborn infants. *Journal of Comparative Psychology*, 1932, **14**, 415–428.

Itil, T. M. and Simeon, J. Computerized EEG in the prediction of outcome of drug treatment in hyperactive childhood behavior disorders. *Psychopharmacology Bulletin*, 1974, **10**, 36.

Jacobs, N. T. A comparison of hyperactive and normal boys in terms of reaction time, motor time, and decision-making time, under conditions of increasing task complexity. *Dissertation Abstracts International*, 1972, **33 (3-A)**, 1045.

James, C. E. Operant conditioning in the management and behavior of hyperactive children: Five case studies. Unpublished manuscript, Orange State College, 1963.

James, M. *Born to Love: Transactional Analysis in the church.* Reading, Mass.: Addison-Wesley, 1973.

Jenkins, J. R., Gorrafa, S., and Griffiths, S. Another look at isolation effects. *American Journal of Mental Deficiency*, 1972, **76**, 591–593.

Johnson, C. F. Hyperactivity and the machine: The actometer. *Child Development*, 1971, **42**, 2105–2110.

Johnson, C. F. Limits on the measurement of activity level in children using ultrasound and photoelectric cells. *American Journal of Mental Deficiency*, 1972, **77**, 301–310.

Jones, K. L., Smith, D. W., Streissguth, A. P., and Myrianthopoulos, N. C. Outcome in offspring of chronic alcoholic women. *Lancet*, 1974, **1**, 1076–1078.

Juliano, D. B. Conceptual tempo, activity and concept learning in hyperactive and normal children. *Dissertation Abstracts International*, 1974, **34A**, 4875.

Kagan, J. *Change and continuity in infancy.* New York: Wiley, 1971.

Kagan, J. and Messer, S. B. A reply to "Some misgivings about the Matching Familiar Figures Test as a measure of reflection-impulsivity." *Developmental Psychology,* 1975, **11**, 244–248.

Kagan, J., Pearson, L., and Welch, L. The modifiability of an impulsive tempo. *Journal of Educational Psychology,* 1966, **57**, 359–365.

Kahn, E. and Cohen, L. Organic driveness: A brain stem syndrome and an experience. *New England Journal of Medicine,* 1934, **210**, 748–756.

Kalverboer, A. F., Touwen, B. C., and Prechtl, H. F. Follow-up of infants at risk of minor brain dysfunction. *Annals of the New York Academy of Sciences,* 1973, **205**, 173–187.

Kappelman, M., Roberts, P., Rinaldi, R., and Cornblath, M. The school health team and school health physician: New role and operation. *American Journal of Diseases of Children,* 1975, **129**, 191–195.

Karelitz, S. and Fisichelli, V. R. The cry thresholds of normal infants and those with brain damage. *Journal of Pediatrics,* 1962, **61**, 679–685.

Karlsson, K. A. Hyperactivity and environmental compliance. *Dissertation Abstracts International,* 1973, **34A**, 861–862.

Kaspar, J. C. and Lowenstein, R. The effect of social interaction on activity level in six- to eight-year-old boys. *Child Development,* 1971, **42**, 1294–1298.

Kaswan, J. W., Love, L., and Rodnick, E. The effectiveness of information and consultation. Unpublished manuscript, Ohio State University, 1968.

Kauffman, J. M. and Hallahan, D. P. Control of rough physical behavior using novel contingencies and directive teaching. *Perceptual and Motor Skills,* 1973, **36**, 1225–1226.

Kazdin, A. Effect of vicarious reinforcement on attentive behavior in the classroom. *Journal of Applied Behavior Analysis,* 1973, **6**, 71–78.

Kehne, C. W. Control of the hyperactive child via medication — at what cost to personality development; some psychological implications and clinical interventions. *American Journal of Orthopsychiatry,* 1974, **44**, 237–238.

Kelly, G. A. *The psychology of personal constructs. Vol. II. Clinical diagnosis and psychotherapy.* New York: Norton, 1955.

Kenny, T. J. and Clemmens, R. L. Medical and psychological correlates in children with learning disabilities. *Journal of Pediatrics,* 1971, **78**, 273–277.

Kenny, T. J., Clemmens, R. L., Hudson, B., Lentz, G. A., Jr., Cicci, R., and Nair, P. Characteristics of children referred because of hyperactivity. *Journal of Pediatrics,* 1971, **79**, 618–622.

Keogh, B. K. Hyperactivity and learning problems: Implications for teachers. *Education Digest,* 1971, **37**, 45–47.

Kessen, W., Hendry, L. S., and Leutzendorff, A. Measurement of movement in the human newborn. *Child Development,* 1961, **32**, 95–105.

Kinsbourne, M. Stimulants for insomnia (correspondence). *New England Journal of Medicine,* 1973, **288**, 1129.

Klein, H. A. Behavior modification as therapeutic paradox. *American Journal of Orthopsychiatry*, 1974, **44**, 353–361.

Klein, R. H. and Salzman, L. F. Paradoxical effects of caffeine. *Perceptual and Motor Skills*, 1975, **40**, 126.

Kline, C. L. Prevalence and management of hyperactive children (letter). *New England Journal of Medicine*, 1975, **292**, 536.

Knights, R. M. and Hinton, G. The effects of methylphenidate (Ritalin) on the motor skills and behavior of children with learning problems. *Journal of Nervous and Mental Diseases*, 1969, **148**, 643–653.

Knights, R. M. and Viets, C. A. The effects of pemoline on hyperactive boys. Department of Psychology, Carleton University, Ottawa, Canada, 1973.

Knobel, M. Psychopharmacology for the hyperkinetic child — Dynamic considerations. *Archives of General Psychiatry*, 1962, **6**, 198–202.

Knobel, M., Wolman, M. B., and Mason, E. Hyperkinesis and organicity in children. *Archives of General Psychiatry*, 1959, **1**, 310–321.

Knobloch, H. and Pasamanick, B. Prospective studies on the epidemiology of reproductive casualty: Methods, findings, and some implications. *Merrill-Palmer Quarterly*, 1966, **12**, 27–43.

Knopp, W., Arnold, L. E., Andras, R. L., and Smeltzer, D. J. Predicting amphetamine response in hyperkinetic children by electric pupillography. *Pharmakopsychiatrie Neuro-Psychopharmakologie*, 1973, **6**, 158–166.

Kohl, H. *36 children*. New York: New American Library, 1967.

Kornetsky, C. Psychoactive drugs in the immature organism. *Psychopharmacologia* (Berlin), 1970, **17**, 105–136.

Kounin, J. S. and Gump, P. V. The ripple effect in discipline. *Elementary School Journal*, 1958, **59**, 158–162.

Krager, J. M. and Safer, D. J. Type and prevalence of medication used in the treatment of hyperactive children. *New England Journal of Medicine*, 1974, **291**, 1118–1120.

Kretsinger, E. A. An experimental study of restiveness in preschool educational television audiences. *Speech Monographs*, 1959, **26**, 72–77.

Kubany, E. S., and Sloggett, B. B. Coding procedure for teachers. In E. J. Thomas (Ed.), *Behavior modification procedure: A sourcebook*. Chicago: Aldine, 1974, pp. 174–181.

Kupietz, S., Bialer, I., and Winsberg, B. G. A behavior rating scale for assessing improvement in behaviorally deviant children: A preliminary investigation. *American Journal of Psychiatry*, 1972, **128**, 116–120.

Lacey, J. I. Somatic response patterning and stress: Some revisions of activation theory. In M. H. Appley and R. Trumbull (Eds.), *Psychological stress: Issues in research*. New York: Appleton-Century-Crofts, 1967.

Landrigan, P. J., Gehlbach, S. H., Rosenblum, B. F., et al. Epidemic lead absorption near an ore smelter. *New England Journal of Medicine*, 1975, **292**, 123–129.

Lapouse, R. and Monk, M. A. An epidemiologic study of behavior characteristics in children. *American Journal of Public Health*, 1958, **48**, 1134–1144.

Lasagna, L. Abuse of amphetamines (letter). *New England Journal of Medicine*, 1974, **291**, 800.

Lasagna, L. and Epstein, L. C. The use of amphetamines in the treatment of hyperkinetic children. In E. Costa and S. Garattini (Eds.), *International symposium on amphetamines and related compounds*. New York: Raven, 1970, pp. 849–864.

Laufer, M. W. Cerebral dysfunction and behavior disorders in adolescents. *American Journal of Orthopsychiatry*, 1962, **32**, 501–506.

Laufer, M. W. Long-term management and some follow-up findings on the use of drugs with minimal cerebral syndromes. *Journal of Learning Disabilities*, 1971, **4**, 55–58.

Laufer, M. W. and Denhoff, E. Hyperkinetic behavior syndrome in children. *Journal of Pediatrics*, 1957, **50**, 463–474.

Laufer, M., Denhoff, E., and Solomons, G. Hyperkinetic impulse disorder in children's behavior problems. *Psychosomatic Medicine*, 1957, **19**, 38–49.

Lazarus, A. A. Behavior rehearsal vs. non-directive therapy vs. advice in effecting behavior change. *Behavior Research and Therapy*, 1966, **4**, 209–212.

Lazarus, R. S. A cognitively oriented psychologist looks at biofeedback. *American Psychologist*, 1975, **30**, 553–561.

Leahly, S. R. and Sands, I. J. Mental disorders in children following epidemic encephalitis. *Journal of the American Medical Association*, 1921, **76**, 373–377.

Lennard, H. L., Epstein, L. J., Bernstein, A., and Ransom, D. C. *Mystification and drug misuse*. New York: Harper & Row, 1971.

Lennard, H. L., Epstein, L. J., Bernstein, A., and Ransom, D. C. Hazards implicit in prescribing psychoactive drugs. *Science*, 1970, **169**, 438–441.

Lesser, L. I. Hyperkinesis in children. *Clinical Pediatrics (Philadelphia)*, 1970, **9**, 548–554.

Leuba, C. Toward some integration of learning theories: The concept of optimal stimulation. *Psychological Reports*, 1955, **1**, 27–33.

Levin, G. R., and Simmons, J. J. Response to praise by emotionally disturbed boys. *Psychological Reports*, 1962, **11**, 10.

Levin, I. *The Stepford wives*. New York: Random House, 1972.

Levitis, K. A. Need for medication in minimal brain dysfunction (letter). *Pediatrics*, 1974, **54**, No. 3, 388.

Levitt, E. E. The results of psychotherapy with children: An evaluation. *Journal of Consulting Psychology*, 1957, **21**, 189–196.

Levitt, E. E. Psychotherapy with children: A further evaluation. *Behavior Research and Therapy*, 1963, **1**, 45–51.

Levitt, E. E. Research on psychotherapy with children. In A. E. Bergin and S. L. Garfield (Eds.), *Handbook of psychotherapy and behavior change: An empirical analysis*. New York: Wiley, 1971, pp. 474–494.

Levitt, R. A. An activity measure of sleeping and waking behavior. *Psychonomic Science,* 1966, **5,** 287–288.

Levy, S. M. Post-encephalitic behavior disorder — A forgotten entity. *American Journal of Psychiatry,* 1959, **115,** 1062–1067.

Lewis, M. A. Hyperactivity and variations in prevalence rates for assignment to special classes among black, white, and Spanish surnamed students in twenty-five urban and suburban school districts in New Jersey. *Dissertation Abstracts International,* 1974, **A34,** 4040.

Lilienfeld, A. M., Pasamanick, B., and Rogers, M. Relationship between pregnancy experience and the development of certain neuro-psychiatric disorders in childhood. *American Journal of Public Health,* 1955, **45,** 637–643.

Lindsley, D. B., and Henry, C. E. Effects of drugs on behavior and the electroencephalograms of children with behavior disorders. *Psychosomatic Medicine,* 1942, **4,** 140–149.

Lindy, J. M. Hyperkinetic behavior among kindergarten children. *Dissertation Abstracts,* 1967, **B28,** 341.

Lin-Fu, J. S. Undue absorption of lead among children — a new look at an old problem. *New England Journal of Medicine,* 1972, **236,** 702–710.

Lion, J. R. Conceptual issues in the use of drugs for the treatment of aggression in man. *Journal of Nervous and Mental Diseases,* 1975, **160,** 76–82.

Lipsitt, L. P. and DeLucia, C. An apparatus for the measurement of specific responses and general activity of the human neonate. *American Journal of Psychology,* 1960, **73,** 630–632.

Lobitz, W. C. A simple stimulus cue for controlling disruptive classroom behavior. *Journal of Abnormal Child Psychology,* 1974, **2,** 143–152.

Loney, J. The intellectual functioning of hyperactive elementary school boys: A cross-sectional investigation. *American Journal of Orthopsychiatry,* 1974, **44,** 754–762.

Loney, J., & Ordona, T. T. Using cerebral stimulants to treat MBD. *American Journal of Orthopsychiatry,* 1975, **45,** 564–572.

Lopez, R. E. Hyperactivity in twins. *Canadian Psychiatric Association Journal,* 1965, **10,** 421.

Lovaas, O. I., Freitag, G., Gold, V. J., and Kassorla, I. C. Recording apparatus for observation of behaviors of children in free play settings. *Journal of Experimental Child Psychology,* 1965, **2,** 108–120.

Lovaas, O. I. and Willis, T. Behavioral control of a hyperactive child. Unpublished manuscript referred to in D. P. Cantwell (Ed.), *The hyperactive child.* New York: Spectrum, 1975, p. 134.

Lucas, A. and Weiss, M. Methylphenidate hallucinosis. *Journal of the American Medical Association,* 1971, **217,** 1079–1081.

Luisada, P. V. REM deprivation and hyperactivity in children. *The Chicago Medical School Quarterly,* 1969, **28,** 97–108.

Luria, A. R. *The role of speech in the regulation of normal and abnormal behavior.* New York: Liveright, 1961.

Luria, A. R. The role of speech in the formation of mental processes. In *The role of speech in the regulation of normal and abnormal behavior.* U.S. Department of Health, Education, and Welfare. Public Health Service, National Institutes of Health, Washington, D.C., 1966.

Lytton, G. J. and Knobel, M. Diagnosis and treatment of behavior disorders in children. *Diseases of the Nervous System,* 1958, **20,** 5–11.

Maccoby, E. E., Dowley, E. M., Hagen, J. W., and Degerman, R. Activity level and intellectual functioning in normal preschool children. *Child Development,* 1965, **36,** 761–770.

MacKay, M. C., Beck, L., and Taylor, R. Methylphenidate for adolescents with minimal brain dysfunction. *New York State Journal of Medicine,* 1973, **73,** 550–554.

MacKeith, R. High activity and hyperactivity. *Developmental Medicine and Child Neurology,* 1974, **16,** 513–514.

MacPherson, E. M., Candee, B. L., and Hohman, R. J. A comparison of three methods for eliminating disruptive lunchroom behavior. *Journal of Applied Behavior Analysis,* 1974, **7,** 287–297.

Madsen, C. H., Becker, W. C., Thomas, D. R., Koser, L., and Plager, E. An analysis of the reinforcing function of "sit down" commands. In R. K. Parker (Ed.), *Readings in educational psychology.* Boston: Allyn & Bacon, 1968.

Maletzky, B. M. d-Amphetamine and delinquency: Hyperkinesis persisting? *Diseases of the Nervous System,* 1974, **35,** 543–547.

Malmquist, C. Depressions in childhood and adolescents, II. *New England Journal of Medicine,* 1971, **284,** 955–961.

Manheimer, D. I. and Mellinger, G. D. Personality characteristics of the child accident repeater. *Child Development,* 1967, **38,** 491–513.

Martin, D. M. Hyperkinetic behavior disorders in children. *Western Medicine,* January, 1967, 23–27.

Martin, M., Burkholder, R., Rosenthal, T. L., Tharp, R. G., and Thorne, G. L. Programming behavior change and reintegration into the school milieux of extreme adolescent deviates. *Behavior Research and Therapy,* 1968, **6,** 371–383.

Marwit, S. J. and Stenner, A. J. Hyperkinesis: Delineation of two patterns. *Exceptional Children,* 1972, **38,** 401–406.

Massari, D., Hayweiser, L., and Meyer, W. J. Activity level and intellectual functioning in deprived preschool children. *Developmental Psychology,* 1969, **1,** 286–290.

Matefy, R. E., Solanch, L., and Humphrey, E. Behavior modification in the home with students as co-therapists. *American Journal of Psychotherapy,* 1975, **29,** 212–223.

Mattson, R. H. and Calverley, J. R. Dextroamphetamine-sulfate-induced dyskinesias. *Journal of the American Medical Association,* 1968, **204,** 400–402.

Mausner, J. S. and Bahn, A. K. *Epidemiology.* Philadelphia: W. B. Saunders, 1974.

Maynard, R. Omaha pupils given "behavior" drugs. *Washington Post*, June 29, 1970.

Mayron, L. W., Ott, J., Nations, R., and Mayron, E. Light, radiation, and academic behavior. *Academic Therapy*, 1974, **10**, 33–47.

McArdle, J. Effects of thioridazine and methylphenidate on learning and retention in retardates. Unpublished master's thesis, University of Illinois, 1968.

McCabe, E. R. B. and McCabe, L. Dissociation of learning on stimulant-drug therapy. *New England Journal of Medicine*, 1972, **287**, 825.

McCandless, B. R. *Behavior and development*. New York: Holt, Rinehart, & Winston, 1967.

McClearn, G. E. Genetic influences on behavior and development. In P. H. Mussen (Ed.), *Carmichael's manual of child psychology*. New York: Wiley, 1970, pp. 39–76.

McConnell, J. V. Criminals can be brainwashed — now. *Psychology Today*, 1970, **4**, 14, 16, 18, 74.

McDermott, J. F. A specific placebo effect encountered in the use of dexedrine in a hyperactive child. *American Journal of Psychiatry*, 1965, **121**, 923–924.

McKeown, D., Jr., Adams, H. E., and Forehand, R. Generalization to the classroom of principles of behavior modification taught to teachers. *Behavior Research and Therapy*, 1975, **13**, 85–92.

McLaughlin, T. and Malaby, J. Reducing and measuring inappropriate verbalizations in a token classroom. *Journal of Applied Behavior Analysis*, 1972, **5**, 329–333.

McMahon, S., Deem, M. A., and Greenberg, L. M. The hyperactive child. *Clinical Proceedings of Children's Hospital*, 1970, **26**, 295–316.

McNamara, J. J. Hyperactivity in the apartment bound child. *Clinical Pediatrics*, 1972, **11**, 371–372.

Medical World News. Minimal brain dysfunction: The three million 'other children.' *Medical World News*, 1970, **11**, 30–36.

Medland, M. B. and Stachnik, T. J. Good behavior game: A replication and systematic analysis. *Journal of Applied Behavior Analysis*, 1972, **5**, 45–51.

Meichenbaum, D. Self-instructional methods. In F. H. Kanfer and A. P. Goldstein (Eds.), *Helping people change*. New York: Pergamon Press, 1974.

Meichenbaum, D. H. and Goodman, J. Training impulsive children to talk to themselves: A means of developing self-control. *Journal of Abnormal Psychology*, 1971, **77**, 115–126.

Mendelson, W., Johnson, N., Stewart, M. A. Hyperactive children as teenagers: A follow-up study. *Journal of Nervous and Mental Diseases*, 1971, **153**, 273–279.

Menkes, J. H. A new role for the school physician. *Pediatrics*, 1972, **49**, 803–804.

Menkes, M. M., Rowe, J. S., and Menkes, J. H. A twenty-five year follow-up study on the hyperkinetic child with minimal brain dysfunction. *Pediatrics*, 1967, **39**, 393–399.

Miklich, D. R. Operant conditioning procedures with systematic desensitization in a hyperkinetic asthmatic boy. *Journal of Behavior Therapy and Experimental Psychiatry*, 1973, **4**, 177–182.

Miller, R. G., Palkes, H. S., and Stewart, M. A. Hyperactive children in suburban elementary schools. *Child Psychiatry and Human Development*, 1973, **4**, 121–127.

Miller, S. Use of tranquilizers by city pupils reported increasing. *Baltimore Evening Sun*, October 2, 1970.

Millichap, J. G. Drugs in management of hyperkinetic and perceptually handicapped children. *Journal of the American Medical Association*, 1968, **206**, 1527–1530.

Millichap, J. G. Minimal brain dysfunction: A concensus for chemotherapy. *Hospital Practice*, 1972, **7**, 30–110.

Millichap, J. G. Drugs in management of minimal brain dysfunction. *Annals of the New York Academy of Sciences*, 1973, **205**, 321–334.

Millichap, J. G., Aymat, F., Sturgis, L. H., Larsen, K. W., and Egan, R. A. Hyperkinetic behavior and learning disorders. III. Battery of neuropsychological tests in controlled trial of methylphenidate. *American Journal of Diseases of Children*, 1968, **116**, 235–244.

Millichap, J. G. and Boldrey, E. E. Studies in hyperkinetic behavior. II. Laboratory and clinical evaluations of drug treatments. *Neurology*, 1967, **17**, 467–471, 519.

Millichap, J. G. and Fowler, G. W. Treatment of "minimal brain dysfunction" syndromes. *Pediatric Clinics of North America*, 1967, **14**, 767–777.

Millman, H. L. Minimal brain dysfunction in children: Evaluation and treatment. *Journal of Learning Disabilities*, 1970, **3**, 89–99.

Minde, K. *A parents' guide to hyperactivity in children*. Montreal: Quebec Association for Children with Learning Disabilities, 1971.

Minde, K., Lewin, D., Weiss, G., Lavigueur, H., Douglas, V., and Sykes, E. The hyperactive child in elementary school: A 5 year, controlled, follow-up. *Exceptional Children*, 1971, **38**, 215–221.

Minde, K., Webb, G., and Sykes, D. Studies on the hyperactive child: VI. Prenatal and paranatal factors associated with hyperactivity. *Developmental Medicine and Child Neurology*, 1968, **10**, 355–363.

Minde, K. K. and Weiss, G. C. The assessment of drug effects in children as compared to adults. *Journal of the American Academy of Child Psychiatry*, 1970, **9**, 124–133.

Mischel, W. *Personality and assessment*. New York: Wiley, 1968.

Mofenson, H. C., Greensher, J., and Horowitz, R. Detection of the hyperactive child (letter). *Journal of Pediatrics*, 1972, **80**, 687.

Molitch, M. and Eccles, A. K. Effect of benezedrine sulphate on intelligence scores of children. *American Journal of Psychiatry*, 1937, **94**, 587–590.

Montagu, J. D. and Swarbrick, L. Hyperkinesis: The objective evaluation of therapeutic procedures. *Biological Psychology*, 1974, **2**, 151–155.

Morrison, J. R. and Stewart, M. A. A family study of the hyperactive child syndrome. *Biological Psychiatry*, 1971, **3**, 189–195.

Morrison, J. R. and Minkoff, K. Explosive personality as a sequel to the hyperactive-child syndrome. *Comprehensive Psychiatry*, 1975, **16**, 343–348.

Morrison, J. R. and Stewart, M. A. The psychiatric status of the legal families of adopted hyperactive children. *Archives of General Psychiatry*, 1973, **28**, 888–891.

Morrison, J. R. and Stewart, M. A. Evidence for polygenetic inheritance in the hyperactive child syndrome. *American Journal of Psychiatry*, 1973a, **130:7**, 791–792.

Morrison, J. R. and Stewart, M. A. Bilateral inheritance as evidence for polygenicity in the hyperactive child syndrome. *Journal of Nervous and Mental Diseases*, 1974, **158**, 226–228.

Moss, H. A. and Robson, K. S. The relation between the amount of time infants spend at various states and the development of visual behavior. *Child Development*, 1970, **41**, 509–517.

Moyer, K. E. Allergy and aggression: The physiology of violence. *Psychology Today*, 1975, **9**, 76–79.

Mussen, P. (Ed.), *Handbook of research methods in child development*. New York: Wiley, 1960.

Nadas, A. S. *Pediatric cardiology*, 2nd ed. Philadelphia: Saunders, 1963.

Nader, P. R., Emmel, A., and Charney, E. The school health service: A new model. *Pediatrics*, 1972, **49**, 805–813.

National Center for Education Statistics. *Statistics of trends in education 1963–64 to 1983–84*. U.S. Department of Health, Education, and Welfare, Education Division, January, 1975.

Nazzaro, J. Impressions of special education Soviet style. *Exceptional Children*, 1973, **40**, 111–117.

Needleman, H. L. Lead poisoning in children: Neurologic implications of widespread subclinical intoxication. *Seminars in Psychiatry*, 1973, **5**, 47–53.

Neisser, U. *Cognitive psychology*. New York: Appleton, 1967.

Nelson, A. E. An analysis of communication effectiveness between parents and the hyperactive child. *Dissertation Abstracts International*, 1973, **34B**, 2905.

Nelson, J. A. A comparative study of the perceptual and conceptual development of hyperactive and normal boys. *Dissertation Abstracts International*, 1970, **30B**, 3392–3393.

Newbury, E. Automatic measurement of general activity in time-units. *American Journal of Psychology*, 1956, **69**, 655–659.

Newell, G. R. and Henderson, B. E. Case-control study of Hodgkin's disease. I. Results of the interview questionnaire. *Journal of the National Cancer Institute*, 1973, **51**, 1437–1441.

Ney, P. G. Psychosis in a child, associated with amphetamine administration. *Canadian Medical Association Journal*, 1967, **97**, 1026–1029.

Ney, P. G. Four types of hyperkinesis. *Canadian Psychiatric Association Journal*, 1974, **19**, 543–550.

Ney, P. G. Uses and abuses of operant conditioning. *Canadian Psychiatric Association Journal*, 1975, **20**, 119–132.

Nichamin, S. J. Recognizing minimal cerebral dysfunction in the infant and toddler. *Clinical Pediatrics*, 1972, **11**, 255–257.

Nichamin, S. J. and Comly, H. M. The hyperkinetic or lethargic child with cerebral dysfunction. *Michigan Medicine*, 1964, **63**, 790–792.

Nolan, J. D., Mattis, P. R., and Holliday, W. C. Long-term effects of behavior therapy: A 12-month follow-up. *Journal of Abnormal Psychology*, 1970, **76**, 88–92.

Oberle, M. W. Lead poisoning: A preventable childhood disease of the slums. *Science*, 1969, **165**, 991–992.

Oettinger, L., Jr. Learning disorders, hyperkinesis, and the use of drugs in children. *Rehabilitation Literature*, 1971, **32**, 162–170.

Oettinger, L., Majovski, L. V., Limbeck, G. A., and Gauch, R. Bone age in children with minimal brain dysfunction. *Perceptual and Motor Skills*, 1974, **39**, 1127–1131.

Office of Child Development Report on the Conference on the Use of Stimulant Drugs in the Treatment of Behaviorally Disturbed Young School Children, 1971. Reprinted in *The National Elementary Principal*, 1971, **50**, 53–59.

O'Leary, K. D. and Drabman, R. Token reinforcement programs in the classroom: A review. *Psychological Bulletin*, 1971, **75**, 379–398.

O'Leary, K. D. and O'Leary, S. G. *Classroom management: The successful use of behavior modification.* New York: Pergamon, 1972.

O'Leary, K. D., Pelham, W. E., Rosenbaum, A., and Price, G. H. Behavioral treatment of hyperkinetic children: Adjunctive therapy or alternative to medication. In press, 1975.

O'Malley, J. E. and Eisenberg, L. The hyperkinetic syndrome. *Seminars in Psychiatry*, 1973, **5**, 95–103.

Omenn, G. S. Genetic issues in the syndrome of minimal brain dysfunction. *Seminars in Psychiatry*, 1973, **5**, 5–17.

Ott, J. The eyes' dual function — Part II. *Eye, Ear, Nose, and Throat Monthly*, 1974, **53**, 377–381.

Overton, D. A. Dissociated learning in drug states (state dependent learning). In D. Efron (Ed.), *Psychopharmacology: A review of progress 1957–1967.* Washington, D. C.: U.S. Government Printing Office, Public Health Service Publication No. 1836, 1968, pp. 918–930.

Overton, D. A. Commentary on state-dependency. In J. H. Harvey (Ed.), *Behavioral analysis of drug action.* Glenview, Ill.: Scott-Foresman, 1971, pp. 73–83.

Paine, R. S., Werry, J. S., and Quay, H. C. A study of 'minimal cerebral dysfunction.' *Developmental Medicine and Child Neurology*, 1968, **10**, 505–520.

Palkes, H. and Stewart, M. Intellectual ability and performance of hyperactive children. *American Journal of Orthopsychiatry*, 1972, **42**, 35–39.

Palkes, H., Stewart, M., and Freedman, J. Improvement in maze performance of hyperactive boys as a function of verbal-training procedures. *Journal of Special Education*, 1972, **5**, 337–342.

Palkes, H., Stewart, M., and Kahana, B. Porteus Maze performance of hyperactive boys after training in self-directed verbal commands. *Child Development*, 1968, **39**, 817–826.

Paluszny, M. and Abelson, A. G. Twins in a child psychiatry clinic. *American Journal of Psychiatry*, 1975, **132**, 434–436.

Parry, P. A. and Douglas, V. I. The effects of reward on the performance of hyperactive children. In press, *Journal of Abnormal Child Psychology*.

Pasamanick, B., Rogers, M., and Lilienfeld, A. M. Pregnancy experience and the development of behavior disorder in children. *American Journal of Psychiatry*, 1956, **112**, 613–617.

Patterson, C. J. and Mischel, W. Plans to resist distraction. *Developmental Psychology*, 1975, **11**, 369–378.

Patterson, G. R. An application of conditioning techniques to the control of a hyperactive child. In L. P. Ullman and L. Krasner (Eds.), *Case studies in behavior modification*. New York: Holt, Rinehart & Winston, 1964.

Patterson, G. R. Behavioral intervention procedures in the classroom and in the home. In A. E. Bergin and S. L. Garfield (Eds.), *Handbook of psychotherapy and behavior change*. New York: Wiley, 1971, Chapter 19.

Patterson, G. R., Jones, R., Whittier, J., and Wright, M. A. A behavior modification technique for the hyperactive child. *Behavior Research and Therapy*, 1965, **2**, 217–226.

Patterson, G. R., McNeal, S., Hawkins, N., and Phelps, R. Reprogramming the social environment. *Journal of Child Psychology and Psychiatry*, 1967, **8**, 181–195.

Patterson, G. R., Ray, R. S., and Shaw, D. A. Direct intervention in families of deviant children. *Oregon Research Institute Research Bulletin*, 1968, 8.

Paulus, P., Cox, V., McCain, G., and Chandler, J. Some effects of crowding in a prison environment. *Journal of Applied Social Psychology*, 1975, **5**, 86–91.

Paxton, P. W. Effects of drug-induced behavior changes in hyperactive children on maternal attitude and personality. Doctoral dissertation, University of Minnesota, 1972.

Peacock, L. J. and Williams, M. An ultrasonic device for recording activity. *American Journal of Psychology*, 1962, **75**, 648–652.

Perel, J. M., Black, N., Wharton, R. N., and Malitz, S. Inhibition of imipramine metabolism by methylphenidate. *Federation Proceedings*, 1969, **28**, 418.

Peters, J. E., Romine, J. S., and Dykman, R. A. A special neurological examination of children with learning disabilities. *Developmental Medicine and Child Neurology*, 1975, **17**, 63–78.

Petit, C. Theory on food dyes. *San Francisco Chronicle*, January 7, 1974, p. 2.

Pihl, R. F. Conditioning procedures with hyperactive children. *Neurology*, 1967, **17**, 421–423.

Pincus, J. H. and Glaser, G. H. The syndrome of "minimal brain damage" in childhood. *New England Journal of Medicine,* 1966, **275**, 27–35.

Plotnikoff, N. Pemoline: Review of performance. *Texas Reports on Biology and Medicine,* 1971, **29**, 467–479.

Poresky, R. H. Arousal and learning, and noncontingency detection in one-year-old infants. *Perceptual and Motor Skills,* 1975, **40**, 23–28.

Porges, S. W., Walter, G. F., Korb, R. J., & Sprague, R. L. The influence of methylphenidate on heart rate and behavioral measures of attention in hyperactive children. *Child Development,* 1975, **46**, 727–733.

Poser, E. G. The effect of therapists' training on group therapeutic outcome. *Journal of Consulting Psychology,* 1966, **30**, 283–289.

Postman, L. Short-term memory and incidental learning. In A. W. Melton (Ed.), *Categories of human learning.* New York: Academic Press, 1964, pp. 146–201.

Prescott, J. W. Early social deprivation. In D. B. Lindsley and A. H. Riesen (Eds.), *Perspectives on human deprivation: Biological, physiological, and sociological.* Bethesda, Md.: National Institutes of Child Health and Human Development. DHEW, 1968.

Prescott, J. W. A developmental psychophysiological theory of autistic-depressive and violent-aggressive behaviors. *Psychophysiology,* 1970, **6**, 628–629.

Price, J. M. The effects of crowding on the social behavior of children. Unpublished doctoral dissertation, Columbia University, 1971.

Prinz, R. and Loney, J. Teacher-rated hyperactive elementary school girls: An exploratory developmental study. *Child Psychiatry and Human Development,* 1974, **4**, 246–257.

Pronko, N. H. Biotelemetry: Psychology's newest ally. *Psychological Record,* 1968, **18**, 93–100.

Quay, H. C. and Peterson, D. R. *Manual for the Behavior Problem Checklist.* Champaign, Ill.: Children's Research Center, University of Illinois, 1967.

Quinn, P. O. and Rapoport, J. L. Minor physical anomalies and neurological status in hyperactive boys. *Pediatrics,* 1974, **53**, 742–747.

Quinn, P. O. and Rapoport, J. L. One-year follow-up of hyperactive boys treated with imipramine or methylphenidate. *American Journal of Psychiatry,* 1975, **132**, 241–245.

Quitkin, F. and Klein, D. F. Two behavioral syndromes in young adults related to possible minimal brain dysfunction. *Journal of Psychiatric Research,* 1969, **7**, 131–142.

Ramp, E., Ulrich, R., and Dulaney, S. Delayed time-out as a procedure for reducing disruptive classroom behavior: A case study. *Journal of Applied Behavior Analysis,* 1971, **4**, 235–239.

Randolph, T. G. Allergy as a causative factor of fatigue, irritability and behavior problems in children. *Journal of Pediatrics,* 1947, **31**, 560–572.

Randrup, A. and Mundvak, I. Stereotyped activities produced by amphetamines in several animal species and man. *Psychopharmacologia,* 1967, **11**, 300–310.

Rapoport, J. L. and Benoit, M. The relation of direct home observations to the clinic evaluation of hyperactive school age boys. *Journal of Child Psychology and Psychiatry,* 1975, **16,** 141–147.

Rapoport, J. L., Lott, I. T., Alexander, D. F., and Abramson, A. U. Urinary nonadrenaline and playroom behavior in hyperactive boys. *Lancet,* 1970, **2,** 1141.

Rapoport, J. L., Quinn, P. O., Bradbard, G., Riddle, D., and Brooks, E. Imipramine and methylphenidate treatments of hyperactive boys. *Archives of General Psychiatry,* 1974, **30,** 789–793.

Rapoport, J. L., Quinn, P. O., and Lamprecht, F. Minor physical anomalies and plasma dopamine-beta-hydroxylase activity in hyperactive boys. *American Journal of Psychiatry,* 1974, **131,** 386–390.

Reger, R. Stimulating the distractible child. *The Elementary School Journal,* 1963, **64,** 42–48.

Report of the Conference on the Use of Stimulant Drugs in the Treatment of Behaviorally Disturbed Young School Children. Washington, D. C., Department of Health, Education, and Welfare, 1971.

Repucci, N. D. and Saunders, J. T. Social psychology of behavior modification. Problems of implementation in natural settings. *American Psychologist,* 1974, **29,** 649–660.

Ricks, D. F. Life history research: Retrospect and prospect 1973. In D. F. Ricks, A. Thomas, and M. Roff (Eds.), *Life history research in psychopathology,* Vol. 3. Minneapolis, Minn.: University of Minnesota Press, 1974, pp. 350–370.

Ridberg, E. H., Parke, R. D., and Hetherington, E. M. Modification of impulsive and reflective cognitive styles through observation of film-mediated models. *Developmental Psychology,* 1971, **5,** 369–377.

Rie, H. E. Hyperactivity in children. *American Journal of Diseases of Children,* 1975, **129,** 783–789.

Rimoldi, H. J. A. Personal tempo. *Journal of Abnormal and Social Psychology,* 1951, **46,** 283–303.

Rioch, M. J., Elkes, E., Flint, A. A., Usdansky, B. C., Newman, R. G., and Silber, E. National Institute of Mental Health pilot study in training mental health counselors. *American Journal of Orthopsychiatry,* 1963, **33,** 678–689.

Ritter, B. J. The group treatment of children's snake phobias using vicarious and contact desensitization procedures. *Behavior Research and Therapy,* 1968, **6,** 1–7.

Robbins, L. C. The accuracy of parental recall of aspects of child development and of child rearing practices. *Journal of Abnormal and Social Psychology,* 1963, **66,** 261–270.

Robin, S. S. and Bosco, J. J. Ritalin for school children: The teachers' perspective. *Journal of School Health,* 1973, **43,** 624–628.

Robins, L. N. *Deviant children grown up.* Baltimore: Williams & Wilkins, 1966.

Robins, L. N. Follow-up studies of behavior disorders in children. In H. C. Quay and J. S. Werry (Eds.), *Psychological disorders of childhood.* New York: Wiley, 1972, pp. 414–450.

Rodin, E., Lucas, A., and Simson, C. A study of behavior disorders in children by means of general purpose computers. *Proceedings of the Conference on Data Acquisition and Processing in Biological Medicine,* Oxford: Pergamon, 1963, pp. 115–124.

Rose, H. E. and Mayer, J. Activity, calorie intake, fat storage and the energy balance of infants. *Pediatrics,* 1968, **41**, 18–29.

Ross, A. O. Behavior therapy. In B. B. Wolman (Ed.), *Manual of child psychopathology.* New York: McGraw-Hill, 1970, pp. 900–925.

Ross, D. M. Case study of a hyperactive four-year-old. Unpublished manuscript, Stanford University, 1961.

Ross, D. M. Differential reinforcement with an impulsive six-year-old boy. Unpublished manuscript. Stanford University, 1967.

Ross, D. M. The relationship between intentional learning, incidental learning, and type of reward in preschool, educable mental retardates. *Child Development,* 1970, **41**, 1151–1158.

Ross, D. M. Case study of a mother of a difficult, high active infant. Unpublished manuscript, University of California, 1973.

Ross, D. M. and Ross, S. A. A multisensory approach to inhibitory motor training. Unpublished manuscript, Stanford University, 1971.

Ross, D. M. and Ross, S. A. *An intensive training curriculum for the education of young EMR children.* Final Report. Washington, D. C.: U.S. Office of Education, Bureau of Education for the Handicapped, 1972.

Ross, D. M., Ross, S. A., and Downing, M. L. Intentional training vs. observational learning of mediational strategies in EMR children. *American Journal of Mental Deficiency,* 1973, **78**, 292–299.

Ross, D. M., Ross, S. A., and Evans, T. A. The modification of extreme social withdrawal by modeling with guided participation. *Journal of Behavior Therapy and Experimental Psychiatry,* 1971, **2**, 273–279.

Ross, S. A. Effects of intentional training in social behavior on retarded children. *American Journal of Mental Deficiency,* 1969, **73**, 912–919.

Rost, K. J. and Charles, D. C. Academic achievement of brain injured and hyperactive children in isolation. *Exceptional Children,* 1967, **34**, 125–126.

Rothenberg, M. B. Reactions of children to illness and hospitalization. In D. W. Smith and R. E. Marshall (Eds.), *Introduction to clinical pediatrics.* Philadelphia: W. B. Saunders, 1972.

Rothschild, C. J. and Nicol, H. Allergic reaction to methylphenidate. *Canadian Medical Association Journal,* 1972, **106**, 1064.

Routh, D. K., Schroeder, C. S., and O'Tuama, L. A. Development of activity level in children. *Developmental Psychology,* 1974, **4**, 38–40.

Rubenstein, L. Continuous radio telemetry of human activity. *Nature,* 1962, **193**, 849–850.

Rutter, M., Lebovici, S., Eisenberg, L., Sneznevskij, A. V., Sadoun, R., Brooke, E., and Lin, T-Y. A tri-axial classification of mental disorders in childhood. *Journal of Child Psychology and Psychiatry*, 1969, **10**, 41–61.

Sachs, D. A. The efficacy of time-out procedures in a variety of behavior problems. *Journal of Behavior Therapy and Experimental Psychiatry*, 1973, **4**, 237–242.

Safer, D. J. Drugs for problem school children. *Journal of School Health*, 1971, **41**, 491–495.

Safer, D. J. A familial factor in minimal brain dysfunction. *Behavior Genetics*, 1973, **3**, 175–186.

Safer, D. J. and Allen, R. P. Factors influencing the suppressant effects of two stimulant drugs on the growth of hyperactive children. *Pediatrics*, 1973, **51**, 660–667.

Safer, D. J. and Allen, R. P. Single daily dose methylphenidate in hyperactive children. *Diseases of the Nervous System*, 1973a, **34**, 325–328.

Safer, D., Allen, R., and Barr, E. Depression of growth in hyperactive children on stimulant drugs. *New England Journal of Medicine*, 1972, **287**, 217–220.

Safer, D. J., Allen, R. P., and Barr, E. Growth rebound after termination of stimulant drugs. *Journal of Pediatrics*, 1975, **86**, 113–116.

Safer, D. J. and Krager, J. J. Prevalence and management of hyperactive children (letter). *New England Journal of Medicine*, 1975, **292**, 537.

Sainsbury, P. A method of measuring spontaneous movements by time-sampling motion pictures. *Journal of Mental Science*, 1954, **100**, 742–748.

Sajwaj, T., Twardosz, S., and Burke, M. Side effects of extinction procedures in a remedial preschool. *Journal of Applied Behavior Analysis*, 1972, **5**, 163–175.

Sander, L. W. Issues in early mother-child interaction. *Journal of the American Academy of Child Psychiatry*, 1962, **1**, 141–166.

Sander, L. W. The longitudinal course of early mother-child interaction: Cross-case comparison in a sample of mother-child pairs. In B. M. Foss (Ed.), *Determinants of infant behavior IV*. London: Methuen, 1969, pp. 189–227.

Santostefano, S. and Paley, E. Development of cognitive controls in children. *Journal of Clinical Psychology*, 1964, **20**, 213–218.

Saraf, K. R., Klein, D. F., Gittelman-Klein, R., and Groff, S. Imipramine side effects in children. *Psychopharmacologia*, 1974, **37**, 265–274.

Sarason, S. B. *Psychological problems in mental deficiency*. New York: Harper, 1949.

Satterfield, J. H. EEG issues in children with minimal brain dysfunction. *Seminars in Psychiatry*, 1973, **5**, 35–46.

Satterfield, J. H., Atoian, G., Brashears, G. C., Burleigh, A. C., and Dawson, M. E. Electrodermal studies of minimal brain dysfunction children. In *Clinical use of stimulant drugs in children*. The Hague: Excerpta Medica, 1974, pp. 87–97.

Satterfield, J. H. and Cantwell, D. P. CNS function and response to methylphenidate in hyperactive children. *Psychopharmacology Bulletin*, 1974, **10**, 36–37.

Satterfield, J. H., Cantwell, D. P., Lesser, L. I., and Podosin, R. L. Physiological studies of the hyperkinetic child: I. *American Journal of Psychiatry,* 1972, **128,** 1418–1424.

Satterfield, J. H., Cantwell, D. P., and Satterfield, B. T. Pathophysiology of the hyperactive child syndrome. *Archives of General Psychiatry,* 1974, **31,** 839–844.

Satterfield, J. H., Cantwell, D. P., Saul, R. E., Lesser, L. I., and Podosin, R. L. Response to stimulant drug treatment in hyperactive children, prediction from EEG and neurological findings. *Journal of Autism and Child Schizophrenia,* 1973, **3,** 36–48.

Satterfield, J. H., Cantwell, D. P., Saul, R. E., and Yusin, A. Intelligence, academic achievement, and EEG abnormalities in hyperactive children. *American Journal of Psychiatry,* 1974, **131,** 391–395.

Satterfield, J. H. and Dawson, M. E. Electrodermal correlates of hyperactivity in children. *Psychophysiology,* 1971, **8,** 191–197.

Satterfield, J. H., Lesser, L. I., Saul, R. E., and Cantwell, D. P. EEG aspects in the diagnosis and treatment of minimal brain dysfunction. *Annals of the New York Academy of Sciences,* 1973, **205,** 274–282.

Sauerhoff, M. W. and Michaelson, I. A. Hyperactivity and brain catecholamines in lead-exposed developing rats. *Science,* 1973, **182,** 1022–1024.

Scanlon, J. Umbilical cord blood lead concentration. *American Journal of Diseases of Children,* 1971, **121,** 325–326.

Scarr, S. Genetic factors in activity motivation. *Child Development,* 1966, **37,** 663–673.

Schachter, S. *The psychology of affiliation.* Stanford, California: Stanford University Press, 1959.

Schaefer, J. W., Palkes, H. S., and Stewart, M. A. Group counseling for parents of hyperactive children. *Child Psychiatry and Human Development,* 1974, **5,** 89–94.

Schaffer, H. R. Activity level as a constitutional determinant of infantile reaction to deprivation. *Child Development,* 1966, **37,** 595–602.

Schain, R. J. Minor physical anomalies and hyperactivity (letter). *Pediatrics,* 1974, **54,** 522.

Schain, R. J. and Reynard, C. L. Effects of a central stimulant drug (methylphenidate) in children with hyperactive behavior. *Pediatrics,* 1975, **55,** 709–716.

Schiff, J. L. with Day, B. *All my children.* New York: M. Evans, 1971.

Schleifer, M., Weiss, G., Cohen, N., Elman, M., Cvejic, H., and Kruger, E. Hyperactivity in preschoolers and the effect of methylphenidate. *American Journal of Orthopsychiatry,* 1975, **45,** 38–50.

Schmidt, K. The effect of continuous stimulation on the behavioral sleep of infants. *Merrill-Palmer Quarterly,* 1975, **21,** 77–88.

Schmitt, B. D., Martin, H. P., Nellhaus, G., Cravens, J., Camp, B. W., and Jordan, K. The hyperactive child. *Clinical Pediatrics,* 1973, **12,** 154–169.

Schnackenberg, R. C. Caffeine as a substitute for Schedule II stimulants in hyperkinetic children. *American Journal of Psychiatry,* 1973, **130,** 796–798.

Schofield, W. *Psychotherapy: The purchase of friendship.* Englewood Cliffs, N. J.: Prentice-Hall, 1964.

Schrag, P., & Divoky, D. *The myth of the hyperactive child.* New York: Pantheon, 1975.

Schulman, J. L., Kaspar, J. C., and Throne, F. M. *Brain damage and behavior.* Springfield, Ill.: Thomas, 1965.

Schulman, J. L. and Reisman, J. M. An objective measure of hyperactivity. *American Journal of Mental Deficiency,* 1959, **64,** 455–456.

Schwartz, G. E. Biofeedback as therapy: Some theoretical and practical issues. *American Psychologist,* 1973, **28,** 666–673.

Scott, T. J. The use of music to reduce hyperactivity in children. *American Journal of Orthopsychiatry,* 1970, **40** (4), 677–680.

Sechrest, L. Implicit reinforcement of responses. *Journal of Educational Psychology,* 1963, **54,** 197–201.

Seitz, S. and Terdal, L. A modeling approach to changing parent-child interactions. *Mental Retardation,* 1972, **4,** 39–43.

Serbin, L. A., O'Leary, K. D., Kent, R. N., and Tonick, I. J. A comparison of teacher response to the pre-academic and problem behavior of boys and girls. *Child Development,* 1973, **44,** 796–804.

Shannon, W. R. Neuropathic manifestations in infants and children as a result of anaphylactic reactions to foods contained in their dietary. *American Journal of Diseases in Children,* 1922, **24,** 89–94.

Shelley, E. M. and Riester, A. Syndrome of minimal brain damage in young adults. *Diseases of the Nervous System,* 1972, **33,** 335–338.

Shetty, T. Photic responses in hyperkinesis of childhood. *Science,* 1971, **174,** 1356–1357.

Shores, R. E. and Haubrich, P. A. Effect of cubicles in educating emotionally disturbed children. *Exceptional Children,* 1969, **36,** 21–24.

Silbergold, E. K. and Goldberg, A. M. A lead-induced behavioral disorder. *Life Sciences,* 1973, **13,** 1275–1283.

Silbergeld, E. K. and Goldberg, A. M. Lead-induced behavioral dysfunction: An animal model of hyperactivity. *Experimental Neurology,* 1974, **42,** 146–157.

Simpson, D. D. and Nelson, A. E. Attention training through breathing control to modify hyperactivity. *Journal of Learning Disabilities,* 1974, **7,** 274–283.

Simpson, R. H. The specific meanings of certain terms indicating differing degrees of frequency. *Quarterly Journal of Speech,* 1944, **30,** 328–330.

Sines, J. O., Pauker, J. D., and Sines, L. K. *Missouri Children's Picture Series.* Unpublished test. Iowa City, Iowa, 1971.

Skinner, B. F. *Science and human behavior.* New York: Macmillan, 1953.

Skinner, B. F. *The technology of teaching.* New York: Appleton-Century-Crofts, 1968.

Slater, E. Expectation of abnormality on paternal and maternal sides: A computational model. *Journal of Medical Genetics,* 1966, **3,** 159–161.

Smith, B. S. and Phillips, E. H. Treating a hyperactive child. *Physical Therapy,* 1970, **50,** 506–510.

Smith, G. B. Cerebral accidents of childhood and their relationships to mental deficiency. *Welfare Magazine,* 1926, **17,** 18–33.

Smithsonian Science Information Exchange. Notice of research projects. Title of this search: D110, Hyperkinetic children. Washington, D.C., April, 1975.

Sobotka, T. J. and Cook, M. P. Postnatal lead acetate exposure in rats: Possible relationship to minimal brain dysfunction. *American Journal of Mental Deficiency,* 1974, **79,** 5–9.

Sollenberger, R. T. Chinese-American child-rearing practices and juvenile delinquency. *Journal of Social Psychology,* 1968, **74,** 13–23.

Solomon, P. *Sensory deprivation.* Cambridge, Mass.: Harvard University Press, 1961.

Solomons, G. The role of methylphenidate and dextroamphetamine in children. *Drug Letter* (University of Iowa Hospitals and Clinics), 1971, **10,** 7–9.

Solomons, G. Drug therapy: Initiation and follow-up. *Annals of the New York Academy of Sciences,* 1973, **205,** 335–344.

Sprague, R. L. Psychopharmacology and learning disabilities. Paper presented at Child Development and Child Psychiatry Conference, School of Medicine, University of Missouri, 1971.

Sprague, R. L. Minimal brain dysfunction from a behavioral viewpoint. Paper presented at the Conference on Minimal Brain Dysfunction, New York, March, 1972.

Sprague, R. L., Barnes, K. R., and Werry, J. S. Methylphenidate and thioridazine: Learning, activity, and behavior in emotionally disturbed boys. *American Journal of Orthopsychiatry,* 1970, **40,** 615–628.

Sprague, R. L., Christensen, D. E., and Werry, J. S. Experimental psychology and stimulant drugs. In C. K. Conners (Ed.), *Clinical use of stimulant drugs in children.* The Hague: Excerpta Medica, 1974, pp. 141–164.

Sprague, R. L., Cohen, M., and Werry, J. S. Normative data on the Conners' Teacher Rating Scale and Abbreviated Scale. Technical Report, Children's Research Center, University of Illinois, Urbana, Illinois, November, 1974.

Sprague, R. L. and Sleator, E. K. Effects of psychopharmacologic agents on learning disorders. *Pediatric Clinics of North America,* 1973, **20,** 719–735.

Sprague, R. L. and Sleator, E. K. Drugs and dosages: Implications for learning disabilities. Paper presented at the NATO Conference on the Neuropsychology of Learning Disorders: Theoretical Approaches. Korsør, Denmark, June, 1975.

Sprague, R. L. and Toppe, L. K. Relationship between activity level and delay of reinforcement in the retarded. *Journal of Experimental Child Psychology,* 1966, **3,** 390–397.

Sprague, R. L. and Werry, J. S. Methodology of psychopharmacological studies with the retarded. In N. R. Ellis (Ed.), *International review of research in mental retardation,* Vol. 5. New York: Academic Press, 1971.

Sprague, R. L., Werry, J., and Davis, K. Psychotropic drug effects on learning and activity level of children. Paper presented at the Gatlinburg Conference on Research and Theory in Mental Retardation, March, 1969.

Sprague, R. L., Werry, J. S., Greenwold, W. E., and Jones, H. Dosage effects of methylphenidate on learning of children. Paper presented at the meeting of the Psychonomic Society, St. Louis, November, 1969.

Sprague, R. L., Werry, J. S., Greenwold, W., and Jones, H. Methylphenidate effects on recognition memory of children. Paper presented at the meeting of the Psychonomic Society, San Antonio, Texas, 1970.

Spring, C., Greenberg, L., Scott, J., and Hopwood, J. Electrodermal activity in hyperactive boys who are methylphenidate responders. *Psychophysiology,* 1974, **11,** 436–442.

Sroufe, L. A. Drug treatment of children with behavior problems. In F. Horowitz (Ed.), *Review of child development research,* Vol. 4. Chicago: University of Chicago Press, 1975.

Sroufe, L. A., Sonies, B. C., West, W. D., and Wright, F. S. Anticipatory heart rate deceleration and reaction time in children with and without referral for learning disability. *Child Development,* 1973, **44,** 267–273.

Sroufe, L. A. and Stewart, M. A. Treating problem children with stimulant drugs. *New England Journal of Medicine,* 1973, **289,** 407–413.

Staats, A. W., Minke, K. A., Finley, J. R., Wolf, M., and Brooks, L. O. A reinforcer system and experimental procedure for the laboratory study of reading acquisition. *Child Development,* 1964, **35,** 209–231.

Stein, M. and Ronald, D. Educational psychotherapy of preschoolers. *Journal of the American Academy of Child Psychiatry,* 1974, **13,** 618–634.

Stein, T. J. Some ethical considerations of short-term workshops in the principles and methods of behavior modification. *Journal of Applied Behavior Analysis,* 1975, **8,** 113–115.

Steinberg, G. G., Troshinsky, C., and Steinberg, H. R. Dextroamphetamine-responsive behavior disorder in school children. *American Journal of Psychiatry,* 1971, **128,** 174–179.

Stephens, J. M. *The process of schooling.* New York: Holt, Rinehart, & Winston, 1967.

Stern, W. C. A physiological model of childhood hyperkinesis. Research in progress, Worcester Foundation for Experimental Biology, Shrewsbury, Massachusetts, 1975.

Stevens, D. A., Stover, C. E., and Backus, J. T. The hyperkinetic child: The effect of incentives on the speed of rapid tapping. *Journal of Consulting and Clinical Psychology,* 1970, **34,** 56–59.

Stevens-Long, J. The effect of behavioral context on some aspects of adult disciplinary practice and affect. *Child Development,* 1973, **44,** 476–484.

Stewart, M. A. Hyperactive children. *American Journal of Psychiatry,* 1973, **94,** 577–585.

Stewart, M. A., Mendelson, W. B., and Johnson, N. E. Hyperactive children as adolescents: How they describe themselves. *Child Psychiatry and Human Development,* 1973, **4**, 3–11.

Stewart, M. A. and Morrison, J. R. Affective disorder among the relatives of hyperactive children. *Journal of Child Psychology and Psychiatry,* 1973, **14**, 209–212.

Stewart, M. A. and Olds, S. W. *Raising a hyperactive child.* New York: Harper & Row, 1973.

Stewart, M. A., Palkes, H., Miller, R., Young, C., and Welner, Z. Intellectual ability and school achievement of hyperactive children, their classmates, and their siblings. In D. Ricks, A. Thomas, and M. Roff (Eds.), *Life history research in psychopathology Vol. 3.* Minneapolis, Minn.: University of Minnesota Press, 1974, pp. 68–86.

Stewart, M. A., Pitts, F. N., Craig, A. G., and Dieruf, W. The hyperactive child syndrome. *American Journal of Orthopsychiatry,* 1966, **36,** 861–867.

Stewart, M. A., Thach, B. T., and Freidin, M. R. Accidental poisoning and the hyperactive child syndrome. *Diseases of the Nervous System,* 1970, **31,** 403–407.

Still, G. F. The Coulstonian Lectures on some abnormal physical conditions in children. *Lancet,* 1902, **1,** 1008–1012, 1077–1082, 1163–1168.

Stone, F. B., Wilson, M. A., Spence, M. E., and Gibson, R. C. A survey of elementary school children's behavior problems. Paper presented at the annual meeting of the American Orthopsychiatric Association, New York, 1969.

Stover, L. and Guerney, B. G., Jr. A demonstration technique for interpreting perceptual-motor neurological difficulties to parents and teachers. *Journal of School Psychology,* 1968, **6,** 275–278.

Stover, L. and Guerney, B. G., Jr. The efficacy of training procedures for mothers in filial therapy. *Psychotherapy: Theory Research and Practice,* 1967, **4,** 110–115.

Straughan, J. H. Treatment with child and mother in the playroom. *Behavior Research and Therapy,* 1964, **2,** 37–41.

Strauss, A. A. and Kephart, N. C. *Psychopathology and education of the brain-injured child.* Vol. II. Progress in theory and clinic. New York: Grune & Stratton, 1955.

Strauss, A. A. and Lehtinen, L. E. *Psychopathology and education of the brain-injured child.* New York: Grune & Stratton, 1947.

Strecker, E. A. and Ebaugh, F. Neuropsychiatric sequelae of cerebral trauma in children. *Archives of Neurology and Psychiatry,* 1924, **12,** 443–453.

Stroop, J. R. Studies of interference in serial verbal reactions. *Journal of Experimental Psychology,* 1935, **18,** 643–661.

Stunkard, A. and Pestka, J. The physical activity of obese girls. *American Journal of Diseases of Children,* 1962, **103,** 812–817.

Sturm, I. E. The behavioristic aspect of psychodrama. *Group Psychotherapy,* 1965, **18,** 50–64.

Sullivan, J. P. Effects of benzedrine sulphate on children taking the new Stanford Achievement Test. *American Journal of Orthopsychiatry*, 1937, **7**, 519–522.

Sundby, H. and Kreyberg, P. *Prognosis in child psychiatry*. Baltimore: Williams & Wilkins, 1969.

Switzer, J. Developmental differences in place and name sequence learning in normal, hyperactive, and hypoactive eight and twelve-year-old boys. *Dissertation Abstracts*, 1962, **22**, 2482.

Sykes, D. H., Douglas, V. I., and Morgenstern, G. The effect of methylphenidate (Ritalin) on sustained attention in hyperactive children. *Psychopharmacologia* (Berlin), 1972, **25**, 262–274.

Sykes, D. H., Douglas, V. I., and Morgenstern, G. Sustained attention in hyperactive children. *Journal of Child Psychology and Psychiatry*, 1973, **14**, 213–220.

Taub, S. J. Allergies may lead to minimal brain dysfunction in children. *Eye Ear Nose & Throat*, 1975, **54**, 168–169.

Tec, L. Unexpected effects in children treated with imipramine. *American Journal of Psychiatry*, 1963, **120**, 603.

Tec, L. The staccato syndrome: A new clinical entity in search of recognition. *American Journal of Psychiatry*, 1971, **128**, 647–648.

Tec, L. Hyperkinetic children and the staccato syndrome (letter). *American Journal of Psychiatry*, 1973, **130**, 330.

Tecce, J. J. and Cole, J. O. Amphetamine effects in man: Paradoxical drowsiness and lowered brain activity. *Science*, 1974, **185**, 481.

Terman, L. M. and Merrill, M. A. *Mental and physical traits of a thousand gifted children*. Stanford: Stanford University Press, 1926.

Terman, L. M. and Oden, M. H. *The gifted child grows up: Twenty-five years' follow-up of a superior group*. Stanford: Stanford University Press, 1947.

Terman, L. M. and Oden, M. H. *The gifted group at mid-life: 35 years' follow-up of the superior child*. Stanford: Stanford University Press, 1959.

Thomas, A., Chess, S., and Birch, H. G. *Temperament and behavior disorders in children*. New York: New York University Press, 1968.

Thomas, A., Chess, S., and Birch, H. The origin of personality. *Scientific American*, 1970, **223**, 102–109.

Thomas, A., Chess, S., Birch, H., and Hertzig, M. E. A longitudinal study of primary reaction patterns in children. *Comprehensive Psychiatry*, 1960, **1**, 103–112.

Thomas, A., Chess, S., Sillen, J., and Mendez, O. Cross-cultural study of behavior in children with special vulnerabilities to stress. In D. Ricks, A. Thomas, and M. Roff (Eds.), *Life history research in psychopathology*, Vol. 3. Minneapolis, Minn.: University of Minnesota Press, 1974, pp. 53–67.

Thomas, C. L. (Ed.), *Taber's cyclopedic medical dictionary*. Philadelphia: Davis, 1973.

Thomas, D. R., Becker, W. C., and Armstrong, M. Production and elimination of disruptive classroom behavior by systematically varying teachers' behavior. *Journal of Applied Behavior Analysis,* 1968, **1,** 35–45.

Towbin, A. Central nervous system damage in the human fetus and newborn infant. *American Journal of Diseases of Children,* 1970, **119,** 529–542.

Towbin, A. Organic causes of minimal brain dysfunction. Perinatal origin of minimal cerebral lesions. *Journal of the American Medical Association,* 1971, **217,** 1207–1214.

Trabasso, T. and Bower, G. H. *Attention in learning: Theory and research.* New York: Wiley, 1968.

Tredgold, C. H. *Mental deficiency (amentia)* (1st ed.), New York: Wood, 1908.

Treisman, A. M. Strategies and models of selective attention. *Psychological Review,* 1969, **76,** 282–299.

Triantafillou, M. Pemoline in overactive mentally handicapped children (letter). *British Journal of Psychiatry,* 1972, **121,** 577.

Turnure, J. E. Children's reaction to distractors in a learning situation. *Developmental Psychology,* 1970, **2,** 115–122.

Turnure, J. E. Control of orienting behavior in children under five years of age. *Developmental Psychology,* 1971, **4,** 16–24.

Twardosz, S. and Sajwaj, T. Multiple effects of a procedure to increase sitting in a hyperactive, retarded boy. *Journal of Applied Behavior Analysis,* 1972, **5,** 73–78.

Ullman, L. P. and Krasner, L. *A psychological approach to abnormal behavior.* Englewood Cliffs, N.J.: Prentice-Hall, 1969.

Urban, H. B. and Ford, D. H. Some historical and conceptual perspectives on psychotherapy and behavior change. In A. E. Bergin and S. L. Garfield (Eds.), *Handbook of psychotherapy and behavior change: An empirical analysis.* New York: Wiley, 1971, pp. 3–35.

Vandenberg, S. G. The heredity abilities study: Hereditary components in a psychological test battery. *American Journal of Human Genetics,* 1962, **14,** 220–237.

Van den Daele, L. D. Modification of infant state by treatment in a rocker box. *Journal of Psychology,* 1970, **44,** 161–165.

Van den Daele, L. D. Infant reactivity to redundant proprioceptive and auditory stimulation: A twin study. *Journal of Psychology,* 1971, **78,** 269–276.

Victor, J. B., Halverson, C. F., Inoff, G., and Buczkowski, H. J. Objective behavior measures of first and second grade boys' free play and teachers' ratings on a behavior problem checklist. *Psychology in the Schools,* 1973, **10,** 439–443.

Wade, M. G. and Ellis, M. J. Measurement of free-range activity in children as modified by social and environmental complexity. *American Journal of Clinical Nutrition,* 1971, **24,** 1457–1460.

Wahler, R. G., Sperling, K. A., Thomas, M. R., Teeter, N. C., and Luper, H. T. The modification of childhood stuttering: Some response-response relationships. *Journal of Experimental Child Psychology,* 1970, **9,** 411–428.

Wahler, R. G., Winkel, G. H., Peterson, R. F., and Morrison, D. C. Mothers as behavior therapists for their own children. *Behavior Research and Therapy,* 1965, **3,** 113–124.

Waizer, J., Hoffman, S. P., Polizos, P., and Engelhardt, D. M. Outpatient treatment of hyperactive school children with imipramine. *American Journal of Psychiatry,* 1974, **131,** 587–591.

Waldrop, M. F. and Goering, J. D. Hyperactivity and minor physical anomalies in elementary school children. *American Journal of Orthopsychiatry,* 1971, **41,** 602–607.

Waldrop, M. F. and Halverson, C. F. Minor physical anomalies and hyperactive behavior in young children. In J. Hellmuth (Ed.), *The exceptional infant.* Vol. II. Seattle: Special Child Publications, 1970.

Waldrop, M. F. and Halverson, C. F. Minor physical anomalies: Their incidence and relation to behavior in a normal and a deviant sample. In R. C. Smart and M. S. Smart (Eds.), *Readings in development and relationships.* New York: Macmillan, 1971.

Waldrop, M. F., Pedersen, F. A., and Bell, R. Q. Minor physical anomalies and behavior in preschool children. *Child Development,* 1968, **39,** 391–400.

Walker, S., III. Drugging the American child. We're too cavalier about hyperactivity. *Psychology Today,* 1974, **8,** No. 7, 43–48.

Warren, R. J., Karduck, W. A., Bussaratid, S., Stewart, M. A., and Sly, W. S. The hyperactive child syndrome. *Archives of General Psychiatry,* 1971, **24,** 161–162.

Watzlawick, P., Weakland, J. H., and Fisch, R. *Change: Principles of problem formation and problem resolution.* New York: Norton, 1974.

Weakland, J. H., and Fisch, R. Case study (personal communication, 1975).

Weakland, J. H., Fisch, R., Watzlawick, P., and Bodin, A. M. Brief therapy: Focused problem resolution. *Family Process,* 1974, **13,** 141–168.

Webb, E. J., Campbell, D. T., Schwartz, R. D., and Sechrest, L. *Unobtrusive measures: Nonreactive research in the social sciences.* Chicago: Rand McNally, 1966.

*Webster's New World Dictionary,* College Edition. New York: World Publishing, 1962.

Weiner, A. S. and Berzonsky, M. D. Development of selective attention in reflective and impulsive children. *Child Development,* 1975, **46,** 545–549.

Weiss, B. and Laties, V. G. Enhancement of human performance by caffeine and the amphetamines. *Pharmacological Reviews,* 1962, **14,** 1–36.

Weiss, G. The hyperactive child (letter). *Canadian Medical Association Journal,* 1975, **112,** 803–805.

Weiss, G. The natural history of hyperactivity in childhood and treatment with stimulant medication at different ages. *International Journal of Mental Health,* 1975a, 4, No. 1-2, 213–226.

Weiss, G., Kruger, E., Danielson, U., and Elman, M. Long-term methylphenidate treatment of hyperkinetic children. *Psychopharmacology Bulletin*, 1974, **10,** 34–35.

Weiss, G., Minde, K., Douglas, V., Werry, J., and Sykes, D. Comparison of the effects of chlorpromazine, dextroamphetamine, and methylphenidate on the behavior and intellectual functioning of hyperactive children. *Canadian Medical Association Journal*, 1971, **104,** 20–25.

Weiss, G., Minde, K., Werry, J. S., Douglas, V., and Nemeth, E. Studies on the hyperactive child: VIII. Five-year follow-up. *Archives of General Psychiatry*, 1971, **24,** 409–414.

Weisz, J. R., O'Neill, P., and O'Neill, P. C. Field dependence-independence on the Children's Embedded Figures Test: Cognitive style or cognitive level? *Developmental Psychology*, 1975, **11,** 539–540.

Weithorn, C. J. The relationship between hyperactivity and impulsive responsiveness in elementary school children. *Dissertation Abstracts International*, 1970, **30B,** 3899.

Wender, P. H. *Minimal brain dysfunction in children*. New York: Wiley-Interscience, 1971.

Wender, P. H. *The hyperactive child: A handbook for parents*. New York: Crown, 1973.

Werkman, S. Brain dysfunction in adolescence. IV. Implications of the research. *American Journal of Orthopsychiatry*, 1970, **40,** 336–337.

Werner, E., Bierman, J. M., French, F. E., Simonian, K., Connor, A., Smith, R. S., and Campbell, M. Reproductive and environmental casualties: A report on the 10-year follow-up of the children of the Kauai pregnancy study. *Pediatrics*, 1968, **42,** 112–127.

Werry, J. S. Developmental hyperactivity. *Pediatric Clinics of North America*, 1968, **15,** 581–599.

Werry, J. S. Studies on the hyperactive child. IV. An empirical analysis of the minimal brain dysfunction syndrome. *Archives of General Psychiatry*, 1968a, **19,** 9–16.

Werry, J. S. Some clinical and laboratory studies of psychotropic drugs in children: An overview. In W. L. Smith (Ed.), *Drugs and cerebral function*. Springfield, Ill.: Thomas, 1970.

Werry, J. S., Minde, K., Guzman, A., Weiss, G., Dogan, K., and Hoy, E. Studies on the hyperactive child. VII. Neurological status compared with neurotic and normal children. *American Journal of Orthopsychiatry*, 1972, **42,** 441–451.

Werry, J. S. and Sprague, R. L. Hyperactivity. In C. G. Costello (Ed.), *Symptoms of psychopathology*. New York: Wiley, 1970, pp. 397–417.

Werry, J. S. and Sprague, R. L. Psychopharmacology. *Mental Retardation*, 1972, **4,** 63–79.

Werry, J. S. and Sprague, R. L. Methylphenidate in children — Effect of dosage. *Australian and New Zealand Journal of Psychiatry*, 1974, **8,** 9–19.

Werry, J. S., Weiss, G., and Douglas, V. Studies on the hyperactive child. I. Some preliminary findings. *Canadian Psychiatric Association Journal,* 1964, **9,** 120–130.

Wessel, M. A. Prevalence and management of hyperactive children (letter). *New England Journal of Medicine,* 1975, **292,** 536–537.

Whitehead, P. L. and Clark, L. D. Effect of lithium carbonate, placebo, and thioridazine on hyperactive children. *American Journal of Psychiatry,* 1970, **127,** 824–825.

Wiener, G. Varying psychological sequelae of lead ingestion in children. *Public Health Reports,* 1970, **85,** 19–24.

Wiens, A. N., Anderson, K. A., and Matarazzo, R. G. Use of medication as an adjunct in the modification of behavior in the pediatric psychology setting. *Professional Psychology,* 1972, **Spring,** 157–162.

Wiggins, J. S. and Winder, C. L. The Peer Nomination Inventory: An empirically derived sociometric measure of adjustment in preadolescent boys. *Psychological Reports,* 1961, **9,** 643–677.

Wikler, A., Dixon, J. F., and Parker, J. B. Brain function in problem children and controls: Psychometric, neurological, and electroencephalographic comparisons. *American Journal of Psychiatry,* 1970, **127,** 634–645.

Willerman, L. Activity level and hyperactivity in twins. *Child Development,* 1973, **44,** 288–293.

Willerman, L. and Plomin, R. Activity level in children and their parents. *Child Development,* 1973, **44,** 854–858.

Williams' testimony. Federal involvement in the use of behavior modification drugs on grammar school children on the right to privacy inquiry. Hearing before a Subcommittee of the Committee on Government Operations, House of Representatives, 91st Congress, Second Session, September 29, 1970, U. S. Government Printing Office, Washington, D.C., 1970, No. 52–268–6–23.

Williams, C. D. The elimination of tantrum behaviors by extinction procedures. *Journal of Abnormal and Social Psychology,* 1959, **59,** 269.

Williams, R. H. The clinical investigator and his role in teaching, administration, and the care of the patient. *Journal of the American Medical Association,* 1954, **156,** 127–136.

Wiltz, N. A. and Gordon, S. B. Parental modification of a child's behavior in an experimental residence. *Journal of Behavior Therapy and Experimental Psychiatry,* 1974, **5,** 107–109.

Winchell, C. A. *The hyperkinetic child* (a bibliography). Westport, Conn.: Greenwood Press, 1975.

Winsberg, B. G., Bialer, I., Kupietz, S., and Tobias, J. Effects of imipramine and dextroamphetamine on behavior of neuropsychiatrically impaired children. *American Journal of Psychiatry,* 1972, **128,** 1425–1431.

Winsberg, B. G., Goldstein, S., Yepes, L. E., and Perel, J. M. Imipramine electrocardiographic abnormalities in hyperactive children. *American Journal of Psychiatry,* 1975, **132,** 542–545.

Witt, P. A. Dosage effects of methylphenidate on the activity level of hyperactive children. *Dissertation Abstracts International,* 1972, **A32,** 5631–5632.

Witt, P. A., Ellis, M. J., and Sprague, R. L. Methylphenidate and activity level in hyperactive children. Unpublished manuscript, Children's Research Center, University of Illinois, 1970.

Wolf, C. W. Transactional analysis and the hyperactive child. Paper presented at the American Psychological Association meetings, New Orleans, August, 1974.

Wolf, M. V., Hanley, E. N., King, L. G., and Giles, D. I. The timer-game: A variable interval contingency for the management of out-of-seat behavior. *Exceptional Children,* 1970, **10,** 113–117.

Wolff, P. H. The causes, controls, and organization of behavior in the neonate. *Psychological Issues, Vol. V,* Monograph 17. New York: International Universities Press, 1966.

Wolff, P. H. The natural history of crying and other vocalizations in early infancy. In B. M. Foss (Ed.), *Determinants of infant behavior IV.* London: Methuen, 1969, pp. 81–109.

Wolpe, J. *Psychotherapy by reciprocal inhibition.* Stanford: Stanford University Press, 1958.

Word, T. and Stern, J. A. A simple stabilimeter. *Journal of Experimental Analysis of Behavior,* 1958, **1,** 201–203.

Worland, J., North-Jones, M., and Stern, J. A. Performance and activity of hyperactive and normal boys as a function of distraction and reward. *Journal of Abnormal Child Psychology,* 1973, **1,** 363–377.

World Health Organization. The use of twins in epidemiological studies. Report of the WHO meeting of investigators on methodology of twin studies. *Acta Geneticae Medicae et Gemellologiae,* 1966, **15,** 109–128.

Wray, J. D. Child care in the People's Republic of China — 1973: Part II. *Pediatrics,* 1975, **55,** 723–734.

Yanow, M. (Ed.) A report on the use of behavior modification drugs on elementary school children. In M. Yanow (Ed.), *Observations from the Treadmill.* New York: Viking, 1973.

Zahn, T. P., Abate, F., Little, B. C., and Wender, P. H. Minimal brain dysfunction, stimulant drugs, and autonomic nervous system activity. *Archives of General Psychiatry,* 1975, **32,** 318–387.

Zaporozhets, A. V. The development of voluntary movements. In B. Simon (Ed.), *Psychology in the Soviet Union.* Stanford, Cal.: Stanford University Press, 1957, pp. 108–114.

Zara, M. M. Effects of medication on learning in hyperactive four-year-old children. *Dissertation Abstracts International,* 1973, **A34,** 2407.

Zeilberger, J., Sampen, S., and Sloane, H. Modification of a child's problem behaviors in the home with the mother as therapist. *Journal of Applied Behavior Analysis,* 1968, **1,** 47–53.

Zentall, S. Effects of stimulation on activity and task performance in hyperactive children with learning and behavior disorders. Unpublished Doctoral dissertation, University of Pittsburgh, Pittsburgh, Pa., 1974.

Zentall, S. Optimal stimulation as theoretical basis of hyperactivity. *American Journal of Orthopsychiatry*, 1975, **45**, 549–563.

Zimmerman, E. H. and Zimmerman, J. The alteration of behavior in a special classroom situation. *Journal of Experimental Analysis of Behavior*, 1962, **5**, 59–60.

Zimmerman, F. T. and Burgemeister, B. B. Action of methylphenidylacetate (Ritalin) and reserpine in behavior disorders in children and adults. *American Journal of Psychiatry*, 1958, **115**, 323–328.

Zrull, J. P., McDermott, J. F., and Poznanski, E. Hyperkinetic syndrome: The role of depression. *Child Psychiatry and Human Development*, 1970, **1**, 33–40.

Zuk, G. Over-attention to moving stimuli as a factor in the distractibility of retarded and brain-injured children. *Training School Bulletin* (The Training School, Vineland, N. J.), 1963, **59**, 150–160.

Zupnick, S. A new approach to disturbed children: The Medical College School program. *Psychiatric Quarterly*, 1974, **48**, No. 1, 76–85.

# Author Index

Hawkins, W. F., 17, 50, 70, 198, 306
Hawley, C., 88
Hayes, T. A., 141
Hayweiser, L., 4
Henderson, A. T., 76, 254
Henderson, B. E., 112
Hendry, L. S., 79, 307
Henke, L. B., 148, 150
Henry, C. E., 17, 292
Hentoff, N., 97, 98
Herron, R. E., 3, 309
Hertzig, M. E., 76
Hewett, F. M., 199
Hibi, S., 110
Hinton, G., 104, 105, 111, 127, 128, 129, 130, 131, 132
Hoffman, H., 1
Hoffman, S. P., 104, 127, 128, 140
Hohman, L. B., 15
Hohman, R. J., 186, 209
Holliday, W. C., 160
Holt, J., 189
Homme, L. E., 213
Hopson, B., 216, 217
Hopwood, J., 105
Howell, M. C., 11, 61, 62
Hoy, E., 240
Huddleston, C. M., 201, 210
Hudson, B., 6, 264
Huessy, H. R., 6, 7, 12, 53, 55, 56, 78, 97, 111, 141, 288, 289, 294
Huestis, R. D., 114, 137, 138
Humphrey, E., 169
Hunsinger, S., 97, 120
Hurst, M., 134
Hutchinson, R. R., 154
Hutt, C., 307
Hutt, S. J., 307

Ilg, F. L., 234
Ingram, T. T., 264
Inoff, G., 4
Insel, J., 52, 89, 103, 105, 107
Insua, A., 133
Irwin, O. C., 307

Jacob, R. G., 35
James, C. E., 151
James, M., 183
Jenkins, J. R., 195

Johnson, C. F., 306
Johnson, N. E., 21, 45, 52, 60, 259, 289
Johnson, S. M., 213
Jones, H., 134
Jones, K. L., 90, 91
Jones, R., 6, 40, 151, 207
Jordan, A., 133
Jordan, K., 263

Kagan, J., 34, 37, 300
Kahana, B., 144, 213, 218
Kahn, E., 14
Kalverboer, A. F., 93, 245
Kandel, H. J., 130, 207
Kappelman, M., 260
Karduck, W. A., 68
Karlin, R. A., 221
Kaspar, J. C., 4, 9, 10, 81, 230, 306
Kassorla, I. C., 310
Kastenbaum, R., 154
Kaswan, J. W., 174
Kauffman, J. M., 199, 207
Kazdin, A., 211
Kehne, C. W., 283, 297
Kelly, G. A., 164
Kendall, D. C., 297
Kenny, T. J., 6, 264
Kent, R. N., 222
Keogh, B. K., 213, 225
Kephart, N. C., 17, 18
Kessen, W., 79, 307
Kilpatrick, A. W., 17
King, L. G., 209
Kinsbourne, M., 111
Kittler, F. J., 87
Klein, D. F., 53, 141
Klein, R. H., 116
Kline, C. L., 98
Knights, R. M., 104, 105, 111, 127, 128, 129, 130, 131, 132, 140
Knobel, M., 101, 104
Knobloch, H., 17
Knopp, W., 99, 101, 104, 106, 107, 115
Kohl, H., 189
Korb, R. J., 109, 143, 290
Kornetsky, C., 114, 115
Koser, L., 209
Kounin, J. S., 211
Krager, J. M., 98, 99
Kramer, R. A., 6, 294

# Subject Index

FE

MA